Health Security for All

# Health Security for All

Dreams of Universal Health Care in America

Alan Derickson

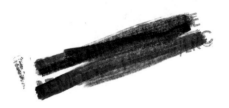

The Johns Hopkins University Press
*Baltimore and London*

The Johns Hopkins University Press
2715 North Charles Street
Baltimore, Maryland 21218-4363
www.press.jhu.edu

*Library of Congress Cataloging-in-Publication Data*

Derickson, Alan.
   Health security for all : dreams of universal health care in America / Alan Derickson.
      p.  ;  cm.
   Includes bibliographical references and index.
   ISBN 0-8018-8081-5 (hardcover : alk. paper)
   1. Right to health care—United States—History.  2. Health services accessibility—United States—History.  3. Insurance, Health—Government policy—United States—History.  4. National health insurance—United States—History.  5. Medical policy—United States—History.  6. Social security—United States—History.
   [DNLM: 1. Health Services Accessibility—history—United States. 2. Universal Coverage—history—United States. 3. Health Policy—history—United States. W 275 AA1 D433h 2005]  I. Title.
   RA395.A3D47 2005
   362.1'0973—dc22
                                                                        2004013499

A catalog record for this book is available from the British Library.

*For Katherine and Elizabeth*

# Contents

# Preface

Our new Economic Bill of Rights should mean health security for all, regardless of residence, station, or race—everywhere in the United States. We should resolve now that the health of this Nation is a national concern; that financial barriers in the way of attaining health shall be removed; that the health of all its citizens deserves the help of all the Nation.

—HARRY S. TRUMAN, 1945

Our . . . goal is high-quality, affordable health care for all Americans.

—GEORGE W. BUSH, 2003

It is well known that the United States entered the twenty-first century as the only affluent nation in the world that does not guarantee its citizens access to basic health care. At the present time, this deficiency has left well over forty million Americans in a precarious state. It is also well known that several attempts to remedy this problem by enacting national health insurance have failed miserably. A series of advertisements that appeared in leading newspapers across the nation in February 2002 trumpeted a fact not so well known. The ads depict a young girl walking down a street by herself—at first glance, a placid image. But the accompanying text presented two contrasting scenarios that shattered the tranquility of this scene. In one scenario, health insurance saves a life and preserves a vital relationship: "Her mom gets cancer. They find the tumor early. Her mom is OK." In the other scenario, disaster strikes: "Her mom gets cancer. She's diagnosed too late. Her mom is gone." The ad goes on to point out that "women with breast cancer are forty-nine percent more likely to die if they're uninsured." The real meaning of health insecurity is not the fears stirred by the lack of a reassuring plastic card in one's wallet or by the humiliation of personal bankruptcy. Instead, lack of insurance means otherwise preventable death, disability, suffering, and loss. People without health insurance receive less care and, as a result, suffer higher rates of morbidity and mortality. According to recent estimates, about fifty Americans die every day from illness or injury because they have no insurance. Beneath the policy jargon and the political rhetoric that often surround this issue is a tragedy of human sacrifice.[1]

Although historians have largely overlooked the topic of universal access to health care, there has been a long history of support for this ideal in America. To be sure, there is a copious historical literature on the failed attempts to pass insurance legislation.[2] The existing literature on health politics does take some notice of inclusive policy formulations, but it does not concentrate on access to care per se. The origins and development of the tenet of universality in American health policy thus remain somewhat obscure. Accordingly, this book focuses on the question of universal access, while leaving aside many other worthy questions. It is not primarily a study in health politics but rather in the imagining and reimagining of a societal ideal and its translation into plans of action. In the course of examining the pursuit of this elusive dream since the turn of the twentieth century, my research has revealed a surprising abundance of plans to reach the goal, a broad array of dreamers and planners involved in the reform process, and a variety of inventive justifications for universalism.

Over the past century, diverse visions of all-inclusive health protection have taken shape. At present, universal access is closely identified with proposals for national health insurance. This study complicates the conventional story by exploring competing possibilities. Social insurance was not always the only policy alternative offered by those who favored a statist approach to reform. Some advocates of health protection for all promoted blueprints for public medicine. At the other end of the ideological spectrum, champions of a voluntarist approach have promoted methods of financing care that left the government little or no role in achieving universal protection. Between these extremes have been a host of pluralistic plans for mixing public and private forms of both insurance and care.

Many different groups of all ideological hues have espoused universalism. During the Progressive Era, an authoritative interpretation of Catholic social doctrine called for health care for all who needed it. The American Medical Association formally endorsed universal access to health care in 1921 and reiterated and refined that position on a number of occasions thereafter. Even before the landmark manifesto by the Committee on the Costs of Medical Care in 1932, leading figures in public health and nursing were outspoken universalists. African-American leaders who might well have been wholly absorbed in efforts to eliminate racial segregation and discrimination in health care have devoted a good portion of their energies since the 1930s to attaining health security for all. Union officials came early to the universalist cause and remained involved with it long after their own members enjoyed negotiated benefits. During the last third of the twentieth century, virtually all of the participants in the national health-policy conversation, including most of the most hard-bitten conservatives, either avowed the virtues or conceded the necessity of an all-inclusive health-care system of some kind. Although some of these advocates have received attention from historians, others, like the religious progressives and the AMA, have been overlooked.

Over the course of the past century, reformers have fashioned a multifaceted rationale for universal health care. Justificatory claims have assumed myriad forms and have attained widely varying levels of sophistication. Reformers relied on three major themes: needs, efficiencies, and rights. The most enduring appeal based on unmet need has been humanitarian. Whether motivated by the values embodied in the biblical tale of the Good Samaritan or other sources, proponents of universalism have stressed the obligation to help fellow human beings who are suffering. Not surprisingly, those closest to the deprivations and sufferings of the needy have been most likely to articulate this perspective. Claims that wider access to health care would lead to a more productive workforce and other efficiencies have long been a weapon in the universalist armamentarium. Proponents of expanded democratic rights have often attempted to reinterpret the Constitution or the Declaration of Independence to encompass an entitlement to health care. Particularly for activists in the militant movements speaking for workers and African Americans, such efforts to extend social rights came naturally. Contentions that full citizenship required the ready accessibility of essential medical services rose to prominence in the 1930s and reached their peak a generation later. Both shifting societal values and the protracted health debate itself have forced partisans of universal health care to rethink the relative importance of needs, efficiencies, and rights over the course of the past century.

Reformers' arguments could shape, but not determine, national policy. A great strength of the universalist position—impassioned advocacy—has sometimes become a weakness. At more than one critical juncture, fervent and long-held commitments to protecting everyone made reformers incapable of accepting alternative paths to universal health protection. As much an impediment to progress as those who held out for too much were those who cared too little. In the thirty years since America reached a consensus in favor of universal care, the ranks of the uninsured have grown significantly. The tendency of professed universalists to give only lip service to the cause should serve as a warning against overreliance on support for health security for all that is widespread but shallow. I wrote this book with the hope that the next cohort of Americans who pursue this noble goal can benefit from a fuller understanding of both the efforts and the errors of their many predecessors.

Health Security for All

# CHAPTER ONE

# A Fertile and Lively Cause of Poverty

The ideal of universal access to health care emerged shortly after the turn of the twentieth century. A number of factors gradually brought this goal into view. The most important was the growing recognition of the wide extent and sad consequences of unmet need for care among the working poor. Progressive investigators disclosed a vicious cycle of poverty and sickness, a cycle too seldom broken by adequate and timely medical care. A searching examination of the predicament of the uninsured and otherwise unprotected confirmed the failure of the prevailing patchwork arrangements to provide for much of the nation's population.

Reformers in the Progressive Era looked to social insurance as the answer to the crisis of unmet need. However, with a few exceptions, the first American proposals for state health insurance aimed to help only a fraction of the neediest wage earners. Critics of "workingmen's insurance" offered other ways to improve access to medical care. By 1920, a handful of intellectuals and activists had gone so far as to embrace universality as a fundamental principle of national health policy. As first formulated, universalism attracted little support, even within Progressive circles. Instead, economists who dominated the social reform network of the time consistently emphasized particularistic plans to insure only those among the needy who were most likely to contribute to economic growth, narrowly defined. Nonetheless, this period of reform fervor did witness the initial stirrings of universalist sentiment with regard to health care.

## Access in Nineteenth-Century America

It is difficult to determine just how accessible health services were to Americans before 1900. (Historians of health care have yet to address this question directly.) Scattered bits of information are contradictory, suggesting both ample supplies of easily available care and significant deprivation. Because most medical education in the nineteenth century was brief and undemanding, physicians were numerous. No medical school required a college degree for admission until Johns Hopkins adopted such a policy in 1893; many other medical schools at that time did not require any collegiate preparation. Alternative approaches to healing proliferated, among them homeopathy and osteopathy. Moreover, by the end of the century, hospital-based schools were training huge numbers of nurses.[1]

A wide array of institutions delivered services. By the turn of the twentieth century, the general acute-care hospital had moved from the periphery of the health system to its center. Thousands of communities had at least one hospital, usually a nonprofit voluntary undertaking. Large cities and many counties maintained public hospitals. As Sandra Opdycke demonstrated in her aptly titled *No One Was Turned Away,* all-inclusive accessibility was the hallmark of New York City's municipal hospitals. Ubiquitous urban dispensaries not only distributed drugs but also delivered a range of outpatient services, often without charge. Special-purpose institutions admitted patients with mental illness, tuberculosis, and other specific conditions.[2]

The scant evidence suggests that health care was more affordable in the nineteenth century. Rudimentary technology, spirited competition among providers, and the persistence of a charity tradition combined to lower financial barriers. Medical fees tended to be modest and adjustable to the patient's perceived ability to pay. The vast majority of hospitals were not intended to be profit-making ventures and operated accordingly. They managed to survive on a mixture of paying patients, philanthropic support from local elites, and casual cross-subsidies for uncompensated care. A significant minority of the population participated in prepaid group health schemes sponsored by employers, unions, fraternal groups, or other community mutual-aid organizations.[3]

Nonetheless, there are signs that the nineteenth century was no golden age of unimpeded access to care. The ethos of medicine was sometimes one of small business rather than of altruistic professionalism. When in 1878 a young immigrant cigar maker named Samuel Gompers attempted to get a neighborhood physician to attend to his wife and newborn son, the doctor refused to comply because Gompers had no money. Only threats of physical violence and the chance discovery of two dollars secured medical attention in this case. As the century drew to a close, hospitals and dispensaries were becoming more vigilant about "charity abuse" and more solicitous of the paying patient. The invention of the means test barred many in the working class from receiving services. Whereas in 1898 New York City had eighteen municipal hospitals with an open-door policy, many other cities had no such refuges at all. No one had health insurance. The limited evidence suggests that access may have been becoming more difficult at the end of the nineteenth century.[4]

Difficulties in obtaining care mattered less when so much of even the best available therapy was relatively ineffective in curing disease. Indeed, advances in medicine constituted an essential condition for the emergence of healthcare access as a societal issue. Progress in biomedical science and technology produced stronger demand for professional treatment, even as it raised its cost. Beginning with the electrifying success of rabies treatment in the 1880s, the American public took (sometimes unwarranted) confidence in the efficacy of health care. "By the late 1890s," Paul Starr discerned, "medicine was making a difference in health."[5]

## A Vicious Partnership

Widespread awareness of the extent and impact of inadequate health care among the lower classes first surfaced only as an indirect object of Progressive concern. Initially, investigations into poverty brought to light the role of ill health as a cause and an effect of impoverishment. A series of American poverty studies conducted at the beginning of the twentieth century fell within a pattern set by British social empiricism. As in Great Britain, no investigator in the United States took the absence of hospital or medical services as the primary subject for study. Nonetheless, thorough exploration of the plight of the poor, and particularly of the dependent poor, invariably led muckrakers, professors, charity workers and other engaged professionals to consider the untreated sick. Although they frequently worked alone or with minimal institutional support, the first wave of investigators managed to illuminate many facets of lives dominated by the intertwined struggles for survival and respectability, struggles often exacerbated by the inaccessibility of health care. Modest inquiries produced narratives of personal and family tragedy, closely observed and often poignantly and unabashedly emotional. At the same time, Progressives explained small events in terms of societal determinants of health status. By both relating intimate stories and carrying out structural analysis, these reformers defended the destitute sick as the worthy poor.[6]

Progressive reformers diligently probed the societal roots of poverty. This was a significant departure from the prevailing perspective of the nineteenth century, which traced poverty to individual deficiencies. Social worker Robert Hunter learned about the urban poor mainly by living and working in such famous settlement houses as Chicago's Hull House, London's Townbee Hall, and New York's University Settlement House. His 1904 book *Poverty* reported that the sick accounted for about one quarter of those so impoverished as to seek charity, a degrading course of action pursued by only a fraction of the destitute. He well understood the lengths to which the disabled went to avoid dependence: "Anyone familiar with the poor knows with what grim determination half-sick workmen labor." Hunter deemed ill health "a fertile and lively cause of poverty, constantly active and supremely powerful." In his sympathetic view, "poverty and sickness form a vicious partnership, each helping the other to add to the miseries of the most unfortunate of mankind."[7]

Hunter's succession of eyewitness accounts of the sick poor seldom mentioned any resort to professional health care. The child dying in a stifling tenement apparently went unattended by any physician and obviously was not admitted to a hospital. The man who collapsed while working on a street-paving crew was simply brought home to share a bed with one of his children. Lower-class women with postnatal fever suffered from a "lack of care."[8]

Hunter's analysis went beyond personal observation of individual predicaments. He estimated that at least ten million Americans lived in poverty. He wondered why we spent "more money than any other nation in the world upon statistical investigations, and yet we know less about the poverty of the people than almost any other great nation of the Western world." Unfortunately, Hunter gave no estimate of how frequently the poor had to forgo the health services they needed. The Progressive settlement worker offered a list of legislative proposals to ameliorate poverty, including sanitary reforms intended primarily to prevent disease by improving living and working conditions. A budding radical, Hunter overstated the mandate for a universalistic health policy: "Socialism is now demanded by everyone to protect the health of the community and to make wise and far-reaching provisions for the physical welfare of all the people." He also recommended a government insurance program, but only in passing. Preoccupied with staving off dependency rather than with assuring the availability of medical care, Hunter presented social insurance as merely a method to "compensate labor for enforced seasons of idleness due to sickness."[9]

Subsequent works elaborated on Hunter's themes. In 1907, Louis More, another settlement house veteran, reviewed the subsistence strategies of two hundred working-class families in New York's Greenwich Village neighborhood. This study confirmed that illness, especially of the breadwinner, caused considerable dependence on private charity and public relief. More found that the poor relied heavily on dispensaries and had grown less wary of hospitals. He did, however, acknowledge that it was "still a common belief that people die if they go there." Edward Devine, professor of social economy at Columbia University and editor of the Progressive weekly *Survey*, drew on his many years as a charity worker to tie lack of health to lack of wealth. In *Misery and Its Causes*, Devine called ill health "perhaps the most constant of the attendants of poverty" and a factor in fully three-fourths of all applications for charitable aid. He concluded that health-related expenditures by low-income families averaged less than ten dollars per year, roughly one percent of family income. He found that those too poor to purchase care relied on free services, but sometimes not in a timely fashion. Rather than advocate enactment of health-insurance legislation, Devine hoped for the day when the incidence of disease would decline because working people were receiving "an income sufficient to provide for the essentials of rational living." Margaret Byington shared Devine's assessment that health care was unaffordable for much of the working class. Based on her exploration of desperate coping in the steel town of Homestead, Pennsylvania, Byington labeled health-care spending a luxury often beyond workers' means. "When, for instance, a child is ill," she maintained, "the state of the pocketbook, no less than the seriousness of the disease, determines whether the doctor is called." Thus, in the first decade of the twentieth century, students of poverty shed light on both the underlying economic determinants of illness and the immediate difficulties in receiving diagnostic and curative services.[10]

## A Healthful Wage

One strain of Progressivism concentrated on higher wages as the key to improving the health of the American working class. Proponents of a living wage delved into its probable implications for health. Notwithstanding its expansiveness and downright vagueness, the very term *living wage* directed attention to physical survival, that is, to a level of income that could sustain life. Arguments for subsistence compensation had arisen repeatedly in the United States throughout the Gilded Age. These earliest formulations occasionally named health care as one of the essential needs that such a wage would meet.[11]

In 1906, John Ryan entered this long discussion with a forceful defense of a pay scale that would enable workers to afford medical care. In *A Living Wage: Its Ethical and Economic Aspects*, Ryan provocatively cast his claims in terms of human rights, an exceptional argument for the time. This activist academic was a Roman Catholic priest, employed as a professor of economics and ethics at St. Paul Seminary. Economist Richard Ely introduced Ryan's work as "the first attempt in the English language to elaborate what may be called a Roman Catholic system of political economy" of which he was aware. Pope Leo XIII's 1891 encyclical *Rerum Novarum* gave Ryan a perspective on the situation of workers in industrializing societies that differed in important ways from that of his predominantly Protestant Progressive colleagues. One obvious distinction was a willingness to base his case directly and openly on religious principles. In contrast, advocates of social protection in this period generally couched moral principles in secular social-scientific language.[12]

Unlike his Protestant and Jewish counterparts, Father Ryan began from the fundamental premise that needs in and of themselves conferred rights. However breathtaking, this leap was only the first step on his path. Whereas settlement-house volunteers and other charity workers argued inductively from their exposure to many cases of deprivation, Ryan reasoned deductively from the Catholic doctrine of natural rights. He outlined an interpretation under which "the individual is endowed by nature, or rather, by God, with the rights that are requisite to a reasonable development of his personality." He maintained that "essential needs" determined the scope of these rights. Ryan recognized that satisfaction of needs, regardless of how essential or even sacred, depended upon the availability of resources. He looked upon America as a prosperous society in which the "natural resources and productive capacity are more than sufficient to furnish the entire population with the requisites of a decent livelihood." This state of affairs gave American wage earners a just claim on the means of subsistence. Ryan contended that this moral right should become a legal one. The state was "morally bound to compel employers to pay a Living Wage whenever and wherever it can" through legislation. He clearly considered moral suasion alone an inadequate force to realize this moral right.[13]

Ryan held that one criterion of a living wage was its capacity to provide for health care as one of the essential human needs. To be sure, his book paid more attention to the contribution of higher pay to preventing disease than to curing it. He approvingly cited this statement from economist William Smart: "Undoubtedly the first moral charge on the national income is such a sum as is necessary to bring up a family, providing for health, education, efficiency of work, and the conditions generally of a moral life." Against the rising national preoccupation with efficiency, he insisted that "the question that we are concerned with is not what a man must have in order to be a profitable producer, but what he ought to have as a human being." From this vantage point, Ryan held that a living wage had to be high enough to allow workers to cope with expenses—including lost income and medical services—entailed by sickness and injury. He sought a "family living wage" that would enable the husband and father to be the sole breadwinner in the household, with wives and daughters provided for as dependents. Ryan did, however, make an allowance for those unable (but apparently not for those unwilling) to secure this standard of living through membership in a male-headed family: "Those women who are forced to provide their own sustenance have a right to what is a Living Wage for them." General adoption of the living wage "would go very far toward removing those plague spots . . . in which thousands upon thousands of human beings are able to obtain only a fraction of the requisites of physical health and comfort." Other Progressives joined Professor Ely in warmly welcoming Ryan's book.[14]

Samuel Gompers shared Father Ryan's assessment of the health-promotive potential of the living wage. Like the Catholic professor, the Jewish labor leader stressed the preventive value of higher wages. As the founding president of the American Federation of Labor (AFL), Gompers drew up a short bargaining agenda that gave top priority to compensation. In a 1914 editorial, he called on those employers truly interested in their subordinates' well-being to prove it by raising pay levels. Thus, even before he took up the battle against government health insurance, Gompers maintained that better wages were crucial to improving the health of wage earners and that unions were the best instrument to achieve this end. In his brand of tightly focused unionism, which dominated labor thinking in the U.S. in the late nineteenth and early twentieth centuries, a higher standard of living became almost a panacea.[15]

## Professors Propose Insurance

Progressive reformers refused to wait for the AFL to organize all American workers and elevate their wages to a level at which illness and injury would pose no financial threat. In the 1910s, middle-class activists mounted a major drive for social insurance to cover health-care expenses. To be sure, this reform initiative may not have sought universal health insurance, but it did represent an important attempt to expand access to health services among the working poor.

European models were important for the American Progressives. As James Kloppenberg and Daniel Rodgers have made abundantly clear, an energetic transatlantic network of reformers exchanged ideas in the late nineteenth and early twentieth centuries. In the area of worker protections, the American Association for Labor Legislation (AALL) served as the chief importer of European legislative innovations in the 1900s and 1910s. From its founding in 1906 as a branch of the International Association for Labor Legislation, the AALL borrowed and adapted statutory language from abroad to craft workers' compensation bills and to win prohibition of workplace exposure to toxic phosphorus, to name just two of a host of labor laws that the group helped bring into existence.[16]

The AALL was led by economists and others trained in the emerging social sciences and employed in the burgeoning research universities. Its first four presidents were professors of economics. John Andrews, a protégé of labor economists John Commons and Richard Ely at Wisconsin, became the secretary of the organization in 1910 and held the position until his death in 1943. With its membership never exceeding three thousand members during the 1910s, the AALL never developed a mass base. Undaunted by its small numbers, the association epitomized Progressive faith in the capacity of scientific expertise to solve social problems through enlightened government intervention. This group firmly believed in its own expertise in designing public policies that would rationally conserve human resources.[17]

In 1912, the AALL Committee on Social Insurance took up state health insurance. The association sought to build on an encouraging precedent of the previous year, the passage of Britain's National Insurance Act. It also sought to capitalize on the growing momentum of the campaign for workers' compensation. Many Progressives assumed that compulsory health insurance represented the next step in the inevitable advance of social insurance. After much deliberation, the AALL offered up its "standard bill" for state health insurance in 1915 and began to introduce it in state legislatures the following year. From 1916 to 1920, the plan remained essentially unchanged.[18]

The AALL's standard bill was far from universal in scope. In this regard, it followed the path hewn by the association's workers' compensation legislation, which omitted large numbers of employees at risk of occupational injuries and illnesses. It also reflected the influence of British and German health insurance laws. Physician and actuary Isaac Rubinow, a tireless AALL activist whose many roles in the reform campaign included that of executive secretary of the AMA Social Insurance Committee, estimated that the German and British programs covered only about a third of their populations. The AALL measure was also predisposed against any commitment to universalism by the ideological orientation of its main sponsors, primarily due to their adoration of efficiency. Determined to maximize workers' productivity, Progressive labor economists took little account of anyone not involved in the world of commodity production, such as the elderly and the permanently disabled. In much the same vein, the reformers' commitment to promoting efficiency in government led them to exclude irregularly or informally employed workers, as they were likely to cause inconvenience for administrators. A preliminary set of AALL legislative standards proposed that insurance "should embrace as large a part of the wage working class as can be reasonably included without creating unsurmountable administrative difficulties." Accordingly, the economists' final plan provided that some sick workers earning less than one hundred dollars a month and their "dependents" would be eligible for health-care benefits and for cash benefits to replace a portion of their lost earnings. The AALL measure left out the unemployed, the self-employed, agricultural laborers, domestic servants, workers making more than one hundred dollars a month, and anyone not consistently a part of the paid workforce—all of whom were likely to present administrative difficulties. In effect, like other forms of American social insurance, this plan privileged white male employees, who were most heavily concentrated in steady jobs in the industrial sectors of the economy, such as manufacturing and transportation. In fact, the earliest American formulations of government health insurance were commonly called "workingmen's insurance."[19]

By the mid-1910s, however, proponents had generally discarded "workingmen's insurance" for less restrictive terms like "sickness insurance" or "health insurance." In part, this change in terminology reflected an important substantive departure from the influential German and English models, a departure in the direction of greater inclusion and less gender inequality. Both of the major European programs bestowed benefits on wage earners, the large majority of whom were males, but not on members of their immediate families. Rubinow estimated that in 1911 almost three times as many German males were insured as females; in the United Kingdom the ratio was more than two to one. He shed some light on the pressures that had prompted the move toward equality: "A limitation of the medical benefits to the wageworker alone would be strongly resented by wageworkers as well as by social workers and representatives of public medicine and hygiene. My own experience in . . . California convinces me that it would be impossible to create any general enthusiasm for a law containing any such limitation, that the great value of health insurance in the broad national movement for health conservation would be seriously jeopardized unless the wives and children were included." On the other hand, political pressures drove the AALL to back away from family coverage in two important states. Revised versions of the standard bill introduced in New York and Massachusetts in 1916 dropped family medical benefits, possibly due to fears that the benefits would disproportionately reach the large families of newly arrived immigrant workers. Nonetheless, the predominant American plan generally displayed more gender equality than its European forerunners, albeit mainly by construing women and girls as dependents of male breadwinners.[20]

A peculiar notion of universalism arose in some Progressive quarters. Discussing "Some Fundamental Considerations in Health Insurance" at a major national conference on social insurance in December 1916, Lee Frankel of the Metropolitan Life Insurance Company explained that what the champions of health reform "really desire is *universal* insurance. They hope to satisfy their sense of justice by including in their scheme of protection all individuals engaged in gainful occupation." That the AALL bill was a far cry from even this shrunken definition of universality did not seem to trouble Frankel. The AALL itself usually presented the matter in a more precisely qualified manner. A 1915 flyer summarizing its bill referred to coverage that would be "universal for all manual workers and for others earning less than $100 a month because experience elsewhere has shown that voluntary insurance will not reach the people who most need its protection." On occasion, however, the association and its leaders misleadingly portrayed their proposition as simply universal. This tendency to misuse the concept indicates that real universalism was tangential to the main policy conversation at that point.[21]

Some of those most acutely aware of the limitations in coverage under the AALL proposal pushed to expand its breadth marginally. The effective exclusion of women provoked much of the skirmishing over the boundaries of the covered population. In late 1914, activist Olga Halsey passed along to John Andrews a concern expressed by her mentor at Wellesley College, social scientist Katharine Coman. Pointing to the English experience, Professor Coman urged the AALL to alter its working draft to take in "outworkers and casual laborers." Andrews diplomatically thanked Halsey and Coman, but the AALL Committee on Social Insurance allowed its worries over administrative complications to override the needs of these workers. Little more than a year later, after Halsey had joined the association's staff with the sterling pedigree of a graduate thesis on British health insurance at the London School of Economics, it was her turn to back away from a wider commitment. In February 1916, she acknowledged to a physician that the bill currently pending in the New York legislature excluded some workers and others outside the paid workforce. Of course, by that time the AALL's well-established priority of administrative rationality had bound Halsey's hands. The association was also criticized for its failure to seek coverage for workers during periods of unemployment. In 1916, Isaac Rubinow cited the Danish policy of broader eligibility for health protection, without going all the way to universal entitlement. Instead, Rubinow vaguely suggested that social insurance "should be extended to all the classes which are in need of it." He also made a case for insuring male workers' families. "Surely," he asserted, "the life and health of wives and of the coming generation are of social value at least equal to the life and health of the laborers."[22]

Despite its severe limitations, the AALL plan did aim to improve significantly the ability of the working poor to get basic health services. Hospital administrator S. S. Goldwater supported a bill before the New York state legislature in 1917 in part "because a large proportion of the industrial workers of the community are without needed medical attendance." A 1915 editorial in the *Journal of the American Medical Association* welcomed further study of compulsory health insurance on the basis of British revelations: "English physicians are expressing their surprise at the mass of suffering which previously was uncared for. The failure of many persons in this country at present to receive medical care constitutes the best argument for a change to the more effectual provision for medical attention offered by health insurance." It was even possible to argue that realization of this form of social insurance would ensure access for the only sizable segment of the nation's population actually deprived of it. After all, the very poorest Americans could generally obtain free charitable care. The middle and upper social strata could purchase still-inexpensive services, including those delivered in hospitals. Thus, in practice, circumscribed compulsory health insurance might achieve a semblance of universal protection. Although none of its advocates appears to have gone so far as to argue that the patchy, segmental protection of the AALL plan would cover the only group denied access, some implied as much. B. S. Warren of the U.S. Public Health Service maintained that compulsory health insurance for low-paid workers would "place adequate medical relief within the reach of all." More realistically, such a program would have extended access to health care to many unserved and underserved members of the working class.[23]

## Debating the AALL Plan

The AALL health-insurance proposal and its variants immediately elicited criticism from all sides. To be sure, much of this opposition had little or nothing to do with the proposed restrictions in the scope of coverage. Physicians feared both a loss of control over the practice of their profession and a loss of income. The insurance industry rejected any government incursion at all into its market. After the United States declared war on Germany in April 1917, the association of state insurance with the German enemy also triggered complaints based on nationalism. In some critiques, these objections combined with concerns about health-care access.[24]

A variety of critics insisted that private alternatives, both real and potential, obviated or would obviate the need for mandatory insurance. Some champions of the living wage held that better pay would not only prevent disease but also enable workers to purchase available insurance. Resentful of what he took to be the ill-informed and patronizing meddling of elite intellectuals, Samuel

Gompers, for his part, relished any opportunity to denounce their statist solutions to workers' problems. In 1916, Gompers testified somewhat testily before a congressional committee that supporters of insurance legislation had overlooked the impact of higher pay on longevity. "No remedy," he told the House Committee on Labor, "is so potent to prolong life and to give help to the individual and to remove poverty as increases in wages." In an editorial about these hearings, he excoriated the AALL as barnacles attached to the labor movement. Unions, he maintained, struggled "to secure to all workers a living wage that will enable them to have sanitary homes, conditions of living that are conducive to good health, adequate clothing, nourishing food and other things that are essential to the maintenance of good health." Needless to say, he mentioned neither the plight of those outside the paid workforce nor the fact that union membership comprised only about ten percent of the American workforce. The AFL president was not alone in his preoccupation with raising wages. In his angry resignation from the AALL, Prudential Insurance executive Frederick Hoffman touted improved wages and working conditions as "a true form of health insurance, infinitely more desirable than a compulsory provision for medical care on the one hand and the payment of proportionate financial benefits on the other."[25]

A living wage would also enable workers to purchase health insurance on their own. Gompers particularly defended one type of voluntary protection. Since the 1870s, he had promoted union health benefits, which indemnified expenses of sickness and forged loyalty to the union. Some in corporate management promoted their own health plans. D. R. Kennedy of the B. F. Goodrich Company put his faith in "the experimentation of broad-minded, philanthropic manufacturers." The business-dominated National Civic Federation held that private insurance was growing and had not yet received a fair trial. Frederick Hoffman, perhaps the only person in America who outdid Gompers in the fervor of his opposition to state provision, cast doubt on claims that voluntarism had proven inadequate. As early as 1913, Hoffman had already begun to argue that expansion of existing private protections would obviate any need for public sickness insurance. Fraternal leaders joined the chorus of private agencies contending that they would soon overcome their shortcomings.[26]

Defenders of public insurance readily agreed on the importance of raising the income of the working poor. B. S. Warren and his PHS colleague Edgar Sydenstricker, among others, heralded "recognition of the principle of a 'living wage' as essential to the healthful standard of living." But reformers like War-

ren and Sydenstricker did not consider the living wage alone sufficient to safeguard the well-being of the working class. Moreover, advocates of compulsory
insurance considered any dramatic elevation in the compensation of all low-
paid employees too distant a prospect. In these circumstances, they reasoned
that state insurance was superior to voluntary insurance by virtue of its obligation to enroll immediately the mass of individuals unacceptable to private
insurers. In his AALL presidential address in 1916, Irving Fisher, professor of
political economy at Yale, asserted that better access to medical care under
state insurance would lift workers' productivity, which, in turn, would push up
their wages. The radical majority report of the U.S. Commission on Industrial
Relations, published the same year, also endorsed the living wage and compulsory health insurance.[27]

Catholic Progressives wanted both higher wages and protective legislation.
In its *Program of Social Reconstruction*, published in 1919, the administrative
committee of the National Catholic War Council accepted government insurance as a stopgap measure. Champions of a "family living wage" that would
keep women and children out of the workforce, the four bishops comprising
this committee acknowledged that this goal was far from realization. Accordingly, they reasoned, in the interim "the worker stands in need of the device of
insurance," so "the state should make comprehensive provision for insurance
against illness, invalidity, unemployment, and old age." The bishops' program
received warm applause from the Catholic community. Archbishop Edward
Hanna in San Francisco, for one, disseminated thousands of copies of the document and based a sermon on it. Non-Catholic reformers welcomed this comprehensive blueprint as well. John Ryan happily catalogued the copious publicity. Indeed, he was probably especially happy: he had drafted the program
for the committee. He described compulsory health insurance as "a logical extension of the living wage principle." Ryan's biographer, Francis Broderick, described the bishops' program as "perhaps the most forward-looking social
document to have come from an official Catholic agency in the United States."
William Kerby, professor of sociology at Catholic University, echoed the program in grounding his support for both the living wage and insurance legislation in ancient church doctrine.[28]

Partisans of state intervention expressed their skepticism about voluntarist
predictions on the promise of private insurance. Irving Fisher reported that
voluntary insurance covered only about five percent of those who needed it.
The AALL leader wrote off the private alternative: "The present insurance fa-

cilities in the United States are, and, as far as we can see, always will be hopelessly inadequate." Edgar Sydenstricker's study of the prevailing system led him to share Fisher's assessment. By 1916, Sydenstricker had already seen enough to predict failure: "The very fact that only a small minority of insurable wage earners are at present insured, even after a large variety of agencies have been available for a number of years, is evidence enough that voluntary insurance in this country . . . will never come up to our expectations." Pauline Newman had helped the International Ladies Garment Workers Union to establish benefit plans, including its own clinics. Yet Newman and her union were committed to state health insurance. "It is well for the moment to forget the organized small minority," she advised the American Nurses Association in 1917, "and think of the great mass of unorganized workers." And Pauline Newman was no isolated maverick. By 1919, twenty-one national unions and eighteen state labor federations formally supported the AALL proposal.[29]

The narrow limits of eligibility under the AALL bill gave opponents a line of attack that resonated in a society uncomfortable with acknowledging cleavages along class lines. Although the primary ideological objection at this moment was the supposedly un-American nature of this scheme, critics also decried compulsory health insurance as "class legislation." Grant Hamilton of the AFL Legislative Committee held that "this new form of charity provides for the division of society into classes, based upon wages received." Hamilton worried that social insurance would "make permanent distinctions between social groups." His colleague Gompers agreed that "governmental regulation tends to fix the citizens of the country into classes, and a long established insurance system would tend to make these classes rigid." The National Industrial Conference Board, a major forum for policy discussion in the business community, observed in 1918 that "no sickness or health insurance program yet offered purports to be available for the benefit of the entire community, or, in fact, for even all of the industrial population." Frederick Hoffman derided the circumscribed New York reform proposition as an inappropriate import that reflected its origins in class-ridden Europe.[30]

## Inquisitive States

Despite all this opposition, the AALL pursued its legislative objective with a sense of certitude. The professorial Progressives knew that state health insurance represented progress; they considered its enactment an inevitability.

They believed that convincing the polity as a whole of the value of compulsory health insurance would depend on their authoritative marshalling of empirical evidence. Revelations of the unpleasant facts of unmet need and lost productivity would, in their rationalistic and optimistic view, play a crucial part in bringing about change. To this end, the AALL political strategy favored the establishment of investigating commissions in those states actively considering the association's standard bill. In contrast to the wave of Progressive inquiry during the previous decade, this time reformers expected public institutions, not private individuals or private groups, to generate knowledge on which to base social policy. Indeed, the AALL never mounted its own major study of the health-care financing situation.[31]

Instead, several states set up commissions to assess the advisability of reform. Given that fields like health services research and health policy studies did not yet exist, the AALL and its network of allies filled a vacuum in terms of expertise. Some of the commissions conducted original investigations into conditions in their state; others only compiled the findings of recent inquiries. These short-lived institutions yielded a wealth of information about the accessibility of health care to workers and the sad consequences of its inaccessibility.[32]

California established the first investigatory body in May 1915. Driven by a sense that "destitution was a growing social disease," state lawmakers ordered the Social Insurance Commission "to make a careful study of European systems of social insurance" and "to determine whether California needed and was ready for a further development of social insurance." The commission concentrated on exploring the need for and the advisability of only one form of social insurance, health insurance. The AALL helped secure the appointment of Barbara Nachtrieb as executive secretary of the commission and the use of Isaac Rubinow as a consultant. These two advocates oversaw a sweeping study of the financial and medical situation of the state's wage earners and dependent poor. The California commission analyzed more than 5,000 applications for charity in Los Angeles and San Francisco. It scrutinized the ability to purchase care of more than 4,000 recipients of free clinic services. It conducted a house-to-house field study of working-class South San Francisco. It mounted a special investigation of more than 1,000 employed women "to find out the burden which sickness has put upon their incomes." It carried out other data-gathering activities too numerous to mention. The commission's report, written by Nachtrieb, appeared in January 1917.[33]

The Social Insurance Commission found that the existing arrangements for paying for health care had deep deficiencies. For many wage-earning households, financing care directly from their own income was out of the question. The commission pointed out the misleading nature of average wage levels and average family medical expenditures, given the extreme range and unpredictable variability of both of these indicators. Wages alone certainly would not suffice when manufacturing employees averaged more than two months of unemployment per year, and over 40 percent of female wage earners made less than nine dollars per week. Five percent of employed women incurred 50 percent of the medical costs. Close comparison of income with the cost of living determined that most workers could not realistically expect to save enough to cope with a significant bout of illness. Moreover, the investigators found that "even those of better incomes who can and do accumulate substantial savings are often unable to meet the heavy bills of protracted illness." Hence, the commission determined that "the problem of making ends meet, even in the normal run of events, is still a real one in the family of the working man or woman of this state. . . . If the ordinary living expenses are greatly enhanced by the necessity of buying costly medical or hospital care, it can be easily seen that the problem of existence becomes a serious one."[34]

This widespread vulnerability had given rise to diverse forms of health insurance and prepaid health care. In almost every case, "health insurance" in California, as elsewhere in this period, covered not the actual expenses of care but rather some of the wages lost during illness, with only the assumption that a portion of these benefits would be spent on health services. Employers, unions, fraternal lodges and other associations offered disability insurance to wage earners. Less commonly, these organizations made available the services of a physician or, much less commonly, the facilities of a hospital. However resourceful, ambitious, and seemingly ubiquitous these provisions may have been, they did not extend nearly widely enough. The Social Insurance Commission concluded its survey with this verdict: "Probably not more than one-third of California wage-workers have voluntarily insured themselves against the hazard of sickness, and these voluntary efforts reach only an extremely small proportion of the people who need it most."[35]

The inadequacy of private health-care funding drove many Californians to medical charities. The commission learned that "a vast amount" of aid was dispensed across the state, either through the delivery of free services or the use of a sliding scale to make doctor's fees affordable. Most patients at urban free clinics were low-paid, full-time workers, not people removed from the workforce and therefore dependent on relief. Men engaged in common labor and women in domestic service resorted to these facilities "despite the instinctive dislike felt by self-respecting working people for dispensation of any sort." Of course, that stigma surely meant that some needy individuals avoided charity altogether or waited too long to seek it. In addition, the commission found that public hospitals did not have nearly enough beds to meet demand. The patchwork of medical charity simply did not cover all the holes left by other methods of health-care financing.[36]

The California commission identified illness as a leading cause of impoverishment, which naturally led to a dependence on charitable relief. Its analysis of 5,296 dependent families found that illness was the primary cause of destitution in more than half the cases. Almost a fifth of these illnesses involved pregnancy. A more probing analysis of 500 families on general relief uncovered numerous instances of health-related financial ruin. A forty-eight-year-old teacher spent her life savings of $3,000 on a series of ineffective operations. These expensive procedures left her "penniless, incapacitated for work and dependent upon charity for the means of mere subsistence." The commission's report did not discuss the extent to which poverty resulted from untreated illness or injury. However, a flier the commission published in 1918 called attention to forgone care: "You all know the girl who would not lay off and go to the doctor until it was too late. You all know the reason why—expense—the cost of the doctor and medicine [and] the loss of wages."[37]

The California commission recommended enactment of compulsory health insurance legislation. Rather than put forward a draft bill, the body delineated basic principles and provisions for future legislation. The nebulous outline did not specify income limits or any other criteria for state health-care coverage eligibility; instead it called for insurance for "wageworkers and other persons of small incomes." Similarly, the recommendations did not clearly state whether health-care benefits would extend to members of wage earners' families or just to the wage earners themselves. However, the commission's estimate that its plan would protect only about one-third of the state's population plainly implied that workers' families were not included.[38]

Subsequent studies in other states amplified the main findings in California. Common methods of funding health services through wages, savings, and voluntary insurance came up short everywhere. Ohio investigators found that about 35 percent of the state's workers had health insurance of any kind.

Moreover, this involved only sick pay, meaning that "practically no medical benefits are given." In Pennsylvania, the Health Insurance Commission estimated that only about 30 percent of employees in the commonwealth had insurance and that families were seldom covered. In Illinois, commissioners augmented their state-wide survey (which, as in Pennsylvania, found approximately 30 percent insured) by intensively canvassing a working-class neighborhood in Chicago. This door-to-door inquiry discovered that less than a quarter of the 2,708 workers' households consulted had any sickness insurance. The Massachusetts Special Commission on Social Insurance admitted that it had failed to calculate the number of uninsured wage earners but was sure that many in the state had no protection. This body also noted that in no European nation had voluntary insurance ever achieved anything like universal coverage.[39]

Across the nation, as in California, scant financial means kept many sick people from receiving health care. AALL leaders John Commons and Arthur Altmeyer advised the Illinois Health Insurance Commission of a Milwaukee survey that found that only 11,000 of 40,000 sick people were under a physician's care. Commons and Altmeyer calculated that under compulsory health insurance more than 25,000 of these individuals would have been eligible to obtain indemnified care. In Massachusetts, investigators discovered that "even in a district as well supplied with medical and hospital facilities as Boston, competent medical service actually fails to reach a substantial portion of the very poor," who supposedly had ready access to charity care. The Pennsylvania commission alerted political leaders to the fact that "approximately a fourth of those actually disabled by illness never receive medical care, and a larger percentage of those ill but still trying to work are without attention." Tracing the downward slide one step further, the Pennsylvania inquiry ascertained that forgone care left many workers with chronic disease. The consistent pattern of deprivation publicized by the commissions was fresh ammunition to reformers everywhere. In New York, where interest in insurance legislation was high but no commission operated, social insurance advocates like Frederick Davenport used the wealth of new information. In a speech to labor and women's activists on August 27, 1919, Davenport, the leading proponent of reform in the New York legislature, called attention to the discovery of "vast uncared for need" in the nation's working population. "There is much neglect of incipient diseases," he warned. "The neglect gives opportunity for the development of a mass of chronic ailments."[40]

The raft of state studies also brought to light other economic and social consequences of the prevailing system. The Pennsylvania and Ohio commissions confirmed that sickness was the main factor leading to dependence. Authorities also discovered financial difficulties short of outright destitution. Ohio investigators estimated that up to half of all indebtedness stemmed from illness. The Illinois study disclosed that major illness sometimes forced beleaguered families to send their children into the workforce at an early age. In an analysis of the Illinois report prepared for the state's labor movement, Olga Halsey noted not only the impact of sickness on child labor but also the willingness of working-class families to take on debt and to "undergo severe hardships" in order to avoid acceptance of charity.[41]

Taken together, the state investigations marshaled a mass of evidence documenting the need for public insurance. As in the previous round of inquiries by conscientious individuals, these studies involved face-to-face contact with the working poor. In addition, ongoing reliance upon charitable agencies for information brought narratives of need to the attention of public officials. Based on these methods, the state continued to present compelling accounts of suffering. Moreover, the commissions continued, to some extent, to use emotionally charged language in portraying that suffering. The Massachusetts commission, for instance, characterized sickness as one of the "gaunt specters of human woe [which] bring a train of misery and evil consequences." Tellingly, anecdotal evidence almost always came forth indirectly, as interpreted by middle-class investigators, not in the voices of those experiencing difficulties.

By the late 1910s, a major transition in policy discourse was already well under way. Quantitative evidence was displacing older forms of qualitative evidence that captured the feelings of humiliation, the sense of loss, the myriad nuances of deprivation. Progressives now deployed stories of hardship primarily to complement the statistical compilations that carried the brunt of the argument. Especially with respect to the problem of access, the more heavily statistical approach certainly had the advantage of more precisely assessing the extent of unmet need, if not the full range of its human ramifications. The economists in the AALL and its circle believed that their numerical rhetoric was far more scientific and, therefore, would be more compelling to political decision makers than the caseworkers' litany of sorrows. As Linda Gordon and others have suggested with respect to the wider trend in American social reform, a male style was challenging a female style of discourse.[42]

The mountains of expert evidence did not, however, produce an unequiv-ocal mandate for reform. Eleven state reports yielded six recommendations in favor of state insurance and four recommendations opposed to it; one report took no position. In fact, the commissions did not even reframe the debate in terms of an imperative need for expanded health care. Instead, criticism of the AALL bill and others like it only intensified amid the nationalistic fervor of World War I and its aftermath, as Ronald Numbers, Beatrix Hoffman, and other historians have made transparently clear. In the political arena, state health insurance propositions everywhere met defeat. Certainly, some of the commissions aborted political deliberation by their refusal to recommend state intervention. In New York and other states where sufficient momentum existed to prompt the introduction of insurance bills, the legislative measures still went nowhere. In California, voters rejected compulsory health insurance in a referendum in November 1918.[43]

## Glimpses of Universalism

In these dreary circumstances, many supporters of state insurance re-treated. On the other hand, a few advocates embraced still more ambitious ideas. Promoting truly universal health protection offered one rejoinder to the charge of "class legislation." At hearings in San Francisco, James Whitney, pro-fessor of medicine at the University of California, told the state Social Insur-ance Commission, "I should like to see everybody, including millionaires, compelled to take out health insurance." In his testimony, state AFL official W. W. Harris agreed: "Organized labor is opposed to being legislated for apart from others." Labor journalist Thomas Mullen testified, "I would favor this in-surance if it were to apply to every citizen in California, but I don't believe in compulsion for one class." The unionists' main underlying concern at this juncture apparently was to gain protection for the unemployed. In the wake of the defeat of the insurance referendum in November 1918, California Progres-sive C. D. Stuart informed John Andrews that the proposition had raised "sus-picion of class legislation." Stuart suggested that future plans might fare better if they were to "include every member of the political body." (Andrews's reply, if any, has not survived.) One less adventurous Progressive dealt with allega-tions of preferential treatment by reasoning that partial programs benefited all members of society. "It is not 'class' legislation in which we are interested," Charles Henderson of the University of Chicago assured the National Conference of Charities and Corrections in 1914. "In protecting the health, the income, and the culture of the toilers we are fortifying the defenses of national vitality, power, and glory." The dialectics of political debate emboldened some reformers more than others.[44]

No one plunged into universalism with more enthusiasm than Rufus Potts, state insurance superintendent in Illinois and chair of the Social Insurance Committee of the National Convention of Insurance Commissioners. Potts had shifted toward a more inclusive position by the time he appeared at congressional hearings in 1916. "Our form of government requires that the sharing of burdens and the sharing of profits shall extend to all," Potts told the House Committee on Labor, while remaining somewhat vague about his preferences regarding the scope of governmental protection. In subsequent statements, however, he unequivocally and even rhapsodically promoted universal provision as a panacea. On one occasion, Potts declared all-encompassing health insurance "an effective method for carrying out Christ's altruistic command to bear one another's burdens." In his assessment, such protection was "urgently needed by everyone not independently wealthy." He presented this remedy as essential to societal progress, promising a "happier world under universal insurance." Moreover, benefits had to come from state intervention, not from private insurance carriers, whom he branded "extortioners [*sic*] and parasites." In light of his fervent moralism, it is somewhat curious that Potts refrained from positing general health security as a moral right.[45]

A few other proponents did set universal provision on a foundation of rights, however. Social rights in Progressive America did not simply follow from citizenship. Instead they had to be earned by a monetary payment or by some other contribution of value. The AALL plan anchored the right in ongoing financial contributions: employees making less than a hundred dollars a month were to pay 40 percent of state health insurance premiums by regular deductions from their wages. (Employers were to match this assessment, with government revenues providing the remaining 20 percent of the financing.) This dollars-and-sense criterion for entitlement forced universalists to think creatively. Socialist physician James Warbasse invented a novel justification in 1914: "Medical knowledge has been won through the sufferings of countless generations of men and women and children. Students of science, long since passed away, have contributed to it. The ancestors of all of us have died to give it to us. It is natural to think of it as social knowledge—the heritage of all—to be denied to none—its benefits to be accessible freely to the descendants of man, all of whom, in due time, must contribute their quota to it." This attempt to get credit for past sacrifice appears to have had no influence on the course of the policy debate. Eden Delphey, a New York physician, turned to the specific precedents of accepted universal public services. After criticizing the exclusion of many groups under the AALL bill, Delphey offered an alternative: "The only way that all these people can be insured and the only way to simplify the insurance [program] is for the State to insure every man, woman, and child whether they are employed or not and whether they pay any share of the cost or not. The State furnishes educational advantages, fire and police protection. Why not furnish this?" This would be among the first of many invocations of the precedent of public education.[46]

Only middle-class supporters of reform made claims of universal entitlement not deriving from the beneficiaries' financial stake. None of the working poor put forward any such arguments. Historian James Patterson took notice of a general reticence: "Although [the poor] aspired to a better life, few thought they had a right to a minimum standard of living—or even to charity. Before 1930 the notion rarely crossed their minds that government would offer much help." Reformers' initial assertions of a right to health care obviously did not succeed in mobilizing mass demands for assistance.[47]

Progressives stressed societal duty over individual right. In 1917, Martha Russell began her explanation of the meaning of state insurance for her fellow nurses with the observation that "during the past twenty years a new recognition of social obligation has grown up in the community." Sociologist William Kerby declared a universal obligation to aid the poor but no corollary entitlement to medical care in his 1921 book *The Social Mission of Charity*. "No one is required to do everything for the poor," Kerby maintained, "but everyone is obliged to do something." His demonstration of the compatibility of Progressive reform with Catholic teachings emphasized dutiful individual initiative as exemplified by the Good Samaritan. At the same time he granted a supplementary role for circumscribed legislation based on human rights. Unprepared to advocate a universal right to health care, Kerby nonetheless put the question in terms compatible with that stance: "Human rights seem shorn of all respect when industry holds life more cheaply than profits, and industrial power absolves itself from the restraints of Christian faith and sympathy in not caring about the helplessness of those who have lost in the competitive struggle." This application of the precepts of the *Rerum Novarum* encyclical to American society would help pave the way for assertions of health rights for all.[48]

During the first twenty years of the twentieth century, health policy discourse in the United States included few suggestions for all-encompassing access to care. In part, the hegemony of particularism reflected European influences. None of the dozen or so European welfare systems already in place had achieved any approximation of universal health coverage. In part, particularism also resulted from the failure of the neediest to join the conversation. It is not unreasonable to conjecture that the marginalized might have made universalistic appeals in order to avoid special pleading. Certainly, union leaders like Pauline Newman, fresh from the ranks of low-paid labor, ventured to offer a more inclusive perspective. However, the main radical political force of the time, the Socialist Party of America, demanded not universal care, but rather only health services for the working class.[49]

In large part, partial forms of health security reflected the limited vision of the leading Progressive reformers. It is especially telling that even in its private deliberations, where more expansive ideas might have been aired, the AALL never seriously entertained either universal protection or any major expansion of health insurance eligibility beyond that inscribed in its standard bill. Instead, the association and its allies were preoccupied with maximizing the productive efficiency of some wage earners. That this tidy prescription entailed the exclusion of many Americans—especially women and minorities—was not yet considered a critical flaw by Progressive intellectuals. But in certain reform circles, that narrow view would soon be overturned.

# CHAPTER TWO

# One of the Most Radical
# Moves Ever Made

Good medical care implies the application of all the necessary services of modern, scientific medicine to the needs of all the people. Judged from the viewpoint of society as a whole, the qualitative aspects of medical care cannot be dissociated from the quantitative. No matter what the perfection of technique in the treatment of one individual case, medicine does not fulfill its functions adequately until the same perfection is within the reach of all individuals.

— ROGER LEE AND LEWIS JONES, 1933

Universal health care became a significant American social policy ideal during the 1920s. Full-fledged arguments for health protection for all citizens replaced the scattered and fleeting references to this distant aim previously put forth. New proponents joined persistent Progressives in imagining pluralist, statist, and voluntarist forms of all-inclusive health protection. Arising in the prosperous twenties, the dream of health care for all certainly reflected the ebullient temper of the times. That this ambitious ideal persisted into the depressed early thirties suggests that it had become more securely embedded in the consciousness of the nation's leading policy architects.

In large part, growing optimism about the value of scientific medicine created interest in distributing its benefits across the population. Advancements in biomedical science—discovering not only the germs that caused disease but also means to treat infection—made many people hopeful. Advances in surgical methods, diagnostic technology, and other services provided by acute-care hospitals gave patients of all classes reason to seek access to sophisticated care. The movement toward physician-controlled childbirth in a hospital setting accelerated after 1920. As community hospitals and other providers further curtailed free services and commodified more of their offerings, the patient of modest or meager income frequently became the ultimate casualty of a consumer society. In the context of apparent medical miracles, inability to purchase services more commonly meant a denial of the means of survival. For some scientistic humanitarians, by the 1920s health care had become too good not to share with all who needed it.[1]

The most fervent champions of universal care came from within the biomedical community itself. Physicians, nurses, and public health practitioners understood most readily and most thoroughly the importance of access in maintaining a decent quality of life, in addition to the more direct benefit of saving lives. Although the social scientists who had dominated the Progressive debate did not disappear from the scene, they did yield leadership to health professionals. As the American Association for Labor Legislation faded into the background, no single advocacy group came forward with an all-encompassing design for reform. Instead, an informal group of elite reformers based in medical and public health schools and health-related foundations led the effort to reshape the policy agenda. Unlike economists predisposed toward promoting productivity by selective investments in human capital, biomedical professionals were familiar with communicable disorders that threatened all members of society and that were often spread by asymptomatic persons. Health workers experienced in battling such infectious conditions understood that it was futile to protect only part of the population. Within the pioneering cohort of biomedical universalists, those from the field of public health were generally the most committed to making medical care accessible to everyone.

Throughout this important period of policy development, there was no consensus as to the optimal way to achieve universal provision. Social insurance, soundly defeated in the 1910s, had lost its allure for many. Indeed, many reformers with medicine and public health backgrounds had never been very enthusiastic about this method, preferring plans that expanded governmental health care. However, during this embryonic period, the predominant style was far from doctrinaire. Most early proponents of universalism envisioned mixed forms of public and private health care delivery and financing.

## Rethinking Prevention

The reformers of the 1910s had promised that social insurance would bring about the prevention of illness and injury. The American Association for

Labor Legislation came to the health-insurance campaign fresh from victories enacting new workers' compensation laws. The financial incentive of lower insurance premiums instantly motivated employers to minimize safety hazards in the workplace. Aiming to repeat this successful formula, the AALL health insurance bill provided for a tripartite financing arrangement that created incentives to minimize disease and nonoccupational injuries. If workers incurred payroll deductions for state health benefits, they would, it was hoped, change their health-endangering habits. Employers' matching contributions would foster workplace health-promotion initiatives. Government funding would presumably lead to further state action to maximize the well-being of the insured. Armed with this rationalistic plan, Progressives made a mantra of prevention. In 1914, in a typical expression of enthusiasm, the AALL's Social Insurance Committee considered it "especially important that sickness insurance be established with emphasis on medical care in order that it shall lead to a campaign of health conservation similar to the 'safety-first' movement resulting from accident compensation." Michael Davis, director of the Boston Dispensary, shared the belief that state insurance would bring "steady economic pressure upon those who have daily opportunity to prevent disease." Progressive reformers thus vigorously promoted the goal of preventing illness.[2]

Attention to prevention shaped policymaking long after the demise of the AALL bills. Opponents of compulsory insurance put forward the alternative of expanded public health work, which directly attacked the causes and spread of illness. In 1918, the National Industrial Conference Board (NICB) maintained that the European experience had yielded no evidence that governmental insurance reduced rates of morbidity. After reminding the public that social insurance sought to cover "only a portion of one class of the population," the board called for the creation of a national commission to design a broader preventive program. The NICB couched its proposal in universalistic terms, referring to disease prevention as "a duty of society to its members." The following year, the business group took this line of thinking one step further. An NICB pamphlet contrasted the insurance bill under consideration in New York, which purportedly covered less than a third of the state's residents, with an expanded public health program with benefits that "could easily be made available for all the people, not merely one small group." When Margaret Stecker testified for the board before the New York legislature on March 31, 1919, she stressed the preventive value of health education and encouraged more funding for the state health department. Other promoters of straightforward prevention within the business community included the National Civic Federation and insurance executive Frederick Hoffman.[3]

Supporters of state insurance agreed that direct prevention of disease was desirable. Beyond a few diehards in the AALL inner circle, Progressives generally stopped looking to social insurance as a panacea by the end of the 1910s. Alice Hamilton perceptively noted that discussions at the 1916 American Public Health Association (APHA) meeting had raised doubts about the ability of insurance alone to curtail disease. British social theorist and activist Sidney Webb advised Olga Halsey that insurance schemes of that sort "are less successful in preventing disease and promoting health than they are in satisfying the ordinary man's desire for a bottle of physic and sick pay." When Webb's Fabian Society inspired proposals for wider social protections in postwar Britain, at least one American sought to borrow the blueprint. In mid-1918, Hornell Hart of the Trounstine Foundation appealed to John Andrews to plan for a whole new social democratic order. Hart drew on the current military mobilization to imagine state intervention reaching far beyond sickness insurance for a minority of Americans: "A vast organization has been built up to protect the health of soldiers at government expense. . . . Medical care should be provided freely by the government for the entire community and the emphasis should be placed, as in the army, on prevention." Andrews wished Hart well and dodged any commitment to expanding public health care. But some of Andrews's closest associates did give some thought to universal public medicine. University of Wisconsin economists John Commons and Arthur Altmeyer included, without comment, "state medical care to provide care for all" in a menu of "counter-suggestions" presented to the commission investigating social insurance in Ohio in 1919. Later that year, Commons, who was Andrews's mentor and predecessor as AALL secretary, speculated to the leaders of the National Tuberculosis Association about expanding the sort of free, comprehensive, and preventively oriented services delivered to students at the University of Wisconsin. "Why," Commons asked, "should not something like this arrangement be extended to the entire population of the state and the nation?" Although Commons must have known that the students received care not through a private insurance arrangement but rather from state-employed health-care providers, he hastened to insist that he still favored state insurance over socialized medicine. The much embattled AALL was not about to risk further denunciations by advocating even more venturesome proposals for governmental intervention in health affairs.[4]

In contrast, some members of the U.S. Public Health Service (PHS) seemed eager to set aside social insurance in favor of extending governmental delivery of health care. Throughout the 1910s, the PHS had mounted a series of probing studies of the health problems besetting the working class and the lack of resources available to solve those problems. Federal investigators initially used their findings to help make the case for state insurance, which Surgeon General Rupert Blue in 1916 called "the next great step in social legislation." But as the prospects of the AALL bill dimmed in the face of staunch opposition, the two leading advocates of reform in the PHS shifted their stance. In an article in the April 18, 1919, issue of *Public Health Reports,* Assistant Surgeon General Benjamin Warren and statistician Edgar Sydenstricker worried about the "probability of sickness insurance acts endangering the very existence of state health departments by absorbing all of the funds available for health work." To meet this potential threat, Warren and Sydenstricker called for the creation of a large cadre of state "medical referees" to certify eligibility for disability benefits and to practice extensive preventive medicine. This corps of state physicians would constitute "a health machine protecting every home" in ways that mere insurance could not. In another article that year in *Public Health Reports,* Warren argued that federal authorities shared with their colleagues in local and state government an interest in "the health of all the people." Hence, he urged greater public coordination in both the prevention and cure of disease. Warren put universal access at the center of his plan for a transformed health system: "In these days of progress in preventive medicine there is some tendency to separate too sharply the preventive from curative medicine. It should not be forgotten that an adequate medical service to the whole people will do more to prevent disease and disability than any other single measure." This belief that the intertwining of prevention and cure warranted universal care would soon become a widely shared viewpoint, but in 1919 it was quite novel in the United States. Understandably, this senior civil servant believed that the virtues of bureaucratic administration made cost no obstacle to reform. Warren declared that "with a proper organization, distribution, and training of the medical and sanitary personnel of the country, and a proper expenditure of the funds now being spent for medical purposes, there would be available, to every person, adequate medical and hospital services and supplies."[5]

## Newsholme Tours America

Whereas Benjamin Warren's suggestion received little attention, a similar analysis imported from abroad generated much interest. Much as European precedents inspired and guided the American campaign for insurance legislation in the 1910s, the transatlantic exchange continued to shape policy thinking in the following decade. However, after World War I the dominant model was no longer social insurance but rather state medicine. By his forceful advocacy of increased public services, Sir Arthur Newsholme did a great deal to introduce the goal of universal health care into medical and public health circles in this country.

The establishment of the first graduate schools of public health provided a natural institutional vantage point from which to envision, if not launch, a more inclusive system of health services. In 1919, Newsholme arrived from Great Britain on the invitation of William Henry Welch, director of the recently founded School of Hygiene and Public Health at Johns Hopkins University. Welch intended to have his old friend help set up a program in health administration. As he had just retired as principal medical officer of Britain's Local Government Board, where his decade of service culminated a long career in public health, Newsholme came well prepared for the assignment. Of perhaps most relevance at this juncture, he landed in America with a close familiarity with the implementation of national health insurance in his homeland following its enactment in 1911.[6]

The British visitor used his two-year stint at Johns Hopkins to articulate an expansive vision. Described by biographer John Eyler as "a tireless lecturer," Newsholme found many opportunities to proclaim universal health care a central component in future public-health practice. As he put it at the New York Academy of Medicine in 1919, socialization of health services would eventually make "available for every member of the community . . . all the potentialities of preventive and curative medicine." As a first step toward this goal, Newsholme urged extending hospital services to all members of society.[7]

Newsholme justified universalism on several grounds. He stretched the Progressive preoccupation with conserving human resources to cover everyone and threw in a less practical consideration: "We are all concerned in the efficiency of every member of the community, from an economic as well as a humanitarian standpoint." He appealed to enlightened self-interest with the scarcely substantiated claim that "health is less costly than disease." He asserted that expanded health provision would help stem social unrest. He held that the world war had created a widespread desire to make sacrifices for the general welfare. In a lecture at Yale on January 22, 1920, Newsholme celebrated this fresh "determination to spend and be spent to secure the welfare of all." He alluded to moral obligations imposed by Christian faith and borrowed Robert Burton's seventeenth-century characterization of physicians as "God's intermediate ministers." Not a sophisticated political philosopher, Newsholme seemingly seized upon whatever justification was at hand.[8]

For Newsholme, universalism also followed directly from the inclusive approach that had long guided public health, both in Britain and in the United States—at least in theory. Environmental sanitation, water purification, food inspection, and other governmental interventions took for granted the goal of safeguarding the entire population. At the annual American Public Health Association meeting of 1919, Newsholme dealt with a fundamental question: "What is public health work? It is best defined by stating its object, which is to secure the maximum attainable health of every member of the community." From his perspective, public health officers were best suited for the task of dismantling the barrier between prevention and cure. Building a case for greater public responsibility, Newholme extrapolated from the trend toward greater state involvement in health affairs that he had observed over the course of his own career. He cited the precedents for strong action: "If communal provision has been recognized as a duty for police protection, for sanitation, for elementary education, should it not likewise be admitted for the more subtle and maleficent enemies of health?" Newsholme thus delineated for Americans an inclusive and comprehensive program of care. Despite his emphasis on the crucial role of government health officers like himself, Newsholme expected the private practice of medicine to continue for an indefinite period of time, with a new preventive component. In this interim scenario, "each medical practitioner . . . [would become] a medical officer of health."[9]

Newsholme criticized social insurance at a number of stops on his 1919–20 speaking tour. He advised audiences of the inability of British health insurance either to deliver preventive services or to lead indirectly to the prevention of disease. The celebration of the fiftieth anniversary of the founding of the Massachusetts Board of Health in September 1919 gave Newsholme a chance to remark upon "the absurdity of regarding insurance as anything beyond the possibly useful handmaiden and auxiliary to Public Health." Instead, in his analysis, enactment of national insurance had represented mainly a distraction from real reform, a missed opportunity to develop public medicine. Moreover, he intently attacked the British insurance system for excluding such a large share of the population.[10]

Newsholme's views received considerable notice. The *Survey* reprinted his address to the New York Academy of Medicine, provocatively entitled "The Increasing Socialization of Medicine." His energy, experience, and stature made up for his lack of eloquence. He played a key catalytic role in shifting discussion away from social insurance and toward universal health care, care which he hoped would eventually be delivered by the state. His efforts amplified the handful of expressions of support for universal care already on record in America. These indigenous expressions, from Benjamin Warren, from some representatives of the Socialist Party, and from reformers like Michael Davis (who remained more identified with social insurance), had heretofore remained virtually inaudible in the policy conversation.[11]

## Incrementalists Take Their First Steps

While Newsholme and Warren sketched grand designs, other reformers searched for ways to improve health-care access in the short term. These reform propositions notably gave priority to prevention over cure. They did not seek all-inclusive coverage for the full complement of health services but sought instead either universal access to a narrow range of services or fairly broad access to a wider range of services.

In 1920, Hermann Biggs spelled out a plan to help New York counties to establish health centers. As state commissioner of health, Biggs feared that shortages of physicians and other personnel, along with the absence of clinical laboratories and other modern facilities and equipment, were depriving much of the state's population of life-saving assistance, both curative and preventive. Augustus Wadsworth, Biggs's colleague at the New York State Department of Health, stressed the latter, imagining the health centers as sites "from which public health activities could radiate to the surrounding community." Embodied in the Sage-Machold Bill presented in Albany in the 1920 legislative session, the commissioner's remedial plan rested on his famous visionary dictum that public health was purchasable. Although its primary purpose was to bring modern diagnostic services to underserved upstate areas, the Biggs proposition had the potential to cover all New Yorkers. Certainly, its inventor conceived of it in universalistic terms, declaring its purpose to be "to provide for the residents of rural districts, for industrial workers and all others in need." His lieutenant Wadsworth agreed that "obviously all the people must be taken care of, and there is no provision for this at present." However, as Milton Terris has pointed out, realizing this bold aim was quite a remote possibility under the Biggs initiative. The bill merely permitted county health units to set up health centers, requiring neither that they do so nor that they deliver anything beyond minimal diagnostic services. These qualifications did not, however, forestall intense opposition from organized medicine, which succeeded in defeating attempts to enact the health-center proposal in 1920 and 1921.[12]

Despite its limitations, the Biggs scheme was seen as the harbinger of all-encompassing state medicine. Journalist Gerald Morgan hailed the introduction of the Sage-Machold measure in a laudatory article in the *New Republic* in 1921. Morgan considered delivery of health services "properly a function of the community, to be available to every member of the community, to be financed partly by fees from those who can pay fees, partly by general taxation." His *Public Relief of Sickness*, published in 1922, developed a fuller proposal that drew heavily on the Biggs model. Morgan unequivocally promoted community health centers to serve everyone with a wide range of services. "Adequate medical treatment ought to be provided not to any particular class, like the working class, for a limited time and while in employment," he maintained, "but at all times to the entire public, since it is beyond the means and beyond the reach of even the so-called well-to-do." By recognizing that access to care was a growing problem for Americans who were neither poor nor residents of underserved rural areas, Morgan signaled an important shift in policy orientation.[13]

On the other side of the debate, representatives of organized medicine in New York and across the nation bristled at what they took to be a dangerous intrusion. At a meeting of the AMA House of Delegates in June 1921, the Medical Society of New Hampshire declared itself "emphatically opposed to 'State Medicine,' and to any scheme for 'Health Centers.'" A year later, the House of Delegates formally avowed its opposition to public provision of care—with specified exceptions, such as care for military personnel, the indigent, and the mentally ill. State medicine had replaced compulsory insurance as the great threat to the profession.[14]

The AMA also resisted a simultaneous attempt to expand health services for mothers and infants. Here, too, proposals to craft a circumscribed public program failed to appease conservatives. To be sure, at least one of the first proponents of public maternal and child health care had cast this issue in open-ended terms that must have disturbed leaders of organized medicine. In 1918, Julia Lathrop, director of the Children's Bureau of the U.S. Department of Labor, took the position that "medical and nursing care at the service of all mothers and infants in this country" was essential to lowering infant mortality. However, Lathrop's bureau subsequently worked closely with a strong and resourceful network of maternalist activists to draft and lobby for a less comprehensive proposition. In November 1921, President Warren Harding signed the Maternity and Infancy Act, whose principal sponsors were Morris Sheppard in the Senate and Horace Towner in the House of Representatives. The Sheppard-Towner Act gave federal funds to state health and welfare agencies to arrange pre- and postnatal services. The law tried to skirt confrontation with the medical establishment by placing a priority on education and diagnosis and not treatment of disease. Nonetheless, opponents of the Sheppard-Towner Act never let up, prevailing upon Congress to kill the outreach program of instruction and care by withholding its funding after June 30, 1929.[15]

Medical leaders also resisted incremental intrusion of the new field of public health nursing into areas beyond maternal and child health. In particular, some medical practitioners were dismayed at the possibility that visiting nurses might venture beyond hygienic instruction to deliver bedside care, especially care not properly supervised by a doctor. Their anxieties were not unfounded. In the 1920s, public nurses often let their sense of universalism override their regard for physicians' authority. On April 12, 1920, Katharine Tucker, president of the National Organization for Public Health Nursing (NOPHN), declared at the convention of the American Nurses' Association that "partisans of every cause are in agreement upon one point—the sick must be taken care of and increasingly the right of all to health is asserted." Reporting on a major study for the Rockefeller Foundation in 1923, Progressive agitator Josephine Goldmark disclosed that public-health nurses had taken on many functions, including some forms of caregiving. Goldmark detected an advantage of public administration over private charity: "Particularly in the West, people feel a genuine satisfaction in having the public health nurse, like the school teacher, a part of the tax-paid town or county government, and rightfully available on equal terms for all." With characteristic perceptiveness, she framed the question not only as a matter of rights but as one of equality as well. She went on to speculate that "the future of public health nursing as an agency of preventive as well as curative science may well be envisaged on a par with public education." The following year, NOPHN leader Sophie Nelson bluntly told a group of doctors that her organization's concern for providing health care for all outstripped its interest in the physician's ability to earn a living. In February 1927, *Public Health Nurse* printed an enthusiastic overview of the Soviet socialist version of universal free medical services, delivered by state-employed physicians, nurses, and other health workers. The article may well have swept aside any lingering doubts among medical conservatives that these subversive women should be prevented from becoming general practitioners to the unserved and underserved.[16]

## The AMA Embraces Universal Access

The American Medical Association did more than merely attack statist initiatives. In the midst of the battles over the Sheppard-Towner and Sage-Machold bills, a prominent AMA leader made a daring and, to some, traitorous proposal. In the February 5, 1921, issue of the *Journal of the American Medical Association* (*JAMA*), Chicago physician Frank Billings, a member of the association's board of trustees, presented an alternative to both compulsory insurance and state medicince. Much as Biggs had done, Billings proposed that counties be allowed to create tax-supported facilities for "the prevention and treatment of all diseases, disabilities and injuries." His immediate objective was to make laboratories and related diagnostic apparatus available to general practitioners, especially in rural locations. However, his proposal also allowed hospital construction and modernization projects. This former AMA president assured *JAMA* readers that it would be private physicians who treated patients in these publicly sponsored clinics and hospitals. Billings's model differed from that of the New York health commissioner in granting governing authority to county medical societies, not to the state health department.[17]

On the other hand, Billings shared Biggs's interest in moving toward universal care. He prefaced his endorsement of new public institutions with the familiar criticism of state health insurance as "class legislation, which usually brings injustice to some other class." He observed that existing legislation allowing Illinois counties to run their own tuberculosis sanatoria benefited not only the poor victims of this disorder but "all of the people." More to the point, his health centers would transcend class distinctions by serving all county residents. His commitment to inclusion led him to accept the possibility that in extreme circumstances government medicine would be necessary. In counties that were too sparsely settled to support a medical practice, the health center could have a salaried medical staff to "care for all the sick and injured." To be sure, Billings was preaching universalism—provided that each individual county remained its own universe.[18]

The Billings design infuriated some of his colleagues. An anonymous circular that traveled widely within the medical fraternity excoriated it, warning that "Health Centers are unquestionably the shortest route possible to 'State Medicine'" and that state medicine was worse than compulsory insurance. The alleged traitor defended himself during the deliberations of the AMA House of Delegates in 1921. Backing away from his qualified endorsement of public medicine for all in thinly populated areas, Billings declared himself categorically opposed to treatment of disease by the state. In no other regard, however, did he retreat from his advocacy of health care for all Americans. He received a unanimous vote of confidence from the house. Later the same day, the delegates reelected Billings as a trustee of the association.[19]

An article by Victor Vaughan in *JAMA* in 1921 was further evidence of a newfound willingness in the medical profession to entertain universalistic notions. After a long and distinguished career in state government and medical academia, Vaughan urged that local authorities be empowered to establish publicly funded and controlled community hospitals equipped with the latest diagnostic technology and other essential resources. Vaughan stated that his scheme "would give to all citizens the benefit of scientific medicine, both preventive and curative." However, he did not go beyond perfunctory endorsement of universal access for patients. Instead, in an appeal likely to receive a better reception from his fellow physicians, Vaughan stressed the aim of placing X-ray equipment, medical libraries, and bacteriological laboratories within the reach of every medical practitioner. Adopting a "lesser of two evils" argument to defend his brand of public financing and public governance of community hospitals, he portrayed his approach as a way to forestall more oppressive forms of state intervention. Vaughan's ideas appear to have elicited no significant criticism from professional leaders.[20]

At the same time, the American Medical Association officially embraced the goal of all-inclusive access for patients. In 1921 the association's Council on Medical Education and Hospitals went beyond its ritualized denunciation of state medicine to delineate a private solution to the access problem. The recent accomplishments of medical science, the promise of further advances, and the lingering possibility that the state would step in to deliver on this promise made the issue a pressing one. Amazingly, the council proclaimed a general entitlement to health services: "The people of our country, rich and poor alike, are entitled to the great benefits of modern medicine and some plan should be devised to secure these for them." As if this weren't a sufficient mandate, the Council on Medical Education and Hospitals challenged the profession to realize that "its most important function is to secure for all the public the benefits of modern medical practice and to develop intelligent practical plans to furnish the best medical service possible in each community." The group recommended that the nation's doctors take steps "to provide the benefit of modern medicine for all the people."[21]

The Council on Medical Education and Hospitals sought to achieve universal protection simply by increasing the number of versatile general practitioners in private practice and the resources available to them. Its outline of a rudimentary supply-side solution urged reform of medical education to emphasize primary care over specialization. The council looked forward to the day when plentiful general practitioners would be "always accessible." Preoccupied with increasing the supply of providers, this proposal made no mention of promoting private insurance or any other means of enhancing the ability of the needy to purchase services.[22]

This mixture of strong principle and weak remedy won the endorsement of the study committee to which it was referred. The House of Delegates, in turn, approved the report of the committee. Thus, on June 7, 1921, the American Medical Association offically placed itself on record as favoring universal access to health care. Although this commitment received little notice from observers of health affairs—and none at all from historians of health policy—it did much to guide AMA involvement in the major debates later in the twenties.[23]

Within the upper echelon of the medical association, Ray Lyman Wilbur picked up where Frank Billings had left off. As the president of Stanford University and a loyal Republican (he would later serve as secretary of the interior in the Hoover administration), Wilbur stood in no danger of being accused of radical subversion. Newly elected as the AMA's president in June 1923, Wilbur used his presidential address to return to the budding question of universalism. He approached the issue by invoking the progressive credo that recent advances portended "almost unlimited possibilities" for medicine. "If applied to the full extent to human need and human development," Wilbur speculated, medical care "would give untold happiness to humanity." The glories of scientific progress were simply too beneficial not to share. A utilitarian criterion warranted an all-encompassing policy: "the maximum of human happiness for the maximum number of men is a universal standard of welfare." A year later, as outgoing president, Wilbur held up the success of American Telephone and Telegraph in approximating all-inclusive service to the nation as an example to follow. Rejecting governmental care for all but traditional wards of the state, he challenged AMA members to improve the distribution of medical knowledge, which, "if it could be directly applied to the benefit of every individual, would prolong life and happiness, and change the whole current of human thought and life."[24]

At the 1926 session of the California Medical Association, Wilbur pressed his fellow physicians harder still. "The problem of extending the health program to reach all the people of our country," he contended, "is not due to lack of funds, lack of existing knowledge, or lack of capacity, but is primarily due to misunderstanding, ignorance, and indifference." By assuming greater social responsibility, the medical profession would secure a privileged place. Wilbur spelled out the terms he expected: "The public must recognize the leadership of the scientifically trained man of medicine. . . . The medical profession must provide the practical means of giving everyone the chance to get what is available." From the contemporary perspective, this smacks of unalloyed elitism. From the perspective of the traditionalists of the day, this understanding reflected only a sense of conscientious professionalism.[25]

## Winslow at the Crossroads

Charles-Edward Amory Winslow early on joined the leadership of the small band of universalists in the biomedical community. When Arthur Newsholme came to New Haven in 1920 to speak about "The Obstacles to and Ideals of Health Progress," he stayed with Winslow, then chair of the Department of Public Health at Yale. The American assured his guest that his visit would "mark an epoch in the public health campaign." However, by that time Winslow had already ventured some distance down the path toward espousing universal protection. In an address given at the American Association for the Advancement of Science just prior to Newsholme's visit, Winslow enlarged upon Biggs's proposition: "I look to see our health departments in the coming years organizing diverse forms of sanitary and medical and nursing and social service in such fashion as to enable every citizen to realize his birthright of health and longevity. I look to see health centers, local district foci for the coordination of every form of health activity, scattered through our cities, as numerous as the school houses of today and as lavishly equipped." At this juncture, he was clearly basing a claim to universal access to care on the compelling rationale of a citizen's rights. His suggestion that the state only organize or coordinate services in some fashion was more oblique. With the same air of ambiguity, he implied that the burgeoning field of public health might expand to encompass more treatment of individual patients.[26]

Winslow shared Newsholme's view that health reform should concentrate on the delivery of medical care, broadly conceived, and not on social insurance. Both men at this moment sought formulations that did not provide for the replacement of earnings lost due to illness. Health professionals generally came to see income maintenance as a discrete problem within the domain of social work. When asked in 1923 to serve on the General Administrative Council of the AALL, Winslow accepted the position but hastened to make known his disagreement with the association's policy of seeking to combine insurance of lost income with insurance of health care.[27]

Like Newsholme, Winslow sometimes employed history to build a case for integrating curative care into public health. His 1923 monograph *The Evolution and Significance of the Modern Public Health Campaign* plotted a line of progress in state activity that culminated in current initiatives in health education and in the detection and early treatment of disease. (The same theme runs through Winslow's biography of Biggs, which appeared six years later.) In projecting trends into the near future, Winslow acknowledged that he shared Newsholme's skepticism regarding the preventive capacity of compulsory sickness insurance. He voiced support for "the gradual expansion of hospital and dispensary and nursing service under public or private auspices." His awareness of the conservatism of American society led him to promote incremental change and to hedge on the public-private division of responsibility. This awareness stemmed in part from an unpleasant encounter with strident antireform forces when he testified on behalf of the New York health-center bill in 1920.[28]

In "Public Health at the Crossroads," his APHA presidential address in 1926, Winslow laid out the three phases—environmental sanitation, bacteriological control of communicable disorders, and education in personal hygiene— through which the field had passed during the preceding half century. He predicted that the next major phase of progress would center on advances in the early diagnosis and treatment of disease. He imagined not just a blurring of the line between public health and clinical medicine but the disappearance of the distinction between prevention and cure. He felt that leadership in this historic project should come from public health workers. His position posed a challenge to his audience at a time when a large share of the association's membership consisted of physicians in private practice who served as municipal or county health officials on a part-time basis.[29]

Winslow's stance was unequivocally universalistic. "In the last analysis," he held, "it will be the duty of the health officer of the future to see that the people under his charge, in city or country, in palace or tenement, have the opportunity of receiving such service as that outlined above and on terms which make it economically and psychologically easy of attainment." Not committed to a governmental takeover of all health care, Winslow considered the function of the community health officer to be complementary to those of other providers. He held that he was not merely advocating compulsory health insurance or "any other panacea." Instead, he called for experimentation that might make use of such devices as state health insurance.[30]

Winslow knew that even this nebulous and qualified proposal for the expansion of public-health activity would meet with strong opposition. Anticipating forthcoming polemics, he warned his audience about the emptiness of catch phrases like "socialized medicine." To that end, he quoted an observation by Royal Meeker, former U.S. commissioner of labor statistics:

Many earnest people are afraid that social insurance will take away from the workingman his independence, initiative, and self-reliance which are so celebrated in song and story and transform him into a mere spoonfed mollycoddle. This would be a cruel calamity. But if the worst comes to the worst, I, for my part, would rather see a race of sturdy, contented, healthful mollycoddles, carefully fed, medically examined, physically fit, nursed in illness, and cared for in old age and at death as a matter of course in recognition of services rendered or for injuries suffered in performance of labor, than to see the most ferociously independent and self-reliant superrace of tubercular, rheumatic, and malarial cripples tottering unsocialistically along the socialized highways, reclining self-reliantly upon the communal benches of the public parks, and staring belligerently at the communal trees, flowers, and shrubbery, enjoying defiantly the social light of the great unsocialized sun, drinking individualistically the socialized water bubbling from the public fountain.

Winslow concluded by leaving his colleagues no room to evade their responsibilities: "No organization is so well fitted as the American Public Health Association to attack this problem from the broad aspect of community well-being."[31]

Despite all of this encouragement, the public-health group was not ready to lead any crusade. As John Duffy has explained so well, the APHA at that time remained fearful of taking any action that might provoke the wrath of the AMA. Public-health officials for the most part maintained a deferential attitude toward fee-based providers throughout the 1920s. Charles Wilinsky's overview of the activities of more than one thousand health centers across the nation, published in 1927, duly noted both government and voluntary sponsorship of community facilities to serve the neediest. But Wilinsky, an APHA fellow who served as deputy health commissioner of Boston, stated flatly that "the private physician is the most important asset in public health work." The interest of this municipal official in treating public-private cooperation and coordination in the vaguest of terms is another indication of the unwillingness to assert authority and, beyond that, the widespread uncertainty about the proper boundary between public and private responsibility in health affairs.[32]

## The One Great Outstanding Question

The small cohort of advocates of universal health care found themselves with a momentous opportunity to develop their views more fully and to disseminate them more widely. In May 1927, two years of discussion culminated in the creation of the Committee on the Cost of Medical Care (CCMC), financed by a consortium of eight philanthropic foundations. In a policy world still quite small, dominated by medical providers, and accustomed to a quasi-corporatist approach, the composition of the CCMC roughly reflected the balance of power among established interests. The final membership of forty-eight included twenty-five men with medical degrees. Each member was explicitly identified as falling into one of five categories: the private practice of medicine (seventeen members), public health (six), the social sciences (six), "institutions and special interests" (ten), and the public (nine). Five women served on the panel. No person of color was part of the group. Ray Lyman Wilbur, whom Daniel Fox aptly described as a "man for all factions," was selected to chair the CCMC. As chair of the executive committee, C.-E. A. Winslow did much to guide its deliberations over the course of five years (during the midst of which, in 1930, the group renamed itself the Committee on the Costs of Medical Care). Operating within a group dominated by clinicians in private practice, Winslow collaborated with progressives like Michael Davis and Edgar Sydenstricker to promote all-inclusive provision.[33]

Two staff appointments in particular bolstered efforts to map universalistic reform. Winslow recruited his former student, Isidore S. Falk, to head the research staff of the CCMC. Trained as a bacteriologist, Falk gained invaluable expertise in the inchoate field of health services research by participating in this venture. However, his technical assignment gave him a crucial role in building a factual case for universalism but little opportunity to promote it per se. In contrast, Falk's immediate superior, Harry Moore, who directed all staff activity, came to the CCMC from the Public Health Service with unabashed partisan tendencies. In *American Medicine and the People's Health,* which appeared just as the committee was being formed, Moore contended that growing public awareness of the value of medical science had brought increased demand for the services it could now provide. He made it plain that universality should be the fundamental principle of health policy. Moore considered opponents of his position to be social Darwinists, who accepted disease as a legitimate test for the survival of the fittest. He encouraged small steps to achieve protection for all and claimed that compulsory health insurance was "not a dead issue." Moore saw to it that every member of the CCMC received a copy of his book.[34]

As it struggled to define its mission, the group committed itself to universal care. Dawning awareness of the full extent of the access problem made it harder to defend partial solutions that targeted only the dependent poor or those on the brink of dependency. From the outset, the men most active in launching the CCMC, the so-called Committee of Five, betrayed a broadly inclusive predisposition. In July 1927, the *American Journal of Public Health* greeted the formation of the CCMC as "a serious attempt to study the fundamental factors in the problem as to how the best medical care can be secured for the whole people at a minimum cost." In February 1928, the Committee on the Cost of Medical Care formally outlined its plan of action. In the foreword to this announcement, Ray Lyman Wilbur diplomatically gave a particular member of his committee much of the credit for setting the course: "The Committee on the Cost of Medical Care has been created to study a problem which, according to the secretary of the American Medical Association, is the one great outstanding question before the medical profession today. This, says

Secretary Olin West, is 'the delivery of adequate, scientific medical service to all the people, rich and poor, at a cost which can be reasonably met by them in their respective stations in life.'" Sensitive to organized medicine's fears that it would be underrepresented in this body, Wilbur shrewdly let the executive officer of the AMA frame the issue. On his own behalf, he stated his hope that, based on its forthcoming studies, the group would produce "recommendations for the provision of more efficient medical service for all the people." Thus, the guiding principle of universality had already emerged prior to the major fact-finding activities of the committee.[35]

Adherence to this key tenet did not imply any preconceived plan. Faced with the suspicion of organized medicine, the leaders of the CCMC attested that they commenced work without any particular policy design in mind. In the spring of 1928, Wilbur told the California Medical Association, "Frankly, we do not know what should be done." His disavowal of quick fixes offered an opportunity to paraphrase Olin West's declaration of the universalist imperative: "The air is full of legislative and other panaceas for the one outstanding social and economic fact, i.e., we have not devised a financial system by which all members of society, regardless of economic status, may receive a full or even a reasonable share of the benefits possible through the practical application of modern medical science." He also asserted that "medicine as a profession has proven itself too valuable for society to allow it to be inadequate or uneven in its service." Wilbur apparently passed up no chance to placate this vital constituency.[36]

Along with several partners commissioned to examine specific issues, the CCMC staff carried out a sprawling research program. During the five years of its existence, it examined the health status of the American people, the quantity and quality of human and capital resources available for delivering services, the types of services actually being provided, and the latest innovations in health organization, as well as the central question of the costs of care. In addition, the committee compiled a great deal of information recently gathered by other investigators. It analyzed this mass of data in more than a score of major research reports, numerous miscellaneous publications, and a landmark final report, adopted on October 31, 1932. In both its assessment of the challenge facing the nation and its contributions to meeting that challenge, the CCMC built a strong case for health services for all.[37]

The committee's studies redefined the social problem of financing health care. Its investigations cogently demonstrated that potential financial difficulties threatened the vast majority of Americans. The central intertwined themes that emerged were the unpredictability of health costs, their highly uneven distribution across the population, and the impossibility of budgeting for them within the family. By the end of the 1920s, medical bills could bankrupt all but the wealthiest citizens. Daunting prices kept people who were not poor from obtaining surgical procedures and other inpatient services. Committee member Michael Davis wondered how to "meet the needs and satisfy the demands of the 'white-collar' people of moderate means." A distillation of the CCMC's findings by Falk and fellow staff members Rufus Rorem and Martha Ring observed that "hospital beds are empty while millions suffer and tens of thousands perish for lack of care." This lengthy account and its companion volumes portrayed as tragic a system of individual financing that worked for only the wealthiest tenth of society. (The majority of the CCMC went quite a bit further in its final report, estimating that 99 percent of American families could not set aside enough money to be assured that they could meet any medical emergency.) Louis Reed's exploration of the ability to afford care found that a sizable share of families could not afford major surgery and other costly services. Reed reported, for example, that when members of households in the lower half of the income range underwent appendectomies, their income, savings, and insurance covered about forty percent of expenses, with insurance reimbursing less than one percent. Middle- and lower-income Americans handled the balance by borrowing money, receiving gifts, and leaving providers unpaid, especially surgeons. A review of previous studies, which, taken together, had examined more than 40,000 loans, found that health-care bills were the leading cause of indebtedness among Americans. A cascade of similar findings on unaffordable medical miracles exploded the Progressive assumption that health policy concerned only the poor. The middle class now became a prominent object—if not the primary object—of consideration for policy architects.[38]

At the same time as its research was shedding light on new concerns, the CCMC turned away from potentially helpful ways of illuminating the issues at hand. The executive committee rejected a proposal to investigate the costs to the community of lack of care. Public medical services in general and preventive public services in particular received relatively little scrutiny. In this regard, it is noteworthy that the committee dropped plans to report on a small study it had undertaken of the Biggs health centers in New York. The notion that basic health care could be largely decommodified, as elementary education had been a century earlier, fell outside the scope of inquiry, despite the expansion of tax-supported services in Europe and Canada occurring at the time. Instead, the nascent specialty of medical economics looked in the opposite direction, toward voluntary insurance and employer-sponsored services. The committee's wide-ranging economic studies made no use of the conceptual tool of the living wage in relating standard of living to the ability to purchase either insurance or care itself. Similarly, fundamental questions of the relation of living standards to the capacity to resist disease were out of bounds. Much exertion went into evaluating the AMA's contention that heavy spending on luxuries, vices, nostrums, and the services of quacks demonstrated that most Americans could really pay for scientific health care but were too ignorant or imprudent to do so.[39]

The CCMC investigations also studiously avoided the question of racial inequality. None of its many research projects concentrated on the health status of African Americans or other minorities. Instead, the committee made passing acknowledgment of conventional wisdom: "It is well known . . . that the ten percent of our population who are colored have health problems which are, on the whole, considerably more serious than those of whites." Similarly, CCMC researchers did not explore the institutional racism pervading the American health-care system. Instead, the committee reductively treated the inadequacies of services as a by-product of black poverty in the South. The plight of other racial and ethnic groups received no real attention in this extensive series of investigations. Because the CCMC enjoyed authoritative stature as an investigative body, its lack of research interest in these matters meant the squandering of an important opportunity to illuminate deep disparities in the accessibility of care.[40]

Although the research staff concentrated on performing its empirical chores, it did occasionally voice support for the sanctioned principle of universality. In their analysis of the elements of adequate medical care, Roger Lee and Lewis Jones invoked "the much-quoted words of Dr. Olin West" on the preeminence of universal access. Lee and Jones then proceeded to smuggle universality into the definition of satisfactory care: "Good medical care implies the application of all the necessary services of modern, scientific medicine to the needs of all the people. Judged from the viewpoint of society as a whole, the qualitative aspects of medical care cannot be dissociated from the quantitative." The executive committee, also responsible for authorizing publications, apparently had no objection to this leap of logic. Falk, Rorem, and

Ring made the same argument in their economic synthesis. They also declared it "eminently desirable that [health care] should be available to everyone." Thus, even technical analysts engaged in the driest dollars-and-cents calculations were able to proclaim the ideal of inclusion.[41]

The Committee on the Costs of Medical Care could not agree upon a course of action to make care accessible to everyone. After much debate, the group splintered. The majority endorsed a set of recommendations that featured voluntary group insurance and community health centers. In this renovation of Biggs's scheme, the centers would become primarily sites for the development of group medical practice. This report encouraged experimentation and further study, mainly at the community level: it did not draw a comprehensive blueprint for reform. Nor did it call for experimental initiatives that targeted the communities of underserved racial and ethnic groups. Within the majority of thirty-five, eight expressed support for governmental insurance for low-income workers and other specific groups, but not for the whole population. A significant minority, based in the leadership of the American Medical Association, opposed any form of group insurance. In addition, the two dentists on the committee submitted their own report, and two members filed individual statements.[42]

Beyond its dissent within the committee, the AMA unleashed a furious public attack on the majority position. An editorial in the December 3, 1932, issue of *JAMA* lambasted the majority proposals as "incitement to revolution" and "utopian fantasies." Another editorial the following week presented the alternatives as "Americanism versus sovietism for the American people." Although the *New England Journal of Medicine*, the *American Journal of Nursing*, and others counseled against alarmism, the AMA had effectively put the reformers on the defensive. Most unfortunately, the subsequent controversy over the proper means of organizing and financing care largely, but not completely, obscured a general agreement among the factions on the necessity of providing health care for all.[43]

In light of their deep disagreements, it might seem remarkable that the motley membership of the CCMC could still manage to agree on universality. In part, this principle survived the stormy voyage because it had been discussed and reaffirmed at so many steps along the way from agenda-setting through final recommendations that no one could abandon his or her position. In late 1929, for example, the executive committee returned to Olin West's by now famous statement about the "one great outstanding question" in reasserting its goal of all-inclusive care. Shortly thereafter, committee member Haven Emerson used West's assertion to frame a set of articles on health policy in the *Survey*. In May 1932, Ray Lyman Wilbur, still searching for common ground, maintained that the committee had been created primarily to deal with the matter of access. Two months later, the *Milbank Memorial Fund Quarterly* published Wilbur's recent address to the fund's board of directors. After thanking the board for its support, he reminded it of the historic import of the committee's work: "Although it is a principle of far-reaching and, perhaps, of revolutionary significance, I think there are few who would deny that our ultimate objective should be to make these benefits available in full measure to all of the people." At least within the network that included the CCMC and its backers, universal provision had become an article of faith.[44]

In fact, by the conclusion of its deliberations, universality remained one of few points of consensus within the sharply divided group. Wilbur's introduction to the final report put forward both an endorsement and a wish: "The report affords for the first time a scientific basis on which the people of every locality can attack the perplexing problem of providing adequate medical care for all persons at costs within their means. It is hoped that the report may thus aid materially in bringing greater health, efficiency, and happiness to all the people." The majority report conveyed the same sense of urgency: "The problem of providing satisfactory medical service to all the people of the United States at costs which they can meet is a pressing one." The majority contingent urged that the nation proceed diligently to make health services more accessible: "It may not be practicable to supply all the people's needs at once, but any plan to be satisfactory must provide for the continuous development of its component services until eventually they cover all the needs of all the people." The section of this report devoted to increased preventive measures also took an inclusive stance. One of the individual dissenters, Yale economist Walton Hamilton, shared the reformers' interventionist approach but felt that the majority did not go far enough toward systematic reform. Hamilton's personal statement advocated sweeping change on economic grounds. "If we are to make the most of our human resources, for work and for life," he contended, "it is necessary that our facilities for health be just as available for all who need them as are the schools and the churches." Hamilton thus concurred with the sizable majority of committee members who not only accepted universality as a goal but advocated immediate concrete steps to reach it.[45]

The minority report by George Follansbee and others in the AMA-dominated group also upheld the universalist ideal. This group of nine averred that it had "tried to keep in mind the main object which called this Committee together, namely to find some solution for the problem of furnishing good medical care to all the people at prices which they can afford." Although primarily devoted to preserving the traditional freedoms and opportunities of physicians and surgeons, the AMA minority did argue that additional training of general practitioners, sponsorship of clinics by county medical societies, increased government care for the indigent, and other initiatives would address the question of access. In essence, organized medicine held to the position it had taken a decade earlier.[46]

The Committee on the Costs of Medical Care forged a consensus in elite circles on the aim of universal protection. In the decade prior to the issuance of its final report, this consensus had been brewing across the ideological spectrum. Encouraging advances in the struggle against disease induced leaders of the biomedical community to view scientific medicine as too valuable to deny to any American. In this context, the preexisting public-health goal of basic services for all members of the community was readily applied to medical services, especially in the realm of preventive care.

The idea of universalism was not instantly translated into a fully wrought plan. Nor was there a political strategy for its realization in 1932. The CCMC submitted its reports, disbanded, and left it to others to pursue the new ideal that it had proclaimed. Nonetheless, the committee, along with the handful of visionaries who preceded it, had invented an important goal in American social policy. The immensity of this departure struck Stewart Roberts, one of the physicians in private practice serving on the CCMC, with particular force. At a meeting in 1931, four working subcommittees had once again affirmed the standard of universal health protection. Roberts pondered the meaning of this unity of purpose: "Each subcommittee has reported that all the people's medical needs should be supplied. That in my mind is one of the most radical moves ever made in the history of American medicine!" No one disagreed with Roberts. Instead, Alphonse Schwitalla, president of the Catholic Hospital Association, indicated that discussion of this principle in his subcommittee had turned on "the fundamental human right that is involved." The Committee on the Costs of Medical Care did not itself declare any fundamental human right to health care, but many others would soon do so.[47]

# CHAPTER THREE

# No Poor-Man's System

Eight days after the Committee on the Costs of Medical Care issued its final report, the nation's voters elected Franklin D. Roosevelt to the presidency. The committee invited the president-elect to address a conference it had organized to publicize its findings and recommendations. Roosevelt, who was still serving as governor of New York, delegated the task to his health commissioner, Thomas Parran. At the National Conference on the Costs of Medical Care, held at the New York Academy of Medicine in Manhattan on November 29, 1932, Parran read the president-elect's message: "I hope that you have arrived at a practical policy for the present emergency whereby more and better medical care may be made available for those in want and for those to whom the disaster of illness would mean destitution. But . . . I hope even more that you have not failed to establish the ideal we should strive for over the next span of years. If you have been able to show us how adequate medical care may be made available for the entire population . . . , then I, as an American citizen, am honored in this occasion to thank you." Parran, a physician who had gone to Albany after more than a decade at the U.S. Public Health Service, also offered his own commentary. "Emergency measures must come first," he acknowledged, "but we need for the future an integrated system of preventive and curative medicine." These statements marked an important transition. The Committee on the Costs of Medical Care had transacted its business with only the most cursory recognition of the unfolding of the Great Depression. The Roosevelt administration, on the other hand, had to evaluate every health initiative in light of the imperative to expedite recovery from the economic collapse.[1]

This episode foreshadowed the Roosevelt administration's approach to health policy during its first three years, beyond its willingness to confront harsh reality. The chief executive himself would be sympathetic but absent from the scene. Thomas Parran and others oriented toward public-health measures would complicate matters by refusing to reduce the issue to one of sickness insurance. The event at which Parran spoke brought together a small, select group and was held at a forbiddingly exclusive medical institution. Perhaps most characteristically, the administration struggled to balance demands to meet exigencies against its desire to undertake sweeping changes in the health-care system.

The framers of the New Deal could not afford to embrace universalism in health affairs. With the nation lost in the depths of a frightening depression, the principle of security overrode all others in setting social policy. A shrinking economy had very limited resources available for health care, a need that competed with other necessities like shelter and nourishment. Hence, interventions to enhance health security had to address the needs of only the most destitute, not the populace as a whole. Economic crisis made the ideal of universal protection seem unreachable to almost everyone involved in designing policy.

Amid this retreat, a few reformers dared to contend for all-encompassing health security. Their arguments blended claims about the value of health to national productivity with assertions regarding the duties of society. At this formative juncture, federal activism led universalists to dwell not so much on the rights of the individual citizen as on the responsibilities of the government to protect all members of society. Nonetheless, the notion of a social right to health care was beginning to appear more frequently as a justification for sweeping protections. Although it is well known that the Social Security Act of 1935 did not include a health-insurance provision, it is less well known that the early days of the New Deal witnessed a good deal of creative thinking on the subject of universal health care.

## The Sickening Economy

The stock market crash of 1929 abruptly ended several years of prosperity and precipitated a disaster that lasted until World War II. During the worst interval, the downward spiral from 1929 to 1933, the American economy contracted by about a third. Countless businesses failed. Unemployment reached a peak of approximately 25 percent in 1933. Despite a mild recovery after 1933, the rate of joblessness remained well above 10 percent for the remainder of the decade. Millions of men, women, and children roamed the nation in search of work. Prisoners chose continued incarceration over parole. Most employers imposed wage and salary cuts on their remaining employees.[2]

The combination of unemployment, underemployment, and pay cuts undermined the standard of living of most Americans. Needless to say, none of the common forms of deprivation was likely to lead to good health. Homelessness became widespread. Many did without heat or utilities. Migratory jobseekers usually had either crude shelter or none at all. Malnutrition became commonplace, and outright starvation occurred. Moreover, family disruption and loss of self-respect plagued the unemployed, millions of whom remained out of work for years. The grim situation forced many to abandon their standards of dignity. Large numbers of Americans survived through such demoralizing practices as begging, thievery, and prostitution. Those fortunate enough to keep their jobs faced deteriorating working conditions and chronic anxiety over employment insecurity. Appalachian coal miners, for example, lived in fear of the "barefootman," the desperate interloper ready to take away their jobs. All these factors exacerbated the risk of physical and mental illness during the Great Depression.[3]

Prolonged periods of increased vulnerability took their toll. The incidence of certain diseases associated with poverty rose after 1929. These were mainly infectious conditions, such as tuberculosis and gastrointestinal disorders, whose incidence had been falling since the turn of the century. A study of more than four thousand working-class families in New York City discovered that the rate of illness among unemployed adults almost doubled and the rate of illness among their children almost tripled between 1930 and 1932. In a 1933 survey of roughly twenty thousand poor whites living in urban areas, the U.S. Public Health Service discovered that disabling illness occurred most frequently among those who had recently become poorer.[4]

Of course, a sizable share of those in need of health care but unable to pay for it went without professional assistance. Investigator Margaret Klem found, for example, that one-fifth of relief recipients in California received no medical care when ill, whereas only 9 percent of sick high-income residents of the state went untreated. Wherever possible, Americans put off expensive surgical procedures. Delays in seeking care due to lack of funds generally only brought more severe consequences. In 1934, Los Angeles health reformer E. T. Remmen estimated that more than two-thirds of Californians could not afford an appendectomy in a private hospital. Recourse to patent medicines and other dubious remedies seldom proved effective.[5]

At the same time, masses of the sick poor continued to seek help from the mainstream health-care system. The demand from these patients placed a stressful burden on providers after 1930. To be sure, as Rosemary Stevens observed, no major American hospital went bankrupt during the depression. Instead, voluntary institutions diverted more of their nonpaying patients to public facilities, which often, but not always, found a way to treat them. Physicians, surgeons, midwives, and other caregivers delivered an enormous amount of free or undercompensated services; they also waited long periods of time to recover charges. One hospital in northern Wisconsin, for example, was paid for handling a case of pneumonia only after the unemployed husband of the patient built a still in the cellar of the family home and sold enough moonshine to cover the bill. The average income of a doctor in private practice in 1933 was about half of what it had been four years earlier. This drop reflected both unpaid services and the absence of patients unwilling to impose on the provider's good will. National expenditures on all forms of health care, which, like doctors' incomes, reflected both the extent of uncompensated care and reduced utilization, declined by 20 percent between 1929 and 1935. Despite the adaptability of both patients and providers in dealing with this crisis, sustained depression caused great suffering among the American people.[6]

## Unreconstructed Progressives

The Roosevelt administration hesitated to tackle the challenge of access to health care. Quite apart from the distractions raised by other pressing issues, the indecisiveness of the CCMC and the acrimony with which the medical profession responded to the CCMC's majority report hardly encouraged the incoming administration to grapple with health reform. However, these in-hibiting circumstances did not discourage the hardiest advocates of social in-surance. After about a dozen years of dormancy, a number of survivors of the 1910s campaign returned to the fray, where they were joined by a few veterans of related struggles of the 1920s. The small progressive coalition managed to reopen policy discussion of health-care financing in ways that the late Com-mittee on the Costs of Medical Care had not.

Barbara Nachtrieb Armstrong waited for neither the CCMC's final report nor Roosevelt's election. After serving as the key staff operative in the Cali-fornia Social Insurance Commission in the 1910s, Armstrong had joined the law faculty of the University of California at Berkeley. In September 1932, Armstrong published *Insuring the Essentials: Minimum Wage Plus Social Insurance—a Living Wage Program*, which confronted the economic crisis at hand and introduced the central theme of security. Armstrong's sensitivity to the impact of the depression led her to attend to the dependent poor as opposed to all citizens. Based on a survey of European and Australasian legis-lation, she concluded that "in western civilization, the burden of support of persons who cannot maintain themselves is an unquestioned social obliga-tion." In contrast to the scientistic humanitarianism of the CCMC, her com-parative perspective led her to frame the issue in terms of societal duty.[7]

Armstrong proposed to redress economic insecurity with a living-wage program. In her interpretation, the living wage became not a strictly pri-vate matter but rather the combination of a legally mandated minimum rate of compensation and a battery of social-insurance plans to deal with sickness, disability, death of the male breadwinner, old age, and unem-ployment. Defending the health-insurance component of her program, she held that the rise in medical costs had made it impossible for any con-ceivable level of wages alone to assure protection. Society would thus meet its obligations by offering a social wage "sufficient to obviate the necessity of public charity."[8]

Armstrong did not share the enthusiasm for governmental delivery of health care that had spread within reform circles over the previous decade. She looked upon the rise of public clinics and other facilities as "a most unwhole-some" trend. Armstrong lamented that "every patient admitted to the clinic's service is carefully examined as to his means, property, and earnings and is left in no doubt that he is receiving charitable assistance." Moreover, socialized medicine would not replace earnings lost during disability.[9]

Instead, Armstrong advocated compulsory insurance. Her endorsement of the far-from-universal standard bill of the American Association for Labor Legislation (AALL) displayed both her own steadfast Progressivism and the lack of fresh thinking on social insurance since 1915. In her characteristically Progressive outlook, the object of attention remained the wage earner and his or her family. Her overview of European legislation yielded no exemplar of universalism but numerous cases of the extension of benefits to the bread-winner's "dependents." Armstrong calculated that Denmark, with slightly more than 60 percent coverage, had the closest approximation to general health insurance. Most other nations on the continent had far less extensive provision. Only about one in seven Swedes, for example, was insured against the expenses of illness. Armstrong did, however, acknowledge that "financial problems that come in the wake of illness strike home to most of the working members of society and to many of the non-workers of moderate incomes as well." This acknowledgment and her close attention to the breadth of popula-tion coverage in Europe suggest that Armstrong's commitment to the AALL model may have been only vestigial at this point.[10]

The AALL returned to the scene shortly after the appearance of Arm-strong's book. The association had avoided the question of financing health care since 1920. But the final report of the Committee on the Costs of Med-ical Care stirred the dormant advocacy organization. On November 16, 1932, John Andrews, still serving as AALL secretary, called upon Isaac Rubinow to "prepare a somewhat slashing criticism of the report" for the group's annual meeting. Rubinow was hesitant to slash at the CCMC majority recommen-dations, especially given the violent criticism they were receiving from the AMA and other conservative parties. Instead, his address to the AALL con-ference on December 30, 1932, adopted a more conciliatory tone. Rubinow held that the committee and the association shared a basic goal: "A compe-tent program of public health, utilization of all existing facilities for preven-tion as well as cure of illness, availability of such facilities to all the people at a cost which they can meet 'without due hardship' . . . —these are things which we all devoutedly [*sic*] pray for, so we shall agree upon the ideal." Differences persisted, of course, on the best means to realize the universalist dream. The grizzled reformer rejected the optimistic position of the CCMC majority on the virtues of voluntarism. He drove home this point by predicting that it would take voluntary health insurance about a century to achieve universal access in the United States. This sense of the inadequacies of the CCMC's preferred remedy did not, however, prompt the AALL to put forth an original alternative to it.[11]

Abraham Epstein had been prodding the AALL to resume the battle for health insurance since 1925. Though primarily identified with the drive for old-age pension legislation, Epstein also became interested in a comprehensive system of social insurance in which health protection would form an integral part. In 1933, his advocacy group changed its name to the American Association for Social Security (AASS) to reflect this broader perspective. The same year, Epstein brought out *Insecurity, a Challenge to America*, a tome that closely examined the issue of health security. The book exuded a passionate partisanship that contrasted sharply with the ambivalence of the CCMC and the lethargy of the AALL. "The function of the student of social problems is not that of a technician observing and recording social phenomena with inhuman detachment," Epstein announced. He derided the "mimicry of the physical sciences" attempted by some policy analysts. Refusal to abide by positivistic standards freed the AASS leader to sketch out unmeasurable parameters of the human meaning of insecurity. Regarding those employees forced into debt to pay health-care bills, he asserted that "nothing so embitters the worker's life as the constant surveillance of the loan shark." At the same time, he pursued the phenomenon of insecurity well beyond the ranks of the wage-earning class, arguing that most farmers, professionals, small business owners, and even corporate executives could not meet major medical expenses. This state of virtually inescapable insecurity stood as his main justification for government intervention. While making no rights claims on his own, he presciently predicted their arrival: "American workers will demand that in addition to theoretical rights to life, liberty and the pursuit of happiness, there be some practical attainment of these ends." He added the ominous warning that the very survival of the social order hinged on realization of social rights.[12]

Epstein performed better as a critic than as an architect. He attributed the "vacuities and contradictions" of the CCMC majority recommendations to "its apparent aim to please everybody." But after ridiculing the CCMC and other proponents of voluntarism, the polemical pension advocate had no plan of his own. Epstein's *Insecurity* merely insisted that only state insurance could curtail health insecurity. Although Epstein offered no specifics on the extent of the population to be protected, his evaluation of recent foreign legislation suggestively mentioned that "the tendency definitely is to extend the circle of persons insured." Moreover, he pointed out the recent move by a few nations to define eligibility for health insurance solely in terms of family income, disregarding occupational categories altogether.[13]

In 1934, another old-guard Progressive filed his own brief for state health insurance. Like Epstein, Isaac Rubinow had all but given up on the AALL but was not prepared to commit to a replacement for the tired standard bill. Instead he focused on identifying the resources indispensable to reaching that end. From his unpleasant experience in the 1910s, Rubinow learned the lesson that victory required a clamorous mass movement of those in need. In hindsight, the Progressive campaign had depended too heavily upon "an academic handful" of reformers. Encouraged by such recent outbursts of militant grassroots activism as the Bonus Army and the Farmers' Holiday Association, he sought to educate the public in general and the working class in particular on the value of compulsory health insurance. In Rubinow's view, the American quest for security in the 1930s would have to engage masses of workers and not merely a few experts.[14]

Rubinow fashioned a rationale for change to arm the potential mass movement. He ambitiously proclaimed that American democratic values entailed "the right of enjoyment of life" and that social insurance represented the best mechanism to attain that right. Unfortunately, he did not go on to explain why democracy, either in America or anywhere else, conferred this grand entitlement. Although such a right would presumably extend to all Americans, the self-described "old advocate" clung to the notion that a universal program only had to cover all the nation's wage earners. On the other hand, departing from the complacent stance that had predominated twenty years earlier, Rubinow avoided the assumption that health protection was the next inevitable step in social evolution. Instead, he tentatively speculated that growing popular interest in state medicine might give the medical profession reason to accept state insurance in order to head off a less palatable outcome.[15]

In general, the Progressive holdovers demonstrated more continuity with the ideas espoused during the 1910s than not. Rubinow's somewhat halfhearted attempt to declare a right to enjoy life notwithstanding, these advocates showed an abiding reluctance to stake out an entitlement to health protection. Moreover, they refused to build on the CCMC's attempt to reconceive the problem—even in the longer term, after the depression had passed—in universalistic terms, on any basis. Most remarkably, they remained fixated on the wage-earning population at a time when so many were earning nothing and so many others had irregular employment. This inflexibility derived from two main factors, both traceable to, if not originating in, the tenets of Progressivism. First, as Alice Kessler-Harris observed, "Gendered economic assumptions led American policy makers to opt for programs tied to wage work rather than to citizenship 'rights.'" Devotion to the ideal of the male breadwinner with the corollary inclusion of women and children only as their dependents had guided health-policy thinking since the heyday of the AALL. Second, a comprehensive approach to safeguarding the working class through various forms of social insurance had characterized Progressivism. Indeed, the compendious works by Armstrong, Epstein, and Rubinow treated illness as one misfortune among many. From this perspective, in the context of the Great Depression, it was natural that these reformers would pay so much attention to unemployment insurance and not as much to rethinking health insurance.[16]

## Formulating an American Plan

One small but influential team of reformers remained singlemindedly devoted to the cause of health reform to the exclusion of unemployment insurance, old-age pensions, and other related matters. Like the hard-core Progressive contingent, the group centered in the Milbank Memorial Fund brought a wealth of experience—and, metaphorically speaking, quite an accumulation of scar tissue—to the question. Unlike their frozen-in-time colleagues, these experts took on the task of designing a system of health insurance that would grant a measure of security to needy citizens who were not members of wage-earning families. Obviously, in the context of the depressed early thirties, such an inclusive approach was especially daring.[17]

The Milbank Memorial Fund was determined both to carry forward and to reinterpret the work of the Committee on the Costs of Medical Care. The fund had a major stake in pursuing this course. In addition to helping to finance the CCMC, two members of the fund's staff had been directly involved with it—Edgar Sydenstricker, as a member of the committee, and Isidore Falk, as associate director of its research staff. In addition, their superior at the Milbank Fund, John Kingsbury, a prominent figure in social welfare and health reform since the 1910s, had a longstanding commitment to extending access to health services. All shared a frustration at the limitations of the CCMC's recommendations and an impatience with the Roosevelt administration's unreadiness to address the worsening health situation. Through its grant-making, brainstorming, barnstorming, and ceaseless networking, this crew of three, with the help of a handful of collaborators, managed to alter the terms of the debate during the early years of the New Deal.

As they set forth to broaden the policy horizons, the staff at the Milbank Fund enjoyed the hearty support of their patron. Less than two weeks after Roosevelt's inauguration, Albert Milbank, chairman of the board of the Borden Company and his family's leader in its philanthropic activities, declared that, far from prohibiting bold initiatives, the depression had created an opening for decisive action. At the fund's annual meeting on March 16, 1933, Milbank contended that Americans at this perilous moment had come to value security above all else. He predicted that the voluntarism promoted by the CCMC would fail and argued that it would take compulsory insurance organized on at least a state-wide basis to achieve health security.[18]

The efforts of Kingsbury and his comrades went well beyond advocacy of renovated individualism. Beginning in the late 1920s, the Milbank Fund had sponsored a series of studies of European health systems by Arthur Newsholme. Upon the publication of the capstone volume of the series in early 1932, Beatrice Webb urged Newsholme to study the Soviet Union as well. Later that year, he and Kingsbury—neither of whom spoke Russian—took a long, Milbank-funded tour of the U.S.S.R. In *Red Medicine*, the partners assessed the progress of universal health protection under socialism. They considered the Soviet Union "the one nation in the world which has undertaken to set up and operate a complete organization designed to provide preventive and curative medical care for every man, woman, and child within its borders." The authors added that this ambitious experiment was by no means complete and might not succeed. Throughout the book, acknowledgment of modest achievements tempered recognition of the Russians' bold objectives. This balanced interpretation resulted from the pairing of the pro-Soviet Kingsbury with the anti-Soviet Newsholme. This odd couple could agree, however, that the Soviet system displayed a strong commitment to both universalism and disease prevention.[19]

Kingsbury believed that the Russian regime and the Roosevelt administration shared a basic principle. Both, in his view, placed the highest importance on maintaining the well-being of their citizens. In light of this commonality of purpose, the stark contrast between Soviet action and American inaction galled this impatient reformer. In November 1933, Kingsbury challenged the New Dealers to get moving. His article in the *Survey* began by invoking the popular president: "If, as President Roosevelt has said, 'the state's paramount concern should be the health of its people,' then, in our magnificent planning for an improved social and economic order, we have neglected something essential in the very basis of our future security—a well-considered plan of health conservation on a nation-wide scale." Rather than perpetuate the Progressive preoccupation with wage earners, he wanted to invent methods of funding care "for the great mass of the population." Health reform should deliver comprehensive services "to all classes of the population in all communities, not merely to the rich and the indigent nor only in some localities or some areas." Future progress required a redefinition of public health to encompass "not merely a limited number of protective measures such as the control of communicable diseases, but all preventive and curative medicine and education in hygiene, as well as efforts to increase the economic security of the people." In a follow-up piece appearing a month later, he broached the possibility that the proper course of action might not be state-level programs but rather a federal program "of national health insurance like those which have been developed in European countries." On January 24, 1934, Kingsbury wrote to Roosevelt, whom he'd known for many years in New York, to report on his meetings with several of the administration's top advisors and to request that the president set up a leadership group to formulate a health plan. He apparently received no reply from the White House.[20]

Undaunted, the Milbank agitators pressed ahead on their own. Isidore Falk began to assist Epstein's AASS with drafting a model health-insurance bill in early 1934. At a forum sponsored by the American Academy of Political and Social Science on February 7, 1934, Edgar Sydenstricker confronted "the socially essential task of providing medical care to all of the people." Sydenstricker dwelt on the nature and implications of pervasive deprivation of care. He advocated what he termed "a pragmatic approach" that extended health care to all needy citizens through a combination of social insurance, welfare medicine, and public medicine. He proposed that the poorest Americans receive care from private providers, who would be reimbursed from the public coffers. For the majority who were not destitute but could not afford expensive services, Sydenstricker recommended a mixture of government insurance and increased public medicine. "We should go beyond the health insurance systems of Great Britain and Europe which provide medical care to employed individuals only," he maintained. Eligibility should extend to "all persons and their families having incomes below an amount sufficient to purchase medical services in any contingency." Indeed, such a severing of the connection between health protection and employment status, openly presented here for the first time, was the principal policy innovation of the Milbank group. Sydenstricker left no doubt regarding the goal of his patchwork plan: "The end of any effective attempt to solve the problem before us should be nothing less than to make it possible for every person to obtain such medical care as we now know how to render." This universalistic proposition challenged the New Deal and vested health interests in a way that the homilies of the CCMC had not.[21]

No one at the Philadelphia meeting took issue with Sydenstricker's framing of the question. A number of other speakers echoed his concerns. Morris Fishbein, the highly conservative editor of *JAMA*, only hedged slightly on his own organization's commitment to all-inclusive care by indicating its willingness to cooperate in attempts to make medical care "possible for the vast majority of our people." Thomas Parran's presentation treated universal access as a matter of consensus. Parran doubted the ability of doctors in private practice "to provide for all the people the minimum essentials of medical care, without adding unbearably to the load of poorly paid and unpaid work they now carry."[22]

Parran looked to government intervention to help both the needy sick and the overburdened medical practitioners. Like Sydenstricker, he envisioned reforms that combined social insurance, public medicine, and related preventive activity. Like Sydenstricker, he identified protection of the health of the nation's population as an essential responsibility of the state. Unlike Sydenstricker, the New York Commissioner of Health staked out an entitlement. Directly linking government duties to citizens' rights, Parran quoted the eminent eighteenth-century British jurist William Blackstone: "The right to the enjoyment of health is a subdivision of the right of personal liberty, one of the *absolute* rights of persons." In his assessment, the current deficiencies in governmental health services, both preventive and curative, reflected "the lack of concern for human rights and lack of confidence in government for protecting human rights, which until recently characterized the popular mind." In light of widespread enthusiasm for the New Deal, this senior public-health official now had a little optimism but no illusions about the cultural obstacles in the way of any attempt to transform the health system of what he described as "a nation of individualists." Unlike some of his fellow liberals, Parran realized that distrust of a statist approach was not confined to a small group of AMA officials.[23]

Other observers took a less nuanced view. E. T. Remmen, former president of the Public Health League of California, saw the prevailing societal attitude toward reform as an irresistible, historic force. Writing in the February 1934 issue of *Western Hospital Review*, Remmen overestimated public enthusiasm for social insurance, citing pent-up demand "that all citizens be provided with the basic necessities of life, even though the idea sets aside our long-cherished ideas of individual initiative." He gave no corroborating evidence for this assessment of the national consciousness. Nonetheless, the Los Angeles physician assured readers that compulsory health insurance was imminent and that universal access would be one of its main benefits. I. S. Falk discerned the same strong outcry. His report to Milbank Fund advisors on March 14, 1934, alluded to "growing public demand for more and better medical care" and an "increasingly impatient" public.[24]

Falk reported that he and his colleagues at the fund had addressed this emergent opportunity by devising a tentative plan based on a set of eighteen principles. Not surprisingly, universality stood at the head of the list. European programs and American formulations that covered only the working poor were summarily dismissed as inadequate. However, at this embryonic phase, the Milbank staff was much clearer about what they did not want than what they did want. Falk posed three alternative limits on eligibility: "Sickness insurance should be compulsory for all families with annual incomes of less than $3,000 (or $5,000), and shall permit the voluntary insurance of families with annual incomes of more than $3,000 (or $5,000); or sickness insurance should be compulsory for all persons in the population." Because the earnings cutoffs at $3,000 or $5,000 represented estimates of the level at which income no longer prohibited purchase of needed care, all three options could be seen as achieving universal access.[25]

Only a modest ideological rationale accompanied this immodest proposal. The report referred in a cursory manner to societal obligation to make care generally available. Falk asserted, without explication, that "provision of good medical care to all of the population is essential to the nation's well-being." The Milbank Memorial Fund's Advisory Council voted unanimously to endorse the staff plan. However, the advisory group suggested deferring the universal insurance option and beginning instead with a program to insure only families making less than $3,000.[26]

The Milbank advisors' conference closed on a rousing note. At a dinner on March 15, Albert Milbank set the tone by declaring that medical care was "not a commodity in the ordinary commercial sense." Milbank held that the pursuit of public health had come to include "medical care of all kinds[,] both preventive and curative[,] for all of the people." Henry Sigerist, director of the Institute of the History of Medicine at Johns Hopkins, distinguished between the early European insurance legislation, which sought to aid the indigent, and contemporary trends. "Society in our day has taken the part of health," Sigerist observed. "It endeavors by all means available to preserve health and to restore it to all its members." The final speaker of the evening was Harry Hopkins, head of the Federal Emergency Relief Administration and Kingsbury's former protégé at the New York Association for Improving the Condition of the Poor. On this occasion, Hopkins showed no inclination to share the Roosevelt administration's hesitation regarding health security. His basic premise was that neighborly mutual aid, community charity, free doctoring, and other voluntarist emergency measures had failed abjectly. His disappointment with the timidity of health leaders and the apparent apathy of the long-suffering public did not dampen his optimism. "I am convinced," he flatly stated, "that with one bold stroke we could carry the American people with us, not only for unemployment insurance but for sickness and health insurance, and that it could be done in the next eighteen months if we only have the courage to go after it and do it." This forceful encouragement of immediate action exploded the conventional wisdom that federal health reform had to wait until after Washington had done much more to aid the unemployed.[27]

No member of the health policy elite followed Hopkins's advice more conscientiously than John Kingsbury, who promptly took the Milbank plan to a wider audience. In an appearance at the Commonwealth Club in San Francisco on April 13, 1934, Kingsbury took a disarmingly humble stance. He disclaimed any prophetic capabilities and characterized the proposal that he and his co-workers had developed as a tentative one. He delineated the alternatives of state health insurance for families with incomes below either $3,000 or $5,000, setting aside the possibility of public insurance for all, as advised. Comparing such schemes to the less inclusive European variants, he held that "we want no poor-man's system in America." He presented no clear-cut arrangements for funding this reform.[28]

Kingsbury's proposal to the Commonwealth Club envisioned the nation as just that—a commonwealth. He reiterated Roosevelt's now well-worn statement that the people's health was the principal concern of government. The state's priorities purportedly mirrored those of American society, which, in turn, combined generosity toward the unfortunate and self-interested fears about the societal burdens imposed by the sick upon the well. Kingsbury reasoned that "the public interest requires that all who are in need of care shall receive it." He buttressed this claim by conveying Arthur Newsholme's view of the basis of modern health policy: "Civilized communities have arrived at two conclusions, from which there will be no retreat. . . . In the first place, the health of every individual is a social concern and responsibility; and secondly, as following from this, medical care in its widest sense for every individual is an essential condition of maximum efficiency and happiness in a civilized community." The American agitator did not discuss any community or nation that had made real this dedication to universalist principles, whether by public insurance or any other means.[29]

In this appeal, the enlightened elements of American society were to bring about a more civilized public policy. If they failed in this endeavor, the threat of state medicine loomed on the horizon. Kingsbury reminded his audience that European-style social insurance was not state medicine, which existed only in the Soviet Union. His brief references to socialist health care in Russia studiously avoided any words of praise. Only a year after the publication of *Red Medicine*, Kingsbury was treating the Soviet experiment as a foil, not a utopia. The strategy was to make compulsory insurance palatable as the lesser of two evils.[30]

A month later, Kingsbury offered a slightly more adventurous version of his proposition to the National Conference of Social Work. The former charities commissioner of New York City understood well the liberal orientation of this group and adapted his message accordingly. Indeed, Kingsbury's paper, "Adequate Health Service for All the People," amounted to a universalist manifesto. He told his colleagues that the rise in health-care costs had made access to services problematic for middle-class Americans even in prosperous times. In the same vein, he prefaced his proposal for state insurance of families earning less than $3,000 or $5,000 with an assertion that undoubtedly provoked some in the audience: "Our primary problem is not how to furnish financial assistance to the poor, but to enable those who cannot buy medical care as individuals to buy it as groups." Stung by what he deemed unfair criticism of his recent speech in San Francisco, Kingsbury denied that he advocated "the socialization of medicine or anything else that a clever person might call it to confuse the issues." Moreover, he underscored the point that the private practitioner would be the central figure in the projected extension of periodic examinations, immunizations, and other preventive services. However, Kingsbury also seemed determined to pick fights with the medical profession.

Certainly, his gratuitous swipes at physicians' lack of skill and his characterization of doctor-patient relations as having "come to grief upon the rocks and shoals of a business world" could only inflame the AMA.[31]

In "Formulating an American Plan of Health Insurance," Isidore Falk continued the Milbank offensive. In June 1934, Falk complemented Kingsbury's broad-brush outline by undertaking both a more highly empirical analysis of the problem at hand and a more detailed, grounded defense of the proposed remedy. From the extensive research in which he had participated with the CCMC and at the fund itself, Falk concluded that "purchased privately and individually, even in the best of times, medical service is in greater or lesser degree beyond the means of seventy-five to ninety percent of the population." The bacteriologist-turned-economist stressed that the unevenness and unpredictability of medical expenses, not their sheer aggregate amount, made this a problem best handled through group insurance. Under an American plan, there would be flexibility regarding the range of benefits, not emulation of any European scheme.[32]

In general, Falk and the other Milbank men took pains to distance themselves from almost all foreign precedents. In effect, they distilled nearly half a century of European experience down to the insight that voluntary systems or mixed voluntary-compulsory systems of health insurance gradually evolved into more thoroughly compulsory ones in response to the inherent limitations of voluntarism. In their haste to downplay the British and continental experience, Kingsbury, Falk, and Sydenstricker failed to take note of the three European nations in which eligibility for insurance depended upon income, not employment in a particular occupation. Instead, these agitators relied upon domestic authorities, especially the Committee on the Costs of Medical Care. However, the Milbank Fund turned the CCMC's call for local voluntary experimentation into a call for national governmental experimentation. The main commonality between these markedly different approaches, of course, was an adherence to universality as a guiding principle.

The Milbank stance vis-à-vis Europe at this juncture squared with that taken by another veteran of the CCMC employed by a progressive foundation. Michael Davis, director of medical services at the Rosenwald Fund, was also anxious to push ahead in forming an innovative, inclusive health plan for the nation. His July 1934 article, "The American Approach to Health Insurance," held that only one in twenty Americans lived in households with sufficient income to enjoy health security. This essay dwelt on the need to break from the

European pattern of combining medical benefits with temporary disability payments. Severing health protection from a complicated and circumscribed income-maintenance program would, in his view, facilitate progress toward universal health care. "The evidence from Europe," Davis warned, "is that we shall interfere with or spoil comprehensive plans for adequate medical care for all the people if we begin by dealing with the wage-loss due to sickness among employed persons." (He also criticized foreign systems for their neglect of preventive services.) Davis thus joined the Milbank militants in promoting expanded access as American exceptionalism.[33]

## Social Security without Health Security

On June 29, 1934, President Roosevelt created the Committee on Economic Security (CES) to develop a comprehensive plan for safeguarding the American people against some of the major risks of life in a volatile industrial society. The committee, comprised of four cabinet members and relief administrator Harry Hopkins, brought University of Wisconsin economist Edwin Witte to Washington to direct its operations. Witte, in turn, assembled an army of experts, both full-time staff and part-time advisors—both to assess the societal damage and concoct solutions. Through an elaborate makeshift jumble of boards, committees, and councils, the CES took up unemployment, old age, disability, child welfare, adverse working conditions, and sickness. Witte brought in Edgar Sydenstricker to head the Technical Committee on Medical Care. At Sydenstricker's request, Falk joined the staff of that committee.[34]

Health insurance faced an uphill battle in the deliberations of the Committee on Economic Security. Sydenstricker and Falk maneuvered to lift health protection to the top tier of proposals dominated by unemployment insurance and old-age pensions. From the outset, they understood that both President Roosevelt and the chair of the CES, Secretary of Labor Frances Perkins, were wary of the issue. This reluctance stemmed from a sense that opposition to government health insurance on the part of the AMA and its allies could sink the whole security plan. Undaunted, Sydenstricker and Falk floated even the option of universal insurance. On August 28, 1934, they sketched out for Witte a range of possibilities for insuring segments of the population. At one end of the spectrum was coverage of "all persons (with payment of premiums by relief agencies for those without means and income)." Such a reference to universality, however brief, was a bold gambit.[35]

The tentative proposal for health insurance immediately encountered opposition from fellow liberals. Thomas Parran, seen as a key figure by virtue of his close association with Roosevelt, responded coolly. On September 24, Parran told Sydenstricker that "it would be most unfortunate for a national program of medical care to be formulated with the major emphasis on general medical care while the more important preventive needs are overlooked." Sydenstricker's rejoinder conceded the primacy of prevention and attempted to subsume curative services under a broad definition of public health. He assured Parran that the president would welcome a public-health component in the reform package and urged him to use his personal influence. "If you could steer his thinking with the conviction that medical care is a public health essential . . . , " Sydenstricker suggested, "you would be doing a great service." Abraham Epstein presented a different challenge. The prickly leader of the AASS averred his continuing support for state health insurance but wanted the New Deal to assist only the unemployed and the elderly in the near term.[36]

Health insurance survived this initial round of criticism. Witte cautiously advised Epstein that since joining the CES, he was "far less sure that health insurance is out of the question as an immediate legislative proposal." By the end of September 1934, the CES staff had made a preliminary recommendation of sickness insurance for all employees earning less than $2,000 per year. They estimated that this was roughly the equivalent of covering all families with annual household incomes under $3,000. In an appendix to the staff report, Sydenstricker and Falk identified their widely inclusive plan with the guiding value of security: "If health insurance is to serve as a system of economic security it should embrace all to whom the costs of ill health—from loss of earnings and from medical service—are serious burdens." They predicted that such an initiative would be very popular. To this end, its sponsors presented this provision as an approximation of universalism. "It can reach almost every home," Sydenstricker and Falk maintained, "and can meet a human and a social need which is profoundly important to all people except those in the high income brackets." The recommendation of public insurance rested upon the assessment that there was "no form of voluntary insurance practiced in the United States which holds promise or has the potentialities of large-scale application." The insurgent New Dealers thus summarily dismissed CCMC voluntarism. At the same time, they recommended funding reform through contributions from employees, employers, and the government. In a sense, this plan, with its emphasis upon employment-based eligibility and contributory financing, constituted only a more capacious version of the AALL approach of the 1910s.[37]

This expansive vision did not survive for long. The Technical Board on Economic Security refused to send it up to the cabinet-level committee. Instead, the senior policy technicians watered down the staff's health proposal by limiting its scope to "the lowest income groups." The board did not specify the limits of this category, but their intention was clearly to rein in any federal responsibility. Their language may have been vague, but the rejection of Sydenstricker and Falk's stance was certainly clear. In their appendix to the staff report, after all, the Milbank activists had declared that "health insurance should not be restricted only to the lowest income groups." In another departure from the staff recommendations, the technical board promoted expansion of public health services for the poor. Witte's optimism about the short-term prospects faded. On October 26, he told Frances Perkins that although he opposed abandonment of the health-insurance proposal at this juncture, he preferred that the final CES report endorse only further study of the subject.[38]

The National Conference on Economic Security, held in Washington on November 14, brought together about two hundred social policy specialists from across the country to discuss all aspects of the administration's master work in progress. The session on medical care featured recitations of the opposing positions staked out within the Committee on the Costs of Medical Care. Livingston Farrand, the president of Cornell University, tried to use his role as chair of the medical session to frame the discussion in terms of the widespread deprivation of care. The AMA rejected this orientation. Nathan Van Etten maintained that expanded governmental care for the truly indigent, not any form of insurance, was sufficient to realize the American people's entitlement to medical services. Both Van Etten and fellow conservative George Follansbee detected little or no popular interest in compulsory health insurance. On the other side of the question, Michael Davis used fresh PHS data to show that the depression had made forgone care a massive problem, not a marginal one. Stewart Roberts, yet another CCMC veteran, joined Davis in returning attention to "the average interest of the average American." Roberts challenged his medical colleagues to address, not trivialize, the situation at hand: "We are on trial, gentlemen; we can obstruct no longer." His plea left the AMA leadership unmoved.[39]

The failure of this widely publicized meeting to achieve any sort of consensus sealed the fate of health insurance. On the day after the conference, Witte suggested to the Advisory Council on Economic Security—yet another ad hoc forum for input from major societal interests, like labor and business, and from recognized authorities from academia and reform organizations—that health insurance merited only additional investigation. Facing a host of other thorny issues regarding the unemployed and the elderly, the council avoided taking a stand for health-care financing.[40]

The protagonists refused to surrender. They prepared a defense of their position and a statement of principles for the Medical Advisory Committee meeting later in November. Not unexpectedly, the first principle of reform remained universal protection: "The availability of good health services and medical care to all of the population is essential." The list of possible courses of action still contained social insurance for the entire population. The preferred alternative was compulsory insurance for all families with incomes of less than either $2,500 or $3,000. Sydenstricker and Falk estimated that if the higher of these income cutoffs were adopted, government health insurance would extend to about three-quarters of the nation's families. Outside the confines of federal policy formulation, Sydenstricker held an even more militant position. In an article in the *Annals of the American Academy of Political and Social Science* that appeared in the midst of this debate, he claimed that Americans had a right to health. Progress toward achieving this right required only "the use of existing scientific knowledge and the application of social common sense." These fervent appeals, however, did nothing to stir the real policymakers. Roosevelt and Perkins listened to the threats of the AMA over the promises of a few policy intellectuals.[41]

All that remained was to arrange a decent burial for the Sydenstricker-Falk initiative. On December 4, the Committee on Economic Security decided to make no firm commitment to health insurance. In the report sent to the president on January 15, 1935, the CES deferred any recommendation on sickness insurance, pending further study, to be completed by March. The committee did, however, note that its staff had produced "a tentative plan of insurance believed adequate for the needs of American citizens with small means and appropriate to existing conditions." The report did little to elaborate on the nature of this plan, indicating nothing of its breadth of population coverage beyond the reference to small means. As a further concession to supporters of more governmental involvement in health affairs, the CES recommended significant expansion of public-health activities and of maternal and child health services. The cabinet secretaries had finessed the explosive issue of health security in order to avoid endangering the larger economic-security plan.[42]

While Congress took up the rest of the Roosevelt administration's package of proposals, Sydenstricker and Falk carried out the additional work promised in the CES report. In the short term, this was another exercise in futility. Further discussion with the doctors uncovered no new receptivity to reform. The budding interest of the California Medical Association and other medical organizations in state insurance was insufficient to budge the AMA leadership. At the Medical Advisory Committee session at the end of January, Thomas Parran discouraged any last-minute rethinking. Parran considered neither the apathetic public nor the prejudiced medical profession ready for transformation. Instead, he argued for the more circumscribed policy of expanded public aid to the very poor and the public provision of selected expensive services for some wage earners. This modest compromise also went nowhere. When Sydenstricker and Falk presented their supplemental report to the CES on March 15, they again urged amendment of the administration bill already under legislative consideration to include a health-insurance section. Frustratingly enough, the cabinet-level officials, still afraid of the AMA, gave this suggestion their sympathy but not their support. On June 15, Perkins finally sent the Sydenstricker-Falk report to the White House. The report never appeared in public view. Barbara Armstrong, who served as a pension expert on the CES staff, believed that the pro-insurance document "was confiscated, sat upon, [and] locked up" by the committee's leaders. Accordingly, Congress gave no serious thought to including a sickness-insurance program in the Social Security Act.[43]

The exclusion of health security from the social policies of the early New Deal illustrates the limits of what Daniel Fox aptly, if uncharitably, termed "coterie politics." A handful of progressive intellectuals dedicated to pursuing social insurance for illness could carry the campaign only so far. Like the AALL in the 1910s, the Milbank crew tried to operate without a supporting movement similar to the massive, grassroots Townsend campaign for old-age pensions. Moreover, they attempted to proceed in the face of vested interests that easily scared off the president and key members of his inner circle. The weakness of the small activist group was further underscored by a devastating attack inflicted upon one of its central figures at a highly inopportune time. John Kingsbury became the object of a campaign of vilification and ostracism just as congressional debate on economic security was heating up. Kingsbury's relentless medical opponents mounted a boycott of the infant formula and other milk products of the Borden Company, the Milbank family's main source of wealth. In March 1935, the Milbank Memorial Fund acceded to this pressure by firing Kingsbury, in what James Rorty described as a "panicky retreat from liberal leadership." With the fund withdrawing from the field of health care studies, Falk departed the following year. (Similarly, three years later the Rosenwald Fund forced out its troublesome director of health programs, Michael Davis.) This episode illuminated both the vulnerability and the scarcity of active supporters of progressive reform. In the next round of agitation for health security, elite activists would profit from this hard lesson by seeking to ally themselves with more substantial social forces, rather than stand off in isolation from the masses in need of assistance.[44]

Their political impotence notwithstanding, the Milbank militants had made a major contribution to the health policy conversation during their brief moment of prominence. They had moved the discussion in the direction of universal protection by advancing two innovative proposals. First and foremost, they had explicitly and repeatedly argued that compulsory health insurance that covered the entire population was one of the viable alternatives available to policymakers. Second, their main proposal for reform aimed to cover the majority of the nation's people, not merely the minority in the industrial working class, as the Progressives had sought to do. The common denominator of these two proposals was a desire to win health protection for the largest possible number of citizens. In less than three years' time, the universalists had replaced the vague voluntarism of the CCMC with detailed plans that made public insurance again the centerpiece of health reform.

In contrast to the preceding generation of advocates of state insurance, this band of activists effectively distanced themselves from foreign models. In their report to President Roosevelt, Sydenstricker and Falk insisted that their proposals "differ in a number of fundamental particulars from the European systems." In large part because the Milbank fund had sponsored thorough studies of foreign health systems, universalists in the United States recognized that none of the capitalist nations most similar to their own had succeeded in achieving any approximation of all-inclusive health protection for its citizens. By accurately characterizing Europe's schemes as "poor man's" plans, the Milbank innovators drew an important distinction between their inclusive proposals and those instituted abroad. At the same time, they defused some criticism by resort to nationalistic tropes—"the American approach" and "an American plan"—that reformists had relied upon since the 1920s. But unlike the Wisconsin economists, whose so-called American plans for unemployment insurance and retirement pensions reinforced certain national values by basing benefits on individual earnings, the Milbank mavericks offered a version of Americanism that featured no ratification of individualism. Benefits were to be uniform; general revenues would fund the participation of those unable to make financial contributions as employees. In this context, "American" mainly meant not European and not unknown in the nation's history, given the precedent of workers' compensation. With the rise of communism and fascism on the continent, health reformers in this country undoubtedly recoiled at the prospect of being associated with any ideological extremes, as they had been during and after World War I. Although this ambitious little group may have miscalculated the probability of immediately winning major reform, they did understand the value of promoting change in exceptionalist terms.[45]

One of these impatient reformers went beyond differentiating indigenous plans from their predecessors across the Atlantic. Stewart Roberts, professor of medicine at Emory University, was the only member of the CES Medical Advisory Committee who refused to sign a letter to Edwin Witte counseling delay on health-insurance legislation. On the eve of the submission of the CES health report to President Roosevelt, this lone dissenter made a final strongly worded appeal for what he identified as "social rights," based on fundamental national values and commitments. Roberts connected the issues at hand to the rights to life, liberty, and the pursuit of happiness proclaimed in the Declaration of Independence: "Many of us believe that economic security for the individual and health security for the individual are also inalienable rights. There is not much liberty without some economic safety and not much happiness without some health and not much life without both." Roberts's perspective was straightforwardly universalistic. He supported state health insurance so that "all may receive adequate medical care." He drew on his clinical experience in the South to underscore his commitment to universalism: "The Negro plowing in the river bottom is as much entitled to adequate medical care as an inalienable right as any of us. The expectant mother in the two-room cabin has an inalienable right to adequate medical care." In the years after 1935, such a sense of entitlement would become much more widespread.[46]

# CHAPTER FOUR

# American Democratic Medicine

After 1935, the nation's health-policy elite faced an insurgency. In the turbulent atmosphere of economic depression, societal unrest, and governmental activism, previously unheard citizens asserted themselves in unprecedented ways. In particular, a militant labor movement instantly became an active force in the field. The union leaders led a coalition that spoke not only for consumers of health services but, more importantly, for those unable to afford to purchase services. Also prominent within this broad-based alliance were organizations representing the long-neglected interests of African Americans. The democratic intrusion emboldened some to take more adventurous positions and shocked others into stiffer resistance to change.

Audacious and novel rights claims became prominent. Reformers traced medical care entitlement to authoritative national and international sources. Interpretations of the Declaration of Independence, the U.S. Constitution, and the Bill of Rights placed health rights on a foundation of national ideals. Important presidential declarations also promoted an inclusive vision of health security. Taken together, these aggressive and often imaginative assertions did much to make the reform movement more legitimate. This new rhetoric of rights effectively threw opponents of universal provision on the defensive.

Insistence on the right to health care fundamentally changed the policy debate. By the 1940s, truly universal formulations had found their way onto the nation's political agenda. Even the less-than-universal Wagner-Murray-Dingell bills, the leading proposals of the period, sought to cover the vast majority of the nation's citizens. Opponents of government intervention had no choice but to speak to the question of how, not whether, to achieve access for all.

## Social Unionists for Health Security

The passage of the Social Security Act lured the American labor movement back into health policymaking. The sharp division within the American Federation of Labor over social insurance during the 1910s had ended in a stalemate. By the mid-1930s, however, much had changed. Samuel Gompers, the most vociferous opponent of state intervention, had died in 1923. The Great Depression had so impoverished millions of wage earners, making medical care less accessible for so many. The economic collapse had devastated union benefit plans. In this context, the Roosevelt administration's plans to use social insurance to protect the elderly and the unemployed encouraged rethinking by labor leaders. Moreover, the prospect that the New Deal would bring about a more humane society kindled hopes throughout the beleaguered working class.[1]

Only two months after the enactment of Social Security, organized labor discarded its longstanding policy of voluntarism in health matters. The AFL convention noted that sickness, more than any other single cause, forced workers to turn to charity. The union leaders identified illness as the second greatest fear of working people (after unemployment) and lamented that the Social Security Act had done nothing about this widespread source of insecurity. Convention delegates voted unanimously to pursue "the enactment of socially constructive health insurance legislation through Congress and the individual states." The AFL Executive Council called upon federal officials to continue "planning for adequate medical care for all."[2]

The unions took their concerns straight into the political arena. In early 1937, Andrew Biemiller, an AFL organizer, presented an insurance bill to his colleagues in the Wisconsin legislature. Accepting the limits set in the Milbank-CES formulations, Biemiller proposed to cover state residents in households with incomes below $3,000 per year. Although this program would take in only those able to purchase little or no health care, organized medicine opposed it. The state medical society and its allies had no trouble defeating this measure.[3]

In a series of editorials in the *American Federationist,* AFL president William Green discussed the issue in terms that would appeal to a broad audience. In February 1937, he contended that an episode of serious illness would leave nine out of ten Americans heavily in debt. Extending Social Security would remove this all-too-common threat. From Green's vantage point, the recent landmark legislation had already established a right to the necessities of life, so adding health insurance to the security system was but a straightforward application of a settled principle of public policy. Five months later, the AFL leader dismissed employment-based benefits as an alternative means to attain universal health protection. Green concluded this editorial by reiterating labor's eagerness to discuss "plans for providing adequate medical services for all." In May 1938, an editorial entitled "Health for All" endorsed further investigation of health-care financing to prepare for "adequate medical, hospital, nursing and diagnostic services for all."[4]

Green's analysis obviously took up more than the interests of the dues-paying members of unions affiliated with the American Federation of Labor. Unlike his predecessor Gompers, Green espoused a wide-ranging social unionism that encompassed varied forms of state action for the common good. This had always been his philosophy. While serving in the Ohio legislature two decades earlier, he sponsored workers' compensation and state health insurance bills. In 1919, he wrote the resolution for compulsory health insurance adopted by his own union, the United Mine Workers of America. His strong convictions on this question led him to take a determined stand against Gompers in the protracted debate within the AFL Executive Council at the end of the 1910s. By the late 1930s, social unionists held prominent positions not only within the AFL, dominated by craft unions, but also within the newborn industrial-union movement of the Congress of Industrial Organizations (CIO). Quite remarkably, the AFL and the CIO were able to work together harmoniously on health reform throughout the bitter internecine warfare that divided the labor movement from the mid-1930s to the mid-1950s.[5]

## Public Medicine Revisited

Exclusion of health insurance from the Social Security Act carried a different meaning for policy insiders than it did for union leaders. In the short term, the resounding defeat of health insurance in the winter of 1935 prompted some to reconsider the alternative of expanding the delivery of health services by public agencies. That the Social Security legislation established new programs for supporting such services suggested the possibility of further development along this line. Particularly encouraging were provisions for federal grants to state health departments for maternal and child health-care initiatives, industrial-hygiene programs, and other public-health activities. These ventures generally emphasized diagnostic work and other practices that spilled over into the realm of clinical services. The fact that the AMA had offered no resistance to this form of governmental encroachment escaped nobody's attention.[6]

Canny advocates of public medicine attempted to capitalize on this apparent opening. In October 1935, Edgar Sydenstricker, who had been promoted to replace Kingsbury at the Milbank Memorial Fund, argued that New Deal initiatives and other recent developments had extended the boundaries of public health. Echoing arguments made a decade earlier by C.-E. A. Winslow and others, Sydenstricker held that public health now involved much more than sewage disposal and other traditional chores. He set the stage for his redefinition by declaring that "the American people are not so healthy as they have a right to be." He claimed that "over a hundred thousand die annually from causes that are preventable through the use of existing scientific knowledge and the application of common social sense." In his view, public-health practice now meant nothing less than efforts to control all the controllable factors in health status. This entailed society's responsibility to guarantee good medical care to every citizen. Sydenstricker took no hard-and-fast position on the optimal means to improve the distribution of services but noted a recent suggestion for a major expansion in public medical care for low- and middle-income families. His willingness to broach the possibility of government health services for the nonindigent population signaled a receptivity not previously associated with Milbank.[7]

The search for a viable way to build on the precedent of federal support for public-health work under Social Security attracted others committed to improving access to care. Like Edgar Sydenstricker, Thomas Parran had spent the formative years of his career on the staff of the U.S. Public Health Service and thus was fully qualified to make the case for public medicine as a legitimate component of public health. "Health Security," his February 25, 1936, speech to the New York Tuberculosis and Health Association, portrayed Social Security as a flexible framework that could accommodate additional initiatives. The state health commissioner made universal protection his standard, insisting that "it must be possible for the whole population to secure medical care if we are to attain any semblance of health security." He categorically rejected state medicine and social insurance as the means to achieve this end. Instead, he proposed a modest extension of the health-care role of governmental agencies —a combination of public assumption of responsibility for low-income patients with especially expensive conditions and increased public funding of health facilities to enhance the productivity of private practitioners. By the time Parran spoke to the American College of Physicians (ACP) on April 4, 1938, he was serving as the surgeon general of the United States. He addressed the meeting in a manner calculated both to disarm distrustful doctors and to alarm them about growing impatience among the laity. Like Sydenstricker, Parran wanted to redefine the mission of public health. Unlike his former PHS colleague, he presented public health as a specialty within medicine. Characterized in this way, public health complemented and thus did not threaten the larger realm of clinical medicine. But beneath this reassurance, Parran sought to take over the treatment of individuals with numerous conditions, like cancer and sexually transmitted diseases: "Public health . . . embraces the prevention and cure of all diseases which because of their wide prevalence, their serious nature, or their costly treatment cannot be dealt with adequately by the individual efforts of the patient." The surgeon general portrayed this expanded mission as a democratic mandate. "The community," he advised fellow ACP members, "is beginning to concern itself with the prevention, alleviation and cure of all sickness, disability and premature death, just as it protects itself against burglaries, embezzlement, arson, and murder." He warned that, in the turbulent context of New Deal activism, this community concern was taking a more aggressive turn. "We have now reached a stage in the evolution of citizenship when all the people, poor and rich alike, are beginning to demand at least a minimum of health protection as a right." Parran invited his colleagues to participate in shaping a health program to meet these popular demands. He hastened to add that in order for such a program to succeed it would have to involve more than insurance alone. In fact, he went much further, announcing that "whether we have health insurance or not makes very little difference, I think, to our great basic problem of saving life and reducing disability." Certainly, many of the physicians present breathed a sigh of relief when a senior health official in the Roosevelt administration trivialized social insurance in this way. Almost as certainly, however, many had to be somewhat uncomfortable about the implications of framing the question of health security in terms of the rights of a demanding citizenry.[8]

Thomas Parran was hardly alone in his unwillingness to reduce the question of access to one of insurance alone. Josephine Roche, the former assistant treasury secretary in charge of the Public Health Service, also favored further public incursions into the world of clinical medicine at the 1937 meeting of the American Public Health Association. Roche described government delivery of health care as "not so much a new function . . . as an extension of the function and services which public health leaders and workers have long claimed as their own." The editor of the *Christian Century* joined those promoting a larger, direct, but ambiguous role of the state in giving care. Michael Davis, no champion of socialized medicine, chose this moment to publish a lengthy survey of the myriad existing forms of governmental health care. Though offered in a noncommittal manner, Davis's account made the point that these activities were already a significant and accepted part of the American scene, not some alien import.[9]

In contrast, some proponents of public medicine wholeheartedly embraced socialization. In 1937, eminent progressive Grace Abbott attacked the Committee on Economic Security's preoccupation with insurance against medical expenses, as well as its intention to fund health insurance by a regressive payroll tax. Abbott preferred "the democratic American principle of medical care supported by general taxes" to what she identified as the European method of social insurance. In justification, she cited the precedent of state care for victims of tuberculosis and mental illness. She argued that "unless some federal-state program for medical care is adopted, we shall still have no care, or inadequate care, for the great army of wage-earners and their families."[10]

Henry Sigerist, a historian of medicine at Johns Hopkins, extolled the wonders of state provision he had seen in two summer tours of Russia. Sigerist's 1937 book *Socialized Medicine in the Soviet Union* challenged the more restrained appraisal presented four years earlier by Arthur Newsholme and John Kingsbury. To the radical physician-historian, the virtues of virtually universal care and a concentration on disease prevention completely overshadowed any shortcomings of the Russian model. Sigerist contrasted the financial impediments to access and the small-business ethos of capitalist health care with the ready accessibility of free services and the enlightened service ethos of socialist care. Even skeptical readers of this uncritical interpretation learned a great deal about the basic principles and workings of a system that was attempting the great leap of decommodifying medicine.[11]

Sigerist took the theme of decommodification further in an essay the following year in the *Yale Review*. He contended that the majority of Americans did not view medical care as a mere commodity, available only to those with the money to purchase it. "Most people," he held, "agree that it is in the interest of society to fight disease and to provide medical care for the whole population regardless of the economic status of the individual." After admitting his argument was utopian, Sigerist outlined an ideal system organized around government-run health centers. In these sophisticated facilities, salaried public employees delivered comprehensive services to all citizens without charge. The only way to reach truly unimpeded access was to offer services without cost to the patient: "If medical care is to be available to all, it must be free of charge like education." This reference to public education helped to make Sigerist's position seem reasonably moderate. However, identifying his approach with the Soviet Union made this a brand of decommodification that many Americans would not buy.[12]

Interest in state medicine after 1935, a phenomenon ignored by historians, illuminates three significant characteristics of American health policy and politics during the New Deal years. First, this resuscitation of interest shows how fluid and unsettled the situation was in the aftermath of the exclusion of sickness insurance from the Social Security Act. Amid political exploration and social ferment, state medicine became one of many objects of curiosity. Even such small beachheads of government intervention as the categorical programs authorized by Social Security could redirect policy thinking. The patchwork experiments of the New Deal encouraged further such improvisation. Second, widespread and well-publicized consideration of state delivery of medical services, especially by reputable individuals not aligned with the far left, made it clear that the American Medical Association and its conservative allies were not simply paranoid. There really was a drive for socialized medicine in the United States. Moreover, some of its champions, like the charismatic and prolific Sigerist (whose picture appeared on the cover of *Time* on January 30, 1939), were indeed infatuated with Soviet socialism. Third and most important, this interlude provides a further reminder that the primary policy objective of the 1930s was expanding access to health care. The state was to step in primarily to fill a void of deprivation in needed curative services and only secondarily to shift the emphasis in services toward disease prevention.[13]

## Vitamin CIO and Vitamin AFL

The Roosevelt administration tried to capitalize on the mounting interest in health reform. Federal officials, especially those at the newly created Social Security Board, also returned to this issue to oppose the free-wheeling advocates of public medicine. To these administrators, social policy still meant social insurance.

The Interdepartmental Committee to Coordinate Health and Welfare Activities, appointed by President Roosevelt in 1935, served as the key institution for refocusing the health debate. Under the leadership of Josephine Roche, the committee commissioned a massive study of the health status of the population and the availability of health resources. The National Health Survey canvassed roughly 800,000 households. The survey authoritatively reaffirmed the assessment rendered by the Committee on the Costs of Medical Care. Lower-income Americans suffered disproportionately from illness and disability and received much less care. The Interdepartmental Committee estimated that "certainly one-third and perhaps one-half of the population is too poor to afford the full cost of adequate medical care." Unlike the CCMC, the federal inquiry collected data on "the colored populations." This newfound attention to diversity did not, however, extend to an exploration of the use of health care by Americans of Asian or Latino ancestry, however. PHS statistician Rollo Britten acknowledged the limitations in the interpretation of survey findings: "The West has been excluded from these comparisons because of the fact that the colored population in the West differs in composition from that in the rest of the country. The present analysis is essentially a comparison between white and Negro populations." Not unexpectedly, the National Health Survey discovered that whites received more care when sick than blacks. The racial disparity was especially striking with respect to hospitalization in the rural South, where African Americans with disabling illnesses were only one-fifth as likely to be hospitalized as whites in similar straits.[14]

In February 1938, the Technical Committee on Medical Care of the Interdepartmental Committee came forward with tentative recommendations for a comprehensive national health program. The centerpiece of this set of proposals was a flexible plan for federal grants to assist the states in enhancing access to care. Individual states would have the option to offer health insurance, public medicine, or both, or neither. The universalistic influence of Martha

Eliot of the Children's Bureau was evident in the recommendation to "make available to mothers and children of all income groups and in all parts of the United States minimum medical services." The assumption that health insurance had to depend on payroll-deduction financing caused familiar anxieties about administering coverage for the self-employed, domestic servants, and farm laborers. In contrast, the bureaucratic group acknowledged that "public medical service is potentially applicable to whole areas and to entire areas, . . . wherever the taxing power of government reaches." The technicians' enumeration of the complications of expanding public medicine did not prevent them from seeing beyond the mechanics of reform. Instead, they stated that "the problems of executing the program must not be permitted to obscure the need for Federal aid in securing to these needy citizens their right to health." The report concluded with a reminder that illness and the associated dependency constituted problems no less pressing than more visible phenomena like mass unemployment and homelessness. "The sick do not gather in crowds on the streets of our cities," the federal officials noted, "but their needs are not less urgent."[15]

The Interdepartmental Committee organized a conference in Washington to discuss its recommendations. The National Health Conference was a wholly extraordinary event. It brought together almost two hundred invited participants for three days of deliberation, beginning on July 18, 1938. The Roosevelt administration brought in leaders from a wide range of groups of consumers and would-be consumers of health services, as well as the providers and other established participants and authorities in the field. Conferees expressed the viewpoints of women and children, industry and agriculture, employees and the unemployed. The AMA and other old-guard elements found themselves greatly outnumbered by new players. This scene impressed Josephine Roche, who chaired the Interdepartmental Committee: "Probably the most significant aspect of the National Health Conference . . . was the make-up of its membership. Here, perhaps for the first time, men and women of the medical and welfare professions were met in open discussion with representatives of the people in need of health care." Isidore Falk remembered the event as a turning point when health policy became "everybody's business." The composition of the conference alone virtually guaranteed that genuinely democratic conversation would supplant the usual elite policy discourse.[16]

The unions led the way in redirecting the discussion. Indeed, this conference marked labor's debut as a major force in the formulation of federal health policy. Workers' organizations comprised the largest contingent in the chorus of previously unheard voices, and the second largest of all delegations present, behind only the providers. As conferee Michael Davis recalled, "The major result of three days' deliberation was to show that, for the first time, a political base had been established for a broad legislative program. This base was the united support manifested by organized labor." This united support came from a mass movement in the midst of a spectacular surge of growth. Between 1933 and 1941, union membership in America tripled. Sitdown strikes, general strikes, and other wild, sometimes violent, tactics colored the organizing drives in major industries. The intrusion of the AFL and the CIO into the staid world of health affairs came at an especially dramatic time.[17]

Militant labor brought a palpable sense of urgency to the conversation at the Mayflower Hotel. It also brought a distinctive unvarnished style. One exchange in particular heralded the arrival of an impatient force to be reckoned with. On the first day of the proceedings, Olin West, secretary of the AMA, urged the ignorant laity to visit the association's headquarters in Chicago to see its expert staff at work safeguarding the nation's well-being. This posture rankled Florence Greenberg, a leader of the women's auxiliaries of the Steel Workers Organizing Committee. "I, too, want to extend an invitation to the delegates here to visit Chicago," Greenberg announced, "but I want to show them another picture. I want to show them a sick Chicago, a Chicago of dirt and filth and tenements." She proceeded to identify ailments afflicting workers in the city and to call attention to the inaccessibility of professional services to diagnose and treat those ailments. She noted that the African-American community had only one hospital, and it was overburdened. She illuminated the difficulties faced by other minorities as well: "The Mexican family whose little girl got double pneumonia twice and finally died of an abscessed lung after three years of suffering knows what lack of hospital facilities for the poor means. She was taken out of Michael Reese Hospital because the relief authorities would not pay for her care any more." To Greenberg, this situation demanded compulsory health insurance. "My people are asking," she reported, "that our Government take health from the list of luxuries to be bought only by money and add it to the list containing the 'inalienable rights' of every citizen." Her invocation of citizens' rights demonstrated a determination to see that universal health security was taken more seriously.[18]

Other labor conferees supported Greenberg's position. Her comrades in the CIO shared her confrontational attitude. Eve Stone of the women's auxiliary of the United Auto Workers called for federal health benefits under the Social Security Act and informed the AMA that it now faced the opposition of "the millions who are in need." Dorothy Bellanca of the Clothing Workers elaborated on the painful implications of the status quo. In an exaggeration calculated to convey her fellow workers' sense of urgency, she held that sickness "deprives its victims of any hope for self-respect and creates a permanent state of despair." CIO attorney Lee Pressman unloaded on "the upper hierarchy of these medical associations that simply refuses to give adequate health service to the people of this country." The American Federation of Labor made the same substantive demands without venturing into arguments involving rights. Instead, it relied on the humanitarian imperative to prevent avoidable suffering. William Green advocated government insurance for "the common people," defined as the 92 percent of the population in households with annual incomes below $5,000.[19]

The Roosevelt administration disavowed any visionary leadership role and presented itself as the obedient instrument of the public will. Presiding over the initial session of the conference, Josephine Roche discerned a democratic mandate for universal protection: "The people of our land are alert and determined that the frequently difficult but ultimately sure and progressive processes of democracy shall serve all the people. We have established the principle that certain insecurities which individuals alone are powerless to withstand must be met through public action, that human conservation is an obligation of government." Thomas Parran told the assemblage that he detected auspicious changes in societal assumptions and values. "People in general," Parran observed, "are beginning to take it for granted that an equal opportunity for health is a basic American right. They are thinking just a little ahead of the lawmakers and even, I fear, ahead of the practitioners of public health and of clinical medicine." In a nationally broadcast radio address during the conference, the Roosevelt administration's senior health official reiterated that many segments of society were pressing for wider availability of health services. Although Parran did his best to present himself as a mere witness of changing public consciousness and not as an angry rebel, one group on the left tried to put him at the head of the reform parade. In her contribution to the conference discussion, Harriet Silverman, a leader of the People's National Health Committee, passed along the surgeon general's recent statement that an American citizen's right to an equal opportunity for health was "coequal with the right to life, liberty, and the pursuit of happiness."[20]

The consensus across the ideological spectrum now favored universal access. Most speakers still avoided the rhetoric of rights. Robert Neff, president of the American Hospital Association, portrayed general entitlement to hospitalization as a condition that a demanding public was about to force upon his industry, not something that hospital administrators themselves reflexively accepted as rightful. AMA President Irvin Abell presented his organization's support for "good medical care for all the people" as a fundamental aim. To reach this objective, Abell advocated extension of health services to the poor through local programs under the control of physicians. This plan drew a skeptical response from the panelist who followed Abell on the program. Dorothy Kahn, director of relief services in Philadelphia, questioned the medical association's fixation on the indigent and its assumption that this was a marginal group at a time when roughly 20 percent of the workforce was unemployed. "Who are the medically indigent?" Kahn asked. "Are we not all more or less medically indigent?" She referred approvingly to the recent recommendation of the American Association of Social Workers that public medical care be extended to the large share of the population that could benefit from it. Leaders of the three-million-member American Farm Bureau Federation stressed rural needs but at the same time promoted general solutions. Louis Wright, chairman of the board of directors of the National Association for the Advancement of Colored People, took an identical approach. Wright, a surgeon, maintained that "the health neglect of colored people represents the ultimate in acute economic, mental, and physical distress." Yet he explicitly disavowed any interest in special pleading, preferring a program for all citizens that gave African Americans equal access and treatment. He hoped that "the American people will begin to realize that the health of the American Negro is not a separate racial problem to be met by separate segregated set-ups or dealt with on a dual standard basis."[21]

Others with medical or public-health credentials joined Wright, dispelling any notion that the AMA led a biomedical monolith. Hugh Cabot of the Mayo Clinic challenged the AMA's authority to assess national needs based on a survey of its members. "I am not clear," Cabot questioned, "by precisely what method physicians are to know about the people whom they never see. The people who get no medical care obviously do not crowd the doctors' offices." Joseph Slavit, chairman of the American League for Public Medicine, upheld the people's right to state care. George Baehr of the New York Academy of Medicine shifted the blame for deprivation to labor and farm leaders, whom he considered "responsible for leading the masses and who have permitted government to ignore the needs of the people." C.-E. A. Winslow gave the same observation a more positive interpretation in rejecting the advice of a medical conferee who compared the reform drive to a frail newborn, to be nurtured slowly. "I think this infant is older than he thinks," Winslow exclaimed, "and I suspect that all it needs is a little administration of vitamin CIO and vitamin AFL and whatever kind of vitamin they make in the Farm Bureau to develop it into a pretty husky child." Obviously, activists like Winslow delighted in the arrival of reinforcements and wanted to move ahead without further delay.[22]

## Toward Universal Insurance

The National Health Conference seemed to generate powerful momentum for reform. Josephine Roche told Roosevelt about the "amazing public support" expressed for the administration's program. The *New England Journal of Medicine* advised its readers that public sentiment had crystallized in favor of immediate government action. This perception of a popular groundswell induced Robert Wagner, a Democratic senator from New York, to introduce the National Health Bill in January 1939. Essentially as outlined in the Interdepartmental Committee's recommendations, this legislation would make federal grants to the states to support either social insurance or public medicine. Other provisions of the measure promoted expansion of traditional public-health activities, construction of health facilities, and development of programs for mothers and children.[23]

The National Health Bill had little potential to expand Americans' access to medical care to any substantial extent. It made grant monies available to the states but did not require them to set up any programs of insurance or care. Wagner assured opponents that his proposition would "not impose a Federal straitjacket upon the development of state plans." He conceded that states could choose to "cover only the relief population." In all likelihood, enactment of the Wagner Bill would have done little or nothing to improve access for residents of many states, especially those in the Deep South. Nonetheless, the plan represented a step in the direction of greater federal responsibility for health security.[24]

The surge of exhilaration from the National Health Conference proved insufficient to bring about immediate change. The AMA and its friends, stung by their embarrassment at the Mayflower Hotel, regrouped and went into an intense mobilization against the proposal. The White House remained afraid of the medical lobby and kept its distance from the National Health Bill. The Roosevelt administration was also increasingly and quite understandably preoccupied with the mounting crisis in Europe. To make matters worse, by the end of the 1930s the domestic political climate had cooled, and the New Deal had largely lost its mandate for social experimentation.[25]

Moreover, the Wagner plan had shortcomings that tempered the enthusiasm of its defenders. Both the AFL and the CIO testified in favor of the bill in Senate hearings but voiced apprehension about the latitude left to individual states. Walter Polakov, representing the United Mine Workers, called the measure "but a modest and inadequate answer to the long-felt need and definitely expressed wish of the masses of the population." Labor's long experience with workers' compensation had shown just how weak social insurance could be in anti-union states. It had also shown them that stronger protections in unionized states sometimes proved disadvantageous when states competed for business. Organized labor also distrusted public-health agencies, which it viewed as controlled by organized medicine. The Wagner Bill gave the PHS a major role in overseeing state medical programs, which in turn would be run by state health departments. This worry immediately reshaped the New Dealers' policy. After 1940, state medicine disappeared from the liberal agenda; compulsory insurance became the preferred method to expand access to health care.[26]

When in December 1941 the U.S. became a direct participant in World War II, discussion of health reform abated only momentarily. The Roosevelt administration grounded an open-ended guarantee of health care in the rights set forth in the Declaration of Independence when it commenced postwar planning. In January 1942, the National Resources Planning Board pledged that "we are intent on winning this war, not only to safeguard our lives and liberties, but also to make possible the 'pursuit of happiness.'" The board then presented an ambitious New Bill of Rights that included entitlement to medical care. In his State of the Union message two years later, President Roosevelt maintained that the rights declared by the Founding Fathers in 1776 had "proved inadequate to assure us equality in the pursuit of happiness." The president sought to repair this deficiency with "a second Bill of Rights under which a basis of security and prosperity can be established for all."[27]

Presidential endorsement, in principle, of a general right to health security helped to stimulate the process of policy reconstruction already under way in the early 1940s. During this brief but formative interval, forces both within the government and outside it launched a drive for a more comprehensive and uniform set of social protections. This meant primarily a shift toward a purely federal system of social insurance, not the federal-state system that dominated under the Social Security Act. The experience of the Social Security Board in funding but not controlling widely varying state programs, such as unemployment insurance, fostered a desire for uniform benefits and eligibility standards. Massive exclusions from protection, especially for women and minorities, under both federal and federally supported state health and welfare programs also bred discontent among the excluded. Under the restrictions in place for the Old Age Insurance program of Social Security, for example, more than 60 percent of employed African Americans could not qualify for a retirement pension. The unveiling in 1942 of a British blueprint for comprehensive protection laid bare the failings of American arrangements. William Beveridge proposed not only social insurance from cradle to grave but also a national health service available to all British citizens. Reformers in this country hoped to import not that sort of socialized medicine but rather the Beveridge report's underlying premise that universal wartime sacrifices warranted universal social benefits. At the same time, America's military mobilization stirred further interest in corrective measures. High rates of disability identified in the course of processing, and often rejecting, draftees illuminated the inaccessibility of health services to much of the nation's population.[28]

The fruit of this rethinking was a purely federal, not federal-state, plan for health security. In June 1943, Robert Wagner, along with James Murray in the Senate and John Dingell in the House of Representatives, introduced a wide-ranging plan to amend the Social Security Act to expand the types of risks underwritten, to enlarge the share of the population eligible for protection, and to increase direct federal control over the system. One section of the Wagner-Murray-Dingell Bill called for a federally administered program of sickness insurance with uniform benefits covering a solid majority of citizens. In its original form, the bill granted hospital and medical insurance benefits not only to industrial workers but also to the self-employed and those employed in domestic service, agriculture, and nonprofit organizations. Eligibility extended to the immediate families of covered employees. Eligibility under the 1943 plan did not extend to retirees, the disabled, the unemployed, government employees, and other Americans not part of the private-sector workforce. Unlike the Milbank proposal of the early 1930s, the New Dealers' proposal did not cut off those in households with income exceeding $3,000 per year. Thus, the Wagner-Murray-Dingell proposal represented a major advance toward universal health security.[29]

The ways in which this proposition fell short of true universality reflected values and assumptions deeply embedded in American social policy. It also reflected the policy designers' steadfast belief that financing through payroll deductions rather than general revenues was crucial to the political viability of reform. One preliminary draft of Wagner-Murray-Dingell stated plainly that eligibility for participation in the health-insurance program would be "based on contributions to the system." Like existing forms of social insurance—unemployment and old-age and survivors' insurance—and a similar initiative for disability insurance also enclosed in this package, national health insurance was fundamentally tied to labor-force participation. The original bill left many of the poorest and sickest Americans to the uncertainties and humiliations of state or local welfare medicine or private charity, a dubious proposition in many parts of the country. The measure perpetuated divisions even among the beneficiaries of national health insurance. Because Wagner-Murray-Dingell assumed that only the performance of paid labor conferred entitlement to care, it defined housewives and minor children as "dependents," rather than simply as citizens.[30]

## The Universalist Coalition

In the immediate aftermath of World War II, the time finally seemed ripe for a transformation in health-care financing. Public opinion supported government action. The Democratic party controlled both houses of Congress. When Harry Truman assumed the presidency upon Franklin Roosevelt's death in April 1945, the attitude of the White House toward national heath insurance became much more enthusiastic. As a county judge in Missouri during the 1920s and 1930s, Truman had had administrative responsibility for the county poorhouse. In this capacity, he had been deeply moved by the sorry spectacle of decent, hard-working members of the community reduced to destitution by medical expenses. With Britain and other advanced democracies constructing elaborate welfare states, the prospect of amending the Social Security Act to take on health insurance seemed a comparatively modest undertaking.[31]

Ever since the National Health Conference, Michael Davis and a few other dedicated activists had worked to enlist the support of diverse groups and individuals. At first, Davis's Committee on Research in Medical Economics filled the void left by the decline of both the American Association for Labor Legislation and the American Association for Social Security. By the end of World War II, a coalition had come together to take advantage of the opportunity to enact health legislation. In February 1946, this network formally coalesced into the Committee for the Nation's Health (CNH), with Davis as its director.[32]

At the forefront of the coalition stood organized labor. Union officials had helped draft the original Wagner-Murray-Dingell proposal. Indeed, Edwin Witte called this "the social security bill of organized labor." The CIO invested considerable time and energy in the issue. Remarkably enough, the more conservative and less politically active AFL put more effort into health reform than its rival, with Nelson Cruikshank emerging as labor's leading spokesperson on this topic. Unionists continued to press the argument that access to care was a right.[33]

By the mid-1940s, the nation's public-health leadership took a more active part in the campaign for reform. This was quite a reversal, given the customary influence of the AMA on the views of physicians who served as state and local health officers. At the National Health Conference, Arthur McCormack, president of the American Public Health Association (APHA) and secretary of the Kentucky Medical Association, staunchly defended the AMA as "the guardian of the health and lives of the people of America." The traditionalist McCormack wanted nothing to do with government insurance of the general population.[34]

However, in the heady atmosphere created by that gathering, many of McCormack's colleagues were ready to pursue the New Deal reforms. At the APHA annual meeting held in October 1938, C.-E. A. Winslow reflected euphorically on the National Health Conference. "It seemed that I had all my life been hearing about democracy," Winslow said, "but that now at last I had seen its face." The arrival of popular forces did not, however, obviate the need for public-health expertise. Winslow held up the health officer as "the only individual in a given community who is primarily responsible for the health of all the people in that community." In his presidential address at this meeting, Abel Wolman, professor of sanitary engineering at Johns Hopkins, maintained that societal responsibilities extended to curative and preventive services for all citizens without prescribing the method for attaining universal access. One year later, Wolman's successor, Edward Godfrey, reminded the association of the plight of the third of the population unable to afford decent care. Godfrey defined and defended an inclusive program of "American democratic medicine" to address this problem. "It must be public health medicine," he insisted, "which means that it is preventive as well as curative medicine; . . . medicine delivered without distinction as to race, creed, occupation, or income." Godfrey's statement encapsulated the two cardinal commitments that the public-health community brought to the reform campaign—its longstanding universalism and its emphasis on prevention.[35]

The Wagner-Murray-Dingell Bill polarized the public-health community. Shortly after its introduction, Social Security administrators pitched the proposition in terms especially attractive to public-health workers: "Except for accidental injuries, the leading causes of death are now the slowly crippling diseases of middle age and old age, often ushered in by long periods of increasing disability. The attack on these forms of ill health cannot be made by mass methods such as chlorinating a water supply. . . . To prevent and curb such causes of disability requires the highly individualized services of physicians, technicians, and laboratories." The Social Security Board (SSB) reasoned that "the direction of progress in health security in the United States lies increasingly in ensuring that all groups in the population can get . . . whatever medical care they need, not only as members of communities but also as individuals." The contention that public health now entailed universal medical care reframed the question of national health insurance for the APHA. The pro-insurance side stressed universality throughout the debate. In October 1944, the association officially resolved that the first objective of national health-care policy should be to "make available to the entire population all essential preventive, diagnostic, and curative services." Unlike the opposition to the AMA mounted by some other biomedical groups, the defection of the highly reputable American Public Health Association from the voluntarist side could not be dismissed as the ideologically driven action of a leftist splinter group. Similarly, Surgeon General Parran's encouragement to the staff of the Public Health Service to promote the Wagner-Murray-Dingell Bill, though highly partisan, still carried the weight of his authority as the nation's top health officer.[36]

The growing involvement of civil rights organizations in the health-rights campaign owed less to a willingness to break with the medical establishment. Prior to the 1940s, the National Medical Association (NMA), the by-product of the professional segregation of African-American physicians and surgeons, displayed deep ambivalence on the question of health-care financing. The editors of the NMA's journal refused either to endorse or to add to the AMA's critique of the majority report of the Committee on the Costs of Medical Care, for example, but reprinted without comment an excoriating (and gratuitously racist) attack on the CCMC by the *Journal of the American Medical Association*. In 1936, the NMA edged away from AMA policy by supporting voluntary insurance. At that year's NMA convention, attorney Raymond Alexander advised African-American physicians of rising universalist sentiment in New Deal America. According to Alexander, "the public believes that medical care should be within the reach of every member of society, whether or not he or she can pay for the services rendered." For practitioners who dealt with a disproportionately poor population, this embryonic sense of entitlement hinted at the prospect of demanding but non-paying patients.[37]

The rebellion against AMA hegemony at the National Health Conference briefly emboldened supporters of health security within the NMA. In August 1938, the African-American association's journal editorialized in favor of independent thought in a manner that left no doubt that this meant primarily independence from the white-dominated medical group. The NMA's Committee on Medical Economics applauded the Roosevelt administration's intention to achieve universal access to health care. However, at a special session of the AMA House of Delegates in September 1938, NMA representatives pledged their solidarity in opposing compulsory health insurance. Four months later, on the eve of the introduction of the Wagner Bill, New Jersey physician John Kenney compared the dilemma of black doctors caught between the AMA and the New Dealers to that of a shipwrecked sailor desperately praying to both God and the devil. Kenney left it to his readers to decide which party was the devil, but soon joined the minority within the NMA openly backing Wagner's proposal.[38]

A number of other prominent African-American groups, on the other hand, faced no such indecision. In December 1938, the board of directors of the National Association for the Advancement of Colored People approved the recommendations floated at the National Health Conference, including governmental health insurance. Board member Louis Wright spoke in favor of the Wagner Bill in Senate hearings in 1939. From its initial engagement with health reform, the NAACP espoused a universalistic position. It did not promote special programs targeting the African-American community and instead sought protection for the general population. At one point in his Senate testimony, Wright reminded Senator Allen Ellender of Louisiana that African Americans were "all American citizens." By the end of the 1930s, NAACP leader

Charles Houston viewed this battle as a chance to "show that the NAACP work with Negroes is work for the whole American people." Although the association unquestionably led the way, it was not the only black organization active on this issue. Both the National Negro Congress and the National Urban League played supporting roles, mainly by underscoring the magnitude of unmet need. As Dona Cooper Hamilton and Charles Hamilton have shown, since the 1930s civil rights groups "have consistently tried to form liberal social welfare policies that would benefit not only blacks but all poor people." In the case of health-care access, they sought to benefit the middle class as well.[39]

Civil-rights activists made a distinctive contribution to the reform campaign at this juncture by drawing attention to racial discrimination as a pervasive obstacle to access. They understood all too well that universalistic reform would be an empty promise for the nation's twelve million African Americans unless the federal government also attacked well-established patterns of segregation and unequal treatment. Activists criticized any plan under which eligibility for benefits depended upon employment that fell within the scope of the Social Security Act. In 1939, John Davis pointed out that two-thirds of African-American females in the paid workforce were domestic servants excluded from Social Security insurance programs. Conversely, five years later, the Urban League's *Opportunity* praised the inclusiveness of the Wagner-Murray-Dingell Bill. In addition, civil rights leaders denounced the unjust patterns of treatment and nontreatment that were widespread throughout the nation and ubiquitous in the South. Davis recounted to senators who were studying the Wagner Bill his own experience in Alabama attempting to aid a black man critically injured in an automobile accident. "We spent at least eight hours going from small town to small town without being able to find a single hospital which would admit this young man." This accident victim died on the way to a hospital in Tennessee. Institutions that did take in African-American patients gave them inferior services. Davis reported seeing three patients sharing a bed in one New Orleans hospital. In the same vein, the NAACP assailed the exclusion and inequality evident throughout the health-care system. On July 30, 1938, Louis Wright told Josephine Roche, "I am heartily in accord with the idea of your Committee to provide adequate health services for all the American people, and this cannot be successfully done if there are to be dual or 'jim crow' set-ups even in the South." The NAACP agitated relentlessly for the addition of antidiscrimination safeguards to federal reform measures. In May 1944, the association set up a National Medical Committee to pursue its interests more systematically. In his capacity as chairman of this commit-tee, Wright induced pathologist W. Montague Cobb to study the actual avail-ability of health care to African Americans.[40]

Forces within the state also constituted an important component of the New Deal/Fair Deal health coalition in their own right. Thomas Parran and a few of his colleagues at the Public Health Service continued to aid the cause, especially with regard to reminding the public and political leaders of the human consequences of neglect. However, of greater significance as the action shifted to the legislative arena was a small cohort of policy designers and po-litical operatives at the Social Security Board, which was led by board chair-man Arthur Altmeyer and included Wilbur Cohen and Robert Ball. Within this group, I. S. Falk stood out as the key figure. In 1936, Falk secured a posi-tion as a medical economist in the brand-new Social Security bureaucracy. Five years later, he was promoted to head the research and statistics office at the board. Surrounded by labor economists whose sole expertise was in income-maintenance programs, Falk became by default the leading health au-thority at SSB. He played both a behind-the-scenes role in shaping the reform agenda and an increasingly prominent one in advancing it. Unlike the more militant union and civil rights agitators of this period, Falk and the other So-cial Security officials largely avoided the rhetoric of rights in favor of the dry statistical language of needs assessment.[41]

The activist bureaucrats' contradictions shaped the development of the con-cept of universal health security in the 1940s. On the one hand, the SSB experts clung to a model of contributory, employment-based insurance that cast a shadow over those not in the sectors of the workforce dominated by white males. Rather than foster an egalitarian sense of national community, the distinction be-tween contributors and noncontributors perpetuated societal divisions. On the other hand, this very emphasis on payroll-deduction financing did confer a measure of legitimacy upon the Wagner-Murray-Dingell plans in America's con-servative culture. Use of this funding mechanism also placed national health in-surance within the framework of the popular Social Security system.

## A Rich Nation

Less than a month after Japan surrendered, President Truman gave Con-gress his administration's blueprint for postwar readjustment, centering on full employment. Truman quoted from Roosevelt's 1944 proposal for an economic Bill of Rights, which contained a "right to adequate medical care and the opportunity to achieve and enjoy good health." On November 19, 1945, the president sent to Capitol Hill a special message solely devoted to his health program, something his predecessor had never done. Truman took the opportunity to declare his universalist aim: "Our new economic bill of rights should mean health security for all, regardless of residence, station, or race—everywhere in the United States."[42]

The president's proposal went beyond total inclusion to full equality of health protection. Rather than continue with a bifurcated approach under which the working population received social insurance and the poorest members of the community received an unreliable mix of government medical services and private benevolence, Truman advocated universal federal health insurance. From his own experience in Missouri, he viewed existing forms of tax-supported institutional care as "insufficient in most of our cities and nearly all of our rural areas." Hence, he sought social insurance for all Americans, with "needy persons and other groups ... covered through appropriate premiums paid for them by public agencies." "We are a rich Nation," the president reminded congressional lawmakers, "and can afford many things. But ill health which can be prevented or cured is one thing we cannot afford." In the context of traditional American social policy, with its entrenched inequalities under which white males received respectable insurance benefits and women and minorities received degrading and inadequate welfare assistance, this was a breathtaking departure. Truman dared to seek a seamless system of protection in which all citizens participated in one program and received identical benefits.[43]

This elegant policy hardly made for elegant politics. Of course, it thrilled reformers. The dormant campaign for national health insurance revived instantly. Wagner, Murray, and Dingell introduced a bill devoted solely to health reform, severing the issue from the far larger and far more complicated effort to amend the Social Security Act. Partisan skirmishing commenced immediately. At a national meeting of officers of state medical societies on December 2, 1945, Arthur Altmeyer rejected as worthless the concept of medical indigence commonly used to consign the needy to welfare medicine, knowing full well that the AMA viewed medical indigence as the primary criterion for determining the appropriateness of government involvement in health care. "Unfortunately," Altmeyer observed, "in the very nature of the unpredictable incidence of sickness, it is impossible to draw a line between those who will and those who will not be able to pay for the health services they need." A unified system of social insurance would erase that line. In an address to the U.S. Conference of Mayors on December 12, Thomas Parran cast the liberal plan as part of a "thoroughly American" effort "to secure for every American citizen the basic rights, political and economic, which our democratic form of government came into being to secure." The *Journal of the American Medical Association* denounced the Democratic initiative as an apocalyptic threat: "Let the people of our country realize that the movement for the placing of American medicine under the control of the federal government through a system of federal compulsory sickness insurance is the first step toward a regimentation of utilities, of industries, of finance and eventually of labor itself. This is the kind of regimentation that led to totalitarianism in Germany and the downfall of that nation." The editorial did not engage the question of universal care.[44]

Hearings before the Senate Committee on Education and Labor in the spring and summer of 1946 provided the main venue for disputing the merits of the Wagner-Murray-Dingell Bill. Even though James Murray himself chaired this committee, his proposal got rough handling throughout its deliberations. On the first day of the hearings, Senator Robert A. Taft interrupted Murray's opening statement to lambaste his plan as "the most socialistic measure that this Congress has had before it." Taft condemned the hearings and stormed out, not to return for any more sessions. His outburst set the tone for the subsequent three months of discussion.[45]

Many progressive groups testified in favor of the Wagner-Murray-Dingell Bill. The hearings featured repeated appeals urging political leaders to recognize additional rights that now defined full democratic citizenship. Maie Lowe, president of the AFL's women's auxiliaries, stated that if this measure became law, "truly we could say, 'We are all Americans.'" Ernst Boas of the Physicians' Forum made universal health care a precondition for freedom: "We believe that in a democracy adequate medical care is a right to which all citizens are entitled. This right is necessary for the enjoyment of all other rights and privileges, for sick people are not free people." Theodore Lawless, representing the Council for Social Action of the Congregational-Christian Churches, looked upon national health insurance as a way to meet the Christian obligation to alleviate suffering. Dr. Lawless insisted that access to care was "the birthright of every citizen." Stephen Wise, president of the American Jewish Congress, based his endorsement of national health insurance on neither his conception of citizenship nor his religious convictions, but rather on his commitment to egalitarianism. At this key moment in the policy discussion, Rabbi Wise, a major figure both in liberal circles reform and Reform Judaism, adhered to the strictly secularist posture that progressive Jewish intellectuals had adopted since the turn of the century. Whereas the NAACP witness, Montague Cobb, stressed unmet needs over ascendant rights, the NMA witness, E. I. Robinson, cited the general welfare clause of the Constitution in his endorsement of Wagner-Murray-Dingell. That the African-American doctors' organization made any commitment at all to this initiative, let alone one based on so grand a premise, was remarkable.[46]

Some strict adherents to the principle of universality counseled the senatorial committee that the Wagner-Murray-Dingell scheme would fall short of complete inclusion. As it had emerged from the process of legislative drafting, President Truman's rough outline of a straightforward plan to insure all Americans had been watered down to conform to the workforce-centered model of contributory insurance. By the time it reached the Committee on Education and Labor, the bill did not cover government employees, religious workers, college students, and most others outside the ranks of paid labor. It did permit state governments and other public authorities to pay insurance premiums for the unemployed, the disabled, any elderly who were ineligible for federal old-age or survivors' pensions, and other excluded persons. However, the Wagner-Murray-Dingell Bill neither required that the lower levels of government do so nor prevented them from using federal funds for establishing or expanding separate medical programs for the needy. These loopholes did not escape criticism. Joseph Mountin of the Public Health Service estimated that the Democratic proposition would insure about 80 percent of the population. Mountin advised legislators that, in the interests of societal equity and administrative simplicity, his agency "would like to see this program assure medical services to 100 percent of the population." Mountin's superior, Surgeon General Parran, along with the leaders of the Children's Bureau, fought behind the scenes for an insurance plan that would include all Americans. Jack McMichael, testifying for the Methodist Federation for Social Service, objected to the perpetuation of the two-track system that both stigmatized recipients of welfare medicine and gave them inferior care. Reverend McMichael stated that his organization favored an insurance program "universally and completely available to all Americans." The conventional version of social insurance was no longer seen in progressive circles as a "natural" approach.[47]

Most proponents of universalism, however, directed their criticisms at the more severe limitations in coverage of the voluntary insurance plans. The wartime growth of the private health programs, especially the Blue Cross hospitalization plans, gave conservatives hope for a constructive alternative to state intervention. Many liberal witnesses concentrated on voluntarism's lack of progress toward universal protection. Senator Claude Pepper maintained that private carriers had already had a century to take care of this problem but had failed to do so. He noted that less than 4 percent of the population had voluntary insurance that covered hospital, surgical, and medical services. Supporters of Wagner-Murray-Dingell also rejected rosy projections of future growth. William Green believed that private coverage was already "reaching the saturation point" and would never extend to the low-income masses. Michael Davis considered "the future of voluntary plans under organized medicine small and dark."[48]

Despite their disadvantage on the question of extent of access, the opponents of federal intervention put up a stout defense. A lengthy roster of witnesses from health professions, health-care institutions, the insurance industry, religious bodies, and other interests articulated objections to the liberal measure. Many witnesses asked for patience while private insurance realized its potential. R. L. Senserich, chairman of the AMA board of trustees, assured the senators that voluntary insurance "will accomplish all the objects of this bill with far less expense." Representatives of major Catholic institutions expressed their commitment to universal protection while noting their preference for voluntary efforts. None of the Catholic officials espoused John Ryan's position that all humans had a right to necessities of life like health care and that government was the final guarantor of that right in modern society. Alphonse Schwitalla, president of the Catholic Hospital Association, maintained that natural law obliged the individual to safeguard his or her own health. Monsignor John O'Grady of the National Conference of Catholic Charities expected private coverage to "grow by leaps and bounds." John Martin, former president of the American Protestant Hospital Association, agreed wholeheartedly, predicting that within about ten years nongovernmental insurance would reach as many people as the proposed governmental alternative. However, Reverend Martin did not indicate what sorts of private insurers would be writing policies for the unemployed, the elderly, the disabled, or the poor. Indeed, none of the enthusiastic testimonials on behalf of voluntarism explained in any depth how the United States would achieve any approximation of universal access without national health insurance. Nonetheless, by complicating the issue and by dragging out the hearings for more than three months, the opposition stalled the Wagner-Murray-Dingell proposal in mid-1946.[49]

## A New Consciousness of Rights

Health-rights advocates were not deterred by their ongoing difficulties in the legislative arena. In the decade preceding the 1946 congressional confrontation, they had succeeded in assembling a diverse coalition to support universal provision. This coalition had begun to articulate a new rationale for undertaking such a transformation. Certainly, older humanitarian and productivist arguments survived. But the big intellectual innovation was the assertion of a right to health security. The late 1930s and early 1940s were, as Alan Brinkley has observed, "an important moment of transition between the reform liberalism of the first third of the twentieth century and the rights-based liberalism that succeeded it." As we might expect during a transitional phase, few of the initial forays into rights-oriented analysis were systematically sustained or theoretically sophisticated. Instead, they usually had a rudimentary and elliptical quality. Nonetheless, taken together, these preliminary rights arguments had a seminal influence on universalist thought.[50]

To be sure, not all rights claims promoted universalism. Fitting state or federal health insurance neatly into the framework of Social Security meant embracing the established system of employee and employer payments. Such arrangements made social insurance just another type of group insurance, with the property rights that followed from paying premiums. This Progressive warranty persisted despite its obvious exclusionary implications. However, by the 1940s this rationale carried less weight than it had a generation earlier.[51]

Forward-looking activists were revitalized by fresh developments outside the United States. The most adventurous universalistic claims stemmed from attempts to adopt a supranational perspective. The first influential formulation of a global human right to health care came in the 1946 constitution of the World Health Organization. On August 21, 1946, Surgeon General Parran discussed the adoption of this historic charter with the National Medical Association, noting that it had proclaimed health "a fundamental right of every human being." The domestic policy implications of the global challenge were imperative: "Those inequalities which we know exist between our citizens must be erased, if we are to stand before the world as leaders without misgivings."

Picking up on this theme, Ernst Boas used his appearance at the NMA meeting to recall that Franklin Roosevelt had spoken out for "basic human rights," such as access to adequate health care, as a worldwide matter.[52]

The ideological stakes raised by the world war led Franz Goldmann to ground universal health care in values that transcended national citizenship. Such an enlightened orientation came more naturally for recent immigrants like Goldmann, who had fled Nazi Germany and found a position in Yale's public-health program. His 1945 book *Public Medical Care* began with this declaration: "Adequate medical care is a fundamental human right. It is as much a necessity of life as food, shelter, clothing, or education. . . . In every civilized country efforts have been made to organize facilities and services necessary to prevent, cure, and mitigate illness." In a 1946 article in *Social Service Review,* the émigré physician hailed the Wagner-Murray-Dingell Bill as the proper means "to secure this human right."[53]

Georges Gurvitch, another academic refugee from fascism, took a similarly cosmopolitan view. Gurvitch, a French sociologist who taught at Columbia, Harvard, and Rutgers during the war, wove together diverse European and American sources to craft a Bill of Social Rights, which he hoped all nations would eventually adopt. These sources included not only Franklin Roosevelt's New Bill of Rights but also a draft of a global bill of social and economic rights put together by the 1944 session of the International Labor Conference. Although Gurvitch's distillation did not enunciate a right to health care per se, it did declare a universal social right to "a minimum of economic security, guaranteed by a system of social insurance against poverty, sickness, incapacity to work, and old age."[54]

Statements from a global perspective were far rarer than invocations of the Declaration of Independence and the U.S. Constitution. Various voices expressed the democratic sentiment that embedded in the founding ideals of the nation was a tacit promise of health security. Reformers drew upon the guarantees of life, liberty, and the pursuit of happiness in the revolutionary declaration as the authoritative source of a national right to care. In a 1946 lecture at Harvard Medical School, Franz Goldmann held that "the words of the Declaration of Independence have been interpreted as including the right to obtain health service." Taking a step beyond a position that was in and of itself quite daring, Goldmann interpreted this right to mean not merely a level of care adequate to sustain life but rather "equal service to all according to need." Journalist James Rorty's reaction to the demands by representatives of unseen patients at the National Health Conference conveyed the shifting terms of the debate: "Did these people have the right—entailed by their citizenship in a progressive democracy—to enjoy the resources of modern medicine, administered and distributed for the benefit of the whole people? Or was this right—involving sometimes the right to liberty, happiness, life itself—a privilege reserved for the rich and the well-to-do?" Rorty traced the history of this right from Thomas Jefferson's declaration back to its roots in the natural rights doctrine of John Locke. Henry Sigerist, too, followed the popular strategy of linking public insurance to the Declaration of Independence. "We do not hesitate to accept the concept of man's right to health or, more correctly, of man's right fully to benefit from all known means for the protection and cultivation of health," Sigerist posited in his 1941 book *Medicine and Human Welfare.* "If we believe that life, liberty, and the pursuit of happiness are inalienable rights of man and that government is instituted to secure these rights, then we must conclude that man has a right to health and is entitled to having this right secured." Unionists, too, ventured into the realm of quasi-constitutional interpretation. Joseph Padway, the AFL's chief lawyer, concluded that the general-welfare clause of the federal constitution allowed measures like the Wagner-Murray-Dingell Bill.[55]

Reformers disinclined to rethink the intent of the Founding Fathers sometimes turned to more recent political developments to confer legitimacy upon health reform. The nation's century-old commitment to universal public schooling still supplied ammunition for activists. Ernest Goodman, a representative of the United Auto Workers, employed this familiar comparison when he reminded Social Security officials of his organization's discomfort with payroll-deduction financing of national health insurance. Goodman pointed out that "many people in this field, and our union originally, took the position that the right of people to medical and hospital care was a right they were entitled to as citizens, just as they were entitled to education for their children, and that the revenue ought to come from general revenues." Reverend McMichael found reason for optimism in the precedent set by educational policy: "It was once regarded as very radical indeed to advocate a system of universal and free education in this country. We now see such a system as an essential and inextricable root of our cherished American democracy. So in the future will it be with universal and freely available medical care." Other activists focused on precedents and pronouncements of the New Deal itself. The key principle of security for the masses, as embodied (however imperfectly) in the Social Security Act, remained a source of inspiration for those seeking to forge a right to health protection. Proposals by both Franklin Roosevelt and Harry Truman for a second Bill of Rights were helpful in this regard.[56]

By the end of World War II, a growing cohort of American reformers had come to see adequate health care, broadly defined to include preventive services, as a right. They had done considerable preliminary work to construct a multifaceted rationale for such a right. Liberal and radical advocates of universal care in this country staked out claims to such an entitlement well before British scholar T. H. Marshall elaborated the influential schema under which access to health care was conceptualized as a social right. Indeed, for more than a decade prior to the publication of Marshall's "Citizenship and Social Class," numerous American universalists were asserting a citizen's right to health services. It is worth noting that, contrary to the tendency for women to speak in terms of needs and men in terms of rights, some of the earliest and most forceful health-rights claims came from women. Florence Greenberg made such an impression on Robert Wagner that he repeated her demand that the government "take health from the list of luxuries . . . , and add it to the list containing the inalienable rights of every citizen," in presenting his National Health Bill in 1939.[57]

At the same time, advocates of universalism also devised ambitious plans to achieve their ultimate goal. After thirty years of looking to state-level social insurance or public medicine, reformers turned to the central government for leadership in resolving the problem of making health care accessible to all. In one form or another, national health insurance would dominate the progressive agenda for the rest of the century.

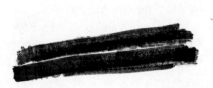

# CHAPTER FIVE

# Well on the Way

Private health insurance in the United States is well on the way toward accomplishing what the "experts" in the field of social security stated on innumerable occasions was impossible, namely, near universal coverage of the whole population.

— RITA R. CAMPBELL AND W. GLENN CAMPBELL, 1960

The health-care rights campaign collapsed in the immediate postwar period. In the fractious atmosphere of the Cold War, national health insurance became identified with subversion. Beginning in 1946, reformers reluctantly but hastily retreated from assertions that a right to medical care was inherent in American citizenship. Although a few diehards stood their ground, the ideal of universal entitlement to care faded from view in the twenty years after World War II.

The appearance of another path to security accelerated the retreat from universalistic state action. The 1940s and 1950s witnessed impressive growth in voluntary forms of health protection. Employment-based insurance benefits comprised the central component of the ascendant private welfare system. Although union negotiators contributed much to forging this protection, enlightened corporate management drove the process of privatization. Despite its advances in enrolling masses of employees and other groups, the voluntarist approach did not attain any semblance of universal coverage. Because no previous historical work has concentrated on health-care access per se, we do not fully appreciate the impact of the spread of private insurance on the ideal of universality and its realization.[1]

## On Defense

As historian James Patterson has observed, a triumphant America entered the postwar era with many grand expectations. Liberals and radicals had ambitious visions of postwar health reform. Supporters of the Truman administration's Fair Deal assumed that national health insurance would be an essential part of this agenda. That didn't mean that anyone assumed that enactment of health-insurance legislation would be anything less than a steep challenge. The harsh treatment meted out to the Wagner-Murray-Dingell Bill in the spring of 1946 constituted further evidence of the intense opposition to government intervention in this area. With strong medical, business, and other conservative resistance unavoidable, no one expected a postwar truce in health politics.[2]

Against this backdrop, the November 1946 congressional elections represented a crucial turning point in the quest for universal health care under federal auspices. The Republican Party won control of both houses of Congress for the first time since 1930. Conservatives of both major parties had the power to block expensive and expansive reform proposals. As historian Alonzo Hamby put it, liberals were "frustrated, beaten, and demoralized." To make matters worse, a spectacular national strike wave in 1945-46 and growing public resentment against the perceived abuses of union power had made the close identification of health reform with organized labor an additional burden. If the window of opportunity had been open even a crack prior to the elections, afterward it had definitely closed. The Wagner-Murray-Dingell Bill had no chance after 1946.[3]

Health activists looked for a viable fallback position. The changing posture of the Public Health Service illustrated the scramble to adapt. On November 6, the day after the electoral rout, Surgeon General Thomas Parran, with the concurrence of Children's Bureau Chief Katharine Lenroot, sent to the Federal Security Administrator a radical proposal fashioned prior to the election. Parran and Lenroot advised that "all persons living within the United States be automatically covered" under the administration's health-insurance proposal to the next session of Congress. Seventeen days later, Parran's assistant Milton Roemer continued to press for a bill "providing comprehensive medical care to the entire population." At the same time, however, Roemer accommodated to the new political reality by recommending two more modest universal programs—either insurance for hospitalization (incorporating the Blue Cross plans) or insurance for the services of physicians delivered outside the hospital. He worried that limiting protection to certain segments of the population would almost certainly entail use of a means test for eligibility and thus create a more stratified health-care system. In contrast, his approach "would serve to build an administrative structure of health services serving all people alike— a structure that could readily be widened to include more and more classes of service until comprehensive care were available for all people." Plainly, the Public Health Service valued universality over comprehensiveness. In hindsight, this sort of compromise to obtain limited benefits for the entire population might have been the last good chance to come to terms with the conservative side.[4]

This proposal for a tactical retreat faced stiff opposition within the reform community, as did similar ones in the years to follow. The main source of obdurate inflexibility throughout the late 1940s was the Social Security Administration (SSA), as the Social Security Bureau was renamed in July 1946. Although they did not have a more optimistic assessment of their immediate legislative prospects, Social Security officials, influenced mainly by I. S. Falk, stuck with a version of national health insurance that covered a comprehensive range of health services for the working population. The Committee for the Nation's Health (CNH) also held fast. Rather than emphasize universal protection, the committee's main adjustment to the political situation was to underscore its commitment to comprehensive benefits, in an attempt to set up a comparison unfavorable to the circumscribed benefit offerings of private insurance.[5]

If the SSA-CNH faction was so concerned with distinguishing social insurance from private insurance, why did they reject the Parran plan for absolute universalism? National health insurance for all Americans as a right of citizenship would have presented a stark alternative to the voluntarist plans. Neither the SSA proposal for 80 percent coverage nor the surgeon general's proposal for full coverage had any possibility of enactment anyway. The Falk-Cohen-Davis group stuck with their less-than-universal formulation and made an issue of comprehensiveness for three reasons beyond their desire to make private benefits look bad. First, they remained devoted to its payroll financing mechanism because it gave contributors and their "dependents" a more defensible rights claim. Second, they valued preventive medicine and believed that only a comprehensive package of benefits would take in such services as periodic examinations and prenatal care.[6]

The third factor in the growing disregard for universalism among the Falk-Cohen-Davis contingent involved its attempts to wrestle with a fundamental dilemma in policy design. With the privatization onslaught well under way, policy intellectuals were hard pressed to explain the proper relationship between private and public protections. Under the prototypical division for retiree income maintenance, the federal Old Age and Survivors Insurance provided basic protection, and private pensions offered supplementary protection. But health protection as it was developing in the 1940s did not conform to the pattern of basic public benefits and supplementary private benefits. As Jacob Hacker has trenchantly observed, with Blue Cross, Blue Shield, and commercial carriers focused on underwriting the risks of hospitalization and surgery, unquestionably the most essential forms of health care at that time, the preferred relationship did not hold. The activist bureaucrats recognized this contradiction and tried to finesse it by calling for public insurance of all services, not just those deemed basic. In a meeting with union officials on December 11, 1946, I. S. Falk conceded the inapplicability of the principle that governed benefits for disability, unemployment, and retirement: "In the case of medical care benefits, the recommendations that we and many others have made are that social security benefits should be quite comprehensive[,] providing all essential services. If such a program were enacted, there would be only a limited need for supplementary provisions." Willing to acknowledge this exception but not its implications, Falk could offer labor negotiators only the vague advice to "take whatever steps are needed to insure . . . that, as far as possible, opportunity is left for these [privately bargained] programs to become supplementary when and if we get the basic protections that are needed under public programs." (Because the primary challenge at that time came from the Blues, which featured service benefits rather than indemnity benefits, Social Security leaders could not escape this predicament by proposing that national health insurance indemnify only a fraction of the cost of designated basic services and that private insurance top off the incomplete public protection.) With the private insurers preempting the ground for basic health security, policy architects maneuvered to outflank the voluntarists by advocating insurance for a comprehensive range of services. In the process, a preoccupation with comprehensiveness diverted attention from the potentially distinctive principle of universality.[7]

Republican leaders in the Eightieth Congress wasted no time in transforming the policy agenda. Senator Robert Taft, who only a year earlier had denounced committee hearings on health reform, was now the new chair for the next round of hearings. Taft's opening statement made a point of equating universalism with socialism. Naturally, the Ohio senator saw to it that the main object of consideration was his own bill, which made no pretense of attaining universal access to medical care. His measure sought to allow limited federal grants to the states either to purchase insurance or deliver care to indigent persons. The unions in particular reacted with outrage to the degradation inherent in welfare medicine. Nelson Cruikshank of the AFL asked rhetorically "whether we shall go backward to the outworn concept of poor laws and provide such care on a charity basis, with the accompanying evils of the means test." Philip Murray, president of the United Steelworkers of America, decried "a charity scheme under which workers would be forced to take an obnoxious means test and pauper's oath."[8]

The senate hearings of 1947–48 also witnessed the culmination of an ugly campaign of vilification against federal officials associated with health reform. The main, but by no means only, object of vilification was Isidore Falk. Throughout the late 1940s, Marjorie Shearon, who had been a subordinate of Falk's at the Social Security Board, mounted a scathing attack on her former boss. In Shearon's imagination, Falk loomed as an evil and powerful genius who was directing a plot to foist an alien system of socialized medicine on a pliable political leadership. Her six days of testimony sought to expose the conspiratorial workings of the "House of Falk," an intricate network of "Collaborationists, Fellow-travelers, Appeasers, Satellites, and Gullible Accepters." The nefarious bureaucrat supposedly used this apparatus to execute socialist plans flowing from International Labor Organization (ILO) headquarters in Geneva. Despite the patent absurdity of many of her allegations, Shearon sat with Taft and fellow inquisitor Forrest Donnell during several months of committee deliberations and helped guide their questioning of witnesses. I. S. Falk, Wilbur Cohen, and other Social Security administrators underwent a grueling marathon of interrogation during the summer of 1947 and the winter of 1948. Shearon's analysis of Falk as the puppet of the ILO failed to explain why he continued to advocate a health plan that was less than all-inclusive well after the labor group had come out in favor of straightforward universalism. In the darkening mood created by the onset of the Cold War, even loosely argued conspiratorial assertions received sustained congressional attention. Rather than advancing efforts to bring health protection to unprotected Americans, loyal public servants were forced to spend their time rebutting unfounded allegations of subversion while enduring a barrage of abusive personal charges and thinly veiled anti-Semitic slurs.[9]

The counteroffensive went far beyond notions of an international conspiracy masterminded by a mid-level bureaucrat. The possibility that social insurance would extend to a large share of the African-American population stoked white supremacist fears of racial equality. The growing likelihood that federal health-insurance legislation would prohibit discrimination in the delivery of care intensified these anxieties even further. (It was one thing to improve minority access to basement wards and other, inferior segregated facilities; it was quite another to underwrite equal access to equal treatment.) In this context, insistence upon decentralized control of health-care financing stood as a bulwark against the threat of nationwide uniform benefits, especially for southern conservatives. By the 1940s, opponents of federal social provision well understood that local and state discretion in setting and interpreting standards of protection allowed white elites to continue to deny assistance to African Americans and other nonwhites. Southerners who bolted the Democratic Party in 1948 to form the States' Rights Party attacked recent proposals to desegregate health care. Dixiecrat home-rule rhetoric carried a coded message whose meaning was unmistakable to its target audience. The Louisiana State Medical Society condemned Wagner-Murray-Dingell in part because it would purportedly abolish states' rights. The Louisiana society believed that enactment of this measure would give the central government an army of 300,000 new bureaucrats in charge of its implementaion. In 1946, Walter Martin, a former president of the Medical Society of Virginia, urged community control over eligibility determination and other administrative matters related to public aid for the medically indigent. "It is the conviction of the medical profession," Martin generalized, "that local situations can be best understood and met on the state and local level." In 1950, Virginia medical leader W. C. Caudill warned that socialized medicine would impose rigid domination by federal "czars in every city, town, and village in the country." One function of these statements on impending centralization was to elide the realities of racism in the Jim Crow health-care system.[10]

Adversaries of universal or nearly universal public insurance confronted rights claims. Blue Cross executive Paul Hawley capitalized on the dedication of Wisconsin labor economists to contributory financing of social insurance in order to attack the Democratic proposal for national health insurance. At a symposium in Madison in 1949 honoring the late John Andrews, Hawley warned that the liberals' plan subtly redefined charity. "Whether or not people contribute anything at all, they will get benefits as a right," he noted. "Now, how can any benefit be other than charity once a person pays none or only a part of its cost?" Hawley put a sharp point on this observation: "If . . . this is merely an effort to redistribute wealth . . . , let's be honest about it." Hospital official John Hayes took on the notion that Americans' right to universal public education warranted a similar entitlement to health care. Hayes considered health care unsuited for government intervention because it was more complicated than education. Of course, the fundamental flaw in this argument was its failure to acknowledge that most reformers did not seek government-delivered services, but rather only a public-insurance program.[11]

Despite its bleak prospects, the Wagner-Murray-Dingell Bill still received strong liberal support. On May 22, 1947, the NAACP's Leslie Perry stated that the association intended to testify on behalf of Wagner's bill even though it did not have "a ghost of a chance" at that time. African-American physician George Cannon brought up Roosevelt's call for a second Bill of Rights in encouraging his colleagues to back a plan that he estimated would benefit 98 percent of the nation's black citizens. Oscar Ewing, head of the Federal Security Agency, assured the AFL that the Truman administration intended to make good on President Roosevelt's promise of a right to health care in order to assure all citizens equality of opportunity. Ewing surrendered not an inch of the high ground: "They screamed about the 'Welfare State.' Now they have another word—'statism.' . . . They talk about liberty. The rich man's son is free to enjoy good health, they say, and the poor man's son is free to be sick." Ideological attacks from the right struck some advocates of health security as simply beside the point. As CNH director Joseph Louchheim put it, "National Health Insurance is as American as apple pie, even though Communists may like apple pie." Louchheim's apology for leftist support suggests the extent to which conservatives had forced his side into a defensive posture.[12]

A few reformers still dared to relate the domestic drive for public insurance to foreign or international standards, the atmosphere of xenophobia and the aversion to ideas associated with multinational organizations prevailing at this time notwithstanding. An editorial in the April 1949 issue of the *American Journal of Public Health* wondered how America could fail to act to increase access to care. This editorial, almost certainly authored by C.-E. A. Winslow, deemed further delay untenable "in a democratic society, to which we have been preaching that—in the words of the WHO [World Health Organization]

Constitution—'the enjoyment of the highest attainable standard of health is one of the fundamental rights of every human being.'" On the other hand, progressives made little, if any, immediate use of the landmark Universal Declaration of Human Rights, promulgated by the United Nations on December 10, 1948. "Everyone," stated Article 25 of the declaration, "has the right to a standard of living adequate for the health and well-being of himself and of his family, including food, clothing, housing and medical care and necessary social services, and the right to security in the event of . . . sickness." That Eleanor Roosevelt headed the working group that created the declaration gave the document more visibility and stature. That her late husband's Four Freedoms obviously provided social-rights benchmarks for the group involved in drafting the proclamation only gave it further authority. The impact of the manifesto may have been diluted because reformers dedicated to statist solutions were uncomfortable with Eleanor Roosevelt's position that these social rights could be achieved by private as well as public action. Perhaps they also sensed that Americans were disinclined to take guidance from foreigners at this moment of postwar triumphalism.[13]

Supporters of state intervention continued to illuminate the vast need for health care and the profound consequences of not meeting that need. Privatizers paid little attention to those aspects of the current situation, except to report that life expectancy had risen since the turn of the century. Faye Stephenson, of the women's auxiliary of the CIO, advised Senator Taft's committee that the nation faced problems more immediate than the machinations of I. S. Falk. Stephenson told the investigators that for working-class women lack of care meant "the bitter experience of seeing our children and our husbands develop physical defects and lifelong handicaps." Oscar Ewing in 1948 defended national health insurance with a provocative estimate of the toll exacted in its absence. "After all," Ewing declared, "we are dealing with human lives and human suffering and anguish. Every year, over 300,000 people die whom we have the knowledge and skills to save." Unfortunately, this senior official of the Truman administration gave little explanation for this startling assertion that the nation could prevent over one-fifth of its mortality. It was also unfortunate that he made almost no effort to corroborate his prediction that private insurance "probably will never be able to cover more than half the total population." However, he left no doubt as to his universalistic aim "that all people shall have access to such health and medical services as they require through a system of insurance covering the entire population." Ewing proposed to reach this goal by phasing in federal protection over an unspecified span of time.[14]

As the prospects for progressive change grew dimmer, there was a final attempt to fashion a plan that made a major advance toward universalism. In January 1949, Harry Becker of the United Auto Workers pleaded with the Federal Security Agency to cut back the bulky Wagner-Murray-Dingell Bill. Becker proposed postponing comprehensive benefits, arguing for national hospitalization insurance for the approximately 80 percent of the population that the administration already intended to insure. Under this approach, other benefits would follow over time. Becker advised federal policymakers that the unions were moving ahead with negotiated insurance protection, and that further progress along this line would undermine any future campaign to protect all members of society. Four months later, C.-E. A. Winslow informed I. S. Falk that the American Public Health Association could not support the elaborate array of benefits in the Wagner-Murray-Dingell Bill. "I do not see how we can possibly jump from nothing to everything," Winslow advised his protégé. "I realize the difficulties of any partial approach, yet I do think some sort of gradualism is essential." In January 1950, he delineated three alternative ways to proceed—limiting protection below a specified income level, conducting experimental programs in a few geographical areas, and limiting the scope of services covered. For the last of these options, he suggested a program that insured only hospital expenses. But Winslow, Becker, and their fellow incrementalists could not move Falk and his colleagues. Opponents of hospital insurance expressed well-grounded apprehension that such an arrangement would lead to inappropriate hospitalization. The Committee for the Nation's Health also refused to retreat to a hospitalization-first position, preferring to wait for the opportunity that it presumed would appear during the next economic depression. The 1949 version of the Wagner-Murray-Dingell Bill retained coverage of a wide range of preventive and curative services.[15]

Leaving nothing to chance, the AMA and its allies in the business community mounted a massive campaign of negative publicity and grassroots pressure against social insurance in 1949 and 1950. The public relations firm of Whitaker and Baxter placed advertisements in more than 10,000 newspapers and distributed more than 50 million pieces of literature. This onslaught devastated what remained of the Fair Deal initiative for national health insurance. The campaign involved more than fierce attacks on "socialized medicine."

Critics of Wagner-Murray-Dingell took the opportunity to intensify efforts to reframe the issue in the public consciousness. Beyond their derogatory themes, a combination of mass-media advertisements, promotional literature, and speeches contended that American medical care was a success, that Americans were healthy people, that America faced no crisis requiring drastic government intervention. The campaign heralded the growth of voluntary insurance. The focus shifted away from the continuing inaccessibility of basic care for tens of millions of the nation's citizens.[16]

## Resurgent Welfare Capitalism

The conservative victories in the 1946 congressional elections changed more than the balance of political power in Washington. They also accelerated a process of privatization of health security that was already under way, but had previously been at a fragile, embryonic stage. On the surface, it appeared that the unions were driving this process. However, in many important, precedent-setting situations, organized labor was only reactively dealing with worker dissatisfaction over preexisting benefit programs initiated by employers. As Sanford Jacoby and other scholars have shown, welfare capitalism in America did not vanish in the turmoil of the 1930s. In some cases, innovative health programs grew out of preexisting practices of corporate paternalism, some of which had begun at the turn of the century. In other cases, nonpaternalistic managers introduced fringe benefits to preempt union demands.[17]

Especially for the industrial unions of the CIO, the 1946 electoral setbacks marked a turning point. Unions knew that they now faced a hostile political environment. Their worst fears were realized within a year with the passage, over President Truman's veto, of the punitive Taft-Hartley Act. The besieged labor movement retrenched on the difficult health-care issue. Ten days after the elections, Walter Reuther told his comrades in the United Auto Workers that "in the immediate future, security will be won for our people only to the extent that the union succeeds in obtaining such security through collective bargaining." (The American Medical Association gleefully reported this announcement in its journal.) To be sure, World War II had already created opportunities to win protection at the bargaining table. The combination of war-induced labor shortages, federal restrictions on wage increases, and favorable tax treatment of employer contributions toward insurance led both labor and management to explore health benefits. Nonetheless, as long as Wagner-

Murray-Dingell remained a viable proposition, relatively little action occurred at the bargaining table. At the end of the war, collective bargaining agreements granted health benefits to well under a million U.S. workers.[18]

The CIO moved swiftly to align policy with emerging practice. At its convention in November 1946, the labor group made only a perfunctory endorsement of the Wagner-Murray-Dingell Bill before taking up a proposal to pursue health and welfare security through collective bargaining. David McDonald of the United Steelworkers declared that his organization could not "wait for perhaps another ten years before the Social Security laws are amended adequately." William Pollock of the Textile Workers concurred, observing that the election results made the probability of enacting the Wagner-Murray-Dingell Bill "almost nil." Convention delegates voted to concentrate on negotiating benefits.[19]

Three major mass-production industries—coal, steel, and auto—led the way to private health insurance. In all three cases, the union forced the issue onto the bargaining agenda. In all three cases, it took dramatic and protracted strikes to gain labor's demands. Nonetheless, in all three cases, labor was mainly reacting to management initiatives that workers and their leaders took to be corporate paternalism. Coal miners rebelled against the longstanding practice of mandatory payroll deductions to support physicians selected by coal operators and facilities run by them. Steel workers resented benefits administered through aid plans that they associated with discredited company unions. Auto workers objected to insurance arrangements unilaterally established and peremptorily altered by management. Robert MacDonald concluded that the UAW "cannot be credited with initiating [health benefits] in the majority of companies." General Motors, for instance, added hospital and surgical insurance in 1939 without consulting the UAW, even though the main source of funding for this benefit was payroll deductions. At the end of the wartime competition to find and keep employees, many firms decided either to cut back health benefits or to require that their employees pay a larger share toward their continuation. Therefore, union leaders in the postwar transition found themselves entangled in established employment-based health programs. With this cumbersome baggage in hand, the United Mine Workers, the United Auto Workers, and the United Steelworkers had little choice but to bring the matter into collective bargaining. By 1950, each had wrested important concessions from their managerial adversaries at the Big Three automakers, in the basic steel industry, and throughout the coalfields. Employees in these basic industries thus came to enjoy contractually guaranteed hospital and surgical protection, along with pensions and other new benefits, in what amounted to private welfare regimes.[20]

The deals struck in the closely watched auto and steel industries became a model for moderate privatization in unionized settings. Perhaps as influential in its own way was the frightening precedent set in the bituminous coal industry. There John L. Lewis controlled a fund that set out not to buy insurance but to deliver care through such ventures as building hospitals and sponsoring group-practice clinics. The specter of the proliferation of health-care facilities featuring statues of union presidents in their lobbies gave American executives nightmares. It certainly made demands for health insurance seem relatively innocuous. Accordingly, organizations affiliated with both the CIO and the AFL quickly made health insurance a commonplace provision in their contracts. As in coal, steel, and autos, union leaders in many situations sought to gain a measure of joint control over health programs that welfarist employers had designed and instituted on their own. In electrical manufacturing, for example, workers' representatives negotiated over the terms of insurance plans that several firms, including General Electric, had put in place unilaterally. By 1950, roughly 80 percent of CIO contracts contained a health-insurance clause. Organized labor and their management counterparts also quickly settled into a routine of refinement through further negotiation, with the unions demanding broader coverage and higher employer contributions toward premium payments.[21]

The privatization drive extended far beyond the unionized workplace. Just as the principal aim of the first generation of welfare capitalists had been to preempt the appeal of unions, a host of nonunion employers adopted and expanded health benefits from the mid-1940s through the 1950s with the intent of heading off a still-growing labor movement. The personnel bureaucracies of sophisticated nonunion companies like Eastman Kodak moved swiftly to deny labor any opening. In this endeavor, they followed the far-sighted minority of their brethren who had already installed plans offering either insurance or health care itself. Of course, many employers offered health protection for reasons other than avoiding unwelcome visits from union organizers. A desire to recruit better workers, humanitarian concerns about employee well-being, and (for a wily few) a strategic interest in stemming growth of the welfare state also impelled American capitalists to shoulder this responsibility. By the end of the 1950s, workers in most sectors of the economy expected to receive at least hospital and surgical insurance for themselves and their families as a standard component of their compensation package.[22]

## The Heyday of Voluntarism

The growth of voluntary health insurance in postwar America resulted from more than the demand generated by labor-management relations. Health-care providers and the insurance industry invented and aggressively marketed remedies for health insecurity. From their modest beginnings as an attempt to protect teachers in Dallas during the depths of the Great Depression, the Blue Cross plans sponsored by the American Hospital Association grew extravagantly. Beginning in 1939 with the California Physicians Service, state medical societies offered medical and surgical coverage under the Blue Shield name. Numerous commercial insurance carriers entered the field to compete against the nonprofit Blues. A willingness to tailor indemnity benefits and premiums for individual employers distinguished the commercial carriers from Blue Cross, which charged uniform premiums across the community and defined its benefits in terms of units of service rendered—that is, days of hospitalization—rather than in terms of dollar amounts of indemnity. By the early 1950s, diverse insurance products existed for groups of employees, as well as for other types of sizable groups. To a lesser but not insignificant extent, individual insurance policies were also sold to many middle-class Americans. Energetic marketing brought these alternatives to everyone's attention. Systematic promotional appeals were inextricably bound up with the publicity campaign attacking national health insurance. At the same time, quiet efforts to court business and union leaders also helped to gain wide acceptance of voluntarism.[23]

New forms of insurance promised access to new forms of care. With life expectancy approaching seventy years by midcentury, Americans worried less about infectious disorders like tuberculosis and influenza than about noninfectious degenerative disorders like cancer and cardiovascular conditions. To meet these rising challenges, health care became increasingly research-based and capital-intensive. The emergence of an enormous biomedical research and training apparatus, driven largely by federal funding through the National Institutes of Health, accelerated medical specialization after World War II. Similarly, federal money made possible the construction and renovation of countless hospitals and clinics under the Hill-Burton Act. Community hospitals added intensive-care units and other technologically advanced facilities and equipment. University-affiliated hospitals and other tertiary-care institutions grew dramatically in scale and sophistication. Glowing reports of medical triumphs amplified the appeal of innovative interventions.[24]

The combination of an expanding supply of health services and a new profusion of insurance options yielded spectacular results. Whereas only about one American in eleven had hospital insurance in 1940, ten years later one in two had it, fully 75 million people. A 1951 Senate study heralded the pattern of growth as nothing less than "one of the most significant social developments of recent years." By 1970, fully three-quarters of the citizenry had health insurance. The Blues led the initial upsurge: Blue Cross enrollment soared from about 4 million at the beginning of the 1940s to about 36 million by the end of the decade. Only a few years later, however, population coverage by commercial carriers surpassed that of Blue Cross and Blue Shield. Rates of health-care utilization immediately rose significantly among the insured.[25]

By midcentury, analysts across the political spectrum agreed that the emerging trend was breathtaking indeed. It was also a matter of consensus that the advance of voluntary insurance and the immediate prospects for further advances had, for the foreseeable future, put to rest any possibility for universal federal insurance. All parties recognized that the large-scale accommodation of the working class through employment benefits had transformed the policy landscape. But beyond these areas of agreement, debate continued throughout the quarter century after World War II over the ultimate potential of private measures to achieve any semblance of universal health care.[26]

The postwar era was a heady time for proponents of voluntarism. At the outset, they radiated confidence about a rosy future, tempered only by fears that the statist juggernaut in Washington would deny them a fair chance to prove the value of their approach. Accordingly, champions of private insurance emphasized the theme of universal protection just beyond the horizon. In the case of the Blue Cross, this grand promise had redemptive significance. Some individuals associated with the Blues had been contending since the 1930s that expansion of their system would kill popular demand for national health insurance. By 1945, thirty-five states had passed legislation that granted the hospital-sponsored plans tax-exempt status and other privileges. Political scientist Deborah Stone has pointed out that "the main justification for this special treatment was their promise to provide health insurance for all people without regard to ability to pay." Blue Cross officials, more than their counterparts in the strictly commercial wing of the insurance industry, had to present their aims in universalist or quasi-universalist terms. Accordingly, they took the lead in imploring political leaders and the society as a whole to give them time to nurture the voluntarist experiment. John Hayes of the American Hospital Association assured the U.S. Chamber of Commerce that his organization wanted "the best hospital and medical service . . . available to all" and that Blue Cross, with its stellar record of growth, was the right tool for the job. "We believe," Hayes stated, "that our government should be actively supporting this program instead of criticizing it because it has not yet covered the entire population." Philadelphia Blue Cross leader E. A. Van Steenwyk was even more strident. In 1951, Van Steenwyk taunted the naysayers and predicted a bright future: "The critics have never been right about Blue Cross and are now being proved wrong about Blue Shield. What is the plans' potential? We say it is unlimited."[27]

The hospitals' partners in organized medicine, who tended to dwell on the dire threat of federal interference, also struck a positive universalistic pose. In 1946, the *Pennsylvania Medical Journal* maintained that "neither the most liberal sociologist nor the most conservative physician would deny medical care to any human being who needs it and seeks it." The journal's editors intended to "meet the evils of compulsory insurance constructively through a comprehensive voluntary medical program." As early as 1944, a champion of insurance sponsored by medical societies proclaimed that it could "be made universally applicable in urban and rural areas, over short or wide distances, in large and small communities, in larger or smaller business units, in upper or lower income groups, the indigent and special governmental groups." In 1949, the *New England Journal of Medicine* noted the swelling membership of Blue Shield and insisted that "voluntary health insurance needs only time to earn the nation's full confidence." As might be expected in an editorial entitled "Still the American Way," the journal patriotically concluded that "until a real majority of the American people may decide otherwise this form of independence and self-reliance must still be considered as a vital part of the American heritage." At the 1947 annual meeting of the Massachusetts Medical Society, Leland McKittrick reminded his colleagues that the society's basic aims included universal access and that attaining this aim would be difficult. Undaunted, McKittrick drew encouragement from the expansion of both Blue Cross and Blue Shield, which he saw as steps in an evolutionary process. In another speech two years later, however, the Boston surgeon qualified his cheery assessment by making clear that he harbored no hopes that voluntary insurance alone would ever cover all Americans. In his view, shared by many others, government assistance would always be necessary to take care of the very poor. (Indeed, Congress in the late 1940s looked into two proposals—the Hill-Aiken Bill and the Flanders-Ives Bill—that featured federal aid to help poor people purchase private insurance. As formulated, however, neither proposal would have produced any approximation of universal health security.)[28]

Commercial insurers and others in and around the business community eagerly joined the campaign to sell their optimistic presentation of their capacities. Earle Muntz of the American Enterprise Association reported that voluntary programs were "springing up at a rate which only a few years ago would have been regarded as virtually impossible." In 1948, A. L. Kirkpatrick, the insurance expert at the U.S. Chamber of Commerce, suggested that "the problem . . . is rapidly being solved through the voluntary action of individuals and employers." When Herbert Northrup, an economist at the National Industrial Conference Board, pointed out the absence of genuine universality from the unfolding pattern of privatization, his candor was extraordinary for this honeymoon period. More typically, the 1952 annual report of the Health Insurance Council celebrated "another striking contribution to the unbroken record of progress," one that reflected "the inherent vitality of the voluntary health movement in this country." Even more impressive than the continued strong gains in hospital and surgical coverage that year was the dramatic 29 percent increase in the number insured for medical expenses, an upsurge mainly attributable to Blue Shield. In 1957, E. J. Faulkner, president of the Health Insurance Association of America (HIAA), calculated that during the previous sixteen years the number of Americans with hospital insurance had grown by 600 percent, with surgical insurance by 1,300 percent, and with medical insurance by 1,700 percent. Faulkner characterized these gains as "some of the most phenomenal social and economic changes in the entire history of our country."[29]

The temptation to extrapolate proved irresistible. The intoxicating rate of expansion in voluntary insurance generated glowing projections. Harry Becker presented this scenario to New England hospital administrators in 1953: "If we make as much progress in the next ten years as in the last ten, with the added advantages of past experience plus today's momentum, we can expect the entire employed population and their dependents—rural workers and self-employed included—to have prepaid hospital protection at benefit levels at least as inclusive as the best now available. The basis for this expectation is the projection of coverage and benefit trends of the past five years." Becker buttressed this assessment by comparing the rate of progress toward universal insurance with the speed at which America had universalized telephone service and running water. A workshop in which Becker participated a month later took an even more positive view, estimating that if voluntary insurance continued to expand at the rate of the previous three years, the whole working population would be safeguarded in less than five years. In early 1954, the Eisenhower administration introduced a very modest plan to promote voluntary insurance by offering federal reinsurance of certain undesirable risks, a proposition with no universalist purpose. Nonetheless, E. Dwight Barnett, professor of hospital administration at Columbia University, welcomed the White House initiative as a positive step in producing a "health system for the people of this country that is really effective for all." Barnett predicted that by 1960 only the disabled and the unemployed would lack private health protection. With the projected advance of voluntarism, "no further question of compulsory governmental health insurance" would remain, in his view. However, the failure of the reinsurance plan to generate much political support, even in conservative quarters, did little to dampen enthusiasm for voluntarism.[30]

In addition to some uncritical projections, postwar exchanges did reshape the debate over paying for health care in important ways. As Rosemary Stevens has demonstrated, an ethos of voluntarism anchored in nonprofit community hospitals and Community Chest charitable ventures had a strong influence in midcentury American health affairs. The benevolent image of these caregiving institutions of civil society gave credibility to Blue Cross directly and to Blue Shield indirectly. A sense that voluntarism was "Still the American Way," as the *New England Journal of Medicine* put it, came naturally to the middle and upper classes. (Many unions also saw the Blues as the lesser of two evils, better than the commercial carriers, and envisaged a major role for themselves in the governance of the community-based Blue Cross plans.) Fuller incorporation of voluntarism into the national identity complemented the hard-edged anticommunist and xenophobic rhetoric attacking the welfare state. The voluntarist campaign also invited popular participation: rhetoric led directly to mobilization. Americans were encouraged to press their employers, fellow employees, and neighbors to establish or enroll in insurance plans. Public relations executive Anson Lowitz in 1949 urged hospital officials to form committees of clubwomen, businessmen, and other community leaders to mount "an intensive, community-wide, house-to-house canvass for Blue Cross membership." Canvassing projects in fact arose in many localities. Voluntarism posed a full-blown alternative to the conception of social citizenship invented in the New Deal and refined in the Fair Deal.[31]

The privatization drive burnished the image of business. Scores of millions of Americans suddenly possessed a sense of security that they generally traced to employers. Under the popular model of corporate providence pioneered by Lemuel Boulware at General Electric, management controlled insurance plans and gained the lion's share of the credit for them. As David Brody has noted, Boulwarism was "designed to show that benefits derived from the company, not the union." An early analysis of employee benefits explained the happy outcomes of corporate welfare: "The benefits available under a group insurance plan give employees a sense of security and freedom from worry, which in turn contributes toward their work and the company. Contented and satisfied workers are usually loyal employees. More cordial relations with employees, better morale, employee good will and satisfaction were listed by cooperating companies as the outstanding advantages of their group insurance plans." The Cold War demanded a moral capitalism. To a great extent, management delivered it.[32]

The conservative intellectual vanguard attempted to reconceptualize the process of obtaining health services. An extended period of prosperity and the formation of a huge middle class set the stage for further commodification of health services. In an affluent society seemingly consumed by consumerism, with the ready availability of insurance products of many varieties, some analysts began to portray gaining access to health services as little more than another routine discretionary purchasing decision by individual shoppers in the marketplace. AMA economist Frank Dickinson in 1949 returned to a theme that conservatives had been exploring since the days of the Committee on the Costs of Medical Care—the unwillingness of many Americans to allocate enough of their income to health services. "We live in a free society where consumers are the dictators," Dickinson stated. "It's not so much a question of what they can afford to spend as . . . what they choose to spend for medical care." Five years later, fellow economist Emerson Schmidt marshaled aggregate spending data to support this line of reasoning. Schmidt noted that national expenditures for health care barely exceeded those for alcohol and tobacco and that consumers eagerly went into debt to purchase cars and television sets, but not to secure surgical procedures or insurance policies. "Failure to meet health needs," Schmidt concluded, "may not be due so much to a lack of 'ability' as to the low priority which many, perhaps most, individuals put on expenditures for health." Like Dickinson, Schmidt saw the consumer as sovereign and, accordingly, opposed potential infringement on this sovereignty. He attacked compulsory health insurance, which necessarily abridged individual decision-making, as antithetical to "the very foundations of our civilization and culture."[33]

The American Medical Association challenged the very concept of need itself. The association bristled at President Truman's creation of the Commission on the Health Needs of the Nation in December 1951 and set out to trivialize its work. The *Journal of the American Medical Association* complained that unmet needs could include "unmet desires, whims, or mere wants." The journal's editor preferred to discard the fuzzy notion of need and substitute for it demand. Within the confines of the market paradigm, human deprivation disappeared and caprice loomed large: "Since persons literally need everything, one cannot say that the unmet needs for a particular service are great, because one does not know 'how great is great' until he knows the unmet needs for many important goods and services." Rather than confront the possibility that some Americans went without valuable health services and suffered as a result, the medical association dismissed unmet needs as an inevitable aspect of life in a free-enterprise society. AMA official George Cooley placed this interpretation directly before the presidential commission in a presentation later that year. "Need, it seems to me, is a very poor term to use," Cooley advised. "All of us have unsatisfied needs and probably for a myriad of services and things. Usually when need is discussed at some detached faraway level, it becomes a subjective version of the rainbow's pot of gold." Beyond their immediate obfuscatory function, such recitations of empty truisms signaled to policymakers just how determined organized medicine was to recast the fundamental issues at stake in the national discussion of access to care.[34]

Medical antagonism to the President's Commission on the Health Needs of the Nation on another sensitive matter further demonstrated the ideological militancy of the period. Although it cautiously endorsed voluntarism as the proper approach for reaching the goal of universal access, the commission placed universality on a foundation that raised objections in some quarters. In enunciating its guiding principles in its report to the White House, the commission declared that "access to the means for the attainment and preservation of health is a basic human right." The *New England Journal of Medicine* heaped scorn on this "pious aspiration" and turned to relativism to discount it: "human rights are only what human beings have declared them to be and may vary, and have varied, from time to time and from place to place and according to the practicability of their attainment." The *Journal of the Louisiana State Medical Society* prefaced its reporting of this human-rights contention with the derisive comment that it appeared within a "carefully built up presentation of the theory of the welfare state." Given the commission's rejection of national health insurance, this interpretation was quite curious.[35]

Less reductive and more important assertions of a consumerist perspective rose to prominence. As third-party payment for health care became widespread, costs began to accelerate steadily. Price inflation and higher rates of utilization set off a spiral of increases in insurance premiums. These increases, in turn, caused conflict over their distribution, especially in the collective-bargaining arena. The evolving situation also had an impact in the realm of public policy. Both the major investigative bodies of the postwar decade—the President's Commission on the Health Needs of the Nation and the Commission on Financing of Hospital Care—used their agenda-shaping authority to elevate cost concerns to greater visibility. Thus, the self-interested priorities of the insured majority had already begun to crowd out the still-unresolved plight of the truly insecure well before this issue took center stage in the policy arena in the 1970s.[36]

Voluntarism also boosted consumerism indirectly. This indirect line of influence was especially important at a time when health care still fit poorly within the market model: almost all the services were undesirable to the typical consumer, purchased under duress of illness or injury after virtually no comparison shopping or data-gathering; major providers did almost no advertising; providers made most of the key decisions about obtaining services. Nonetheless, the explosive growth of private health protection liberated most members of American society from fears that had previously tempered their willingness to make risky purchases on credit. Harry Becker believed that there were "few social programs of greater importance than prepaid health care protection in giving needed confidence to buy goods and services." This newfound and widespread sense of security helped to keep the postwar economy rolling. The private welfare state served the common good, further obviating the need to attend to the plight of the excluded.[37]

## Scattered Skeptics

A small band of dissenters sat out the gala celebration. A few stalwarts, mainly in and around the labor movement, remained unreconstructed advocates of social insurance. In fact, the initial phase of headlong privatization in the late 1940s led to various attempts to have it both ways. Social Security official William Mitchell blithely contended that "perhaps the greatest value of voluntary health insurance has been the experience gained in learning how to operate compulsory health insurance." Some union leaders held that once bargaining forced employers to shoulder the costs of insurance, rather than deducting them from employees' wages, the opposition of the business community to national health insurance would soften. Unions signed contracts that canceled or curtailed benefits upon the enactment of insurance legislation. Labor leaders reasoned that familiarity with private insurance and its manifest deficiencies would stimulate rank-and-file demand for federal action. In 1947, Nelson Cruikshank reassured his comrades that voluntary plans were "temporary stopgaps pending the enactment of a comprehensive national program." Two years later, Cruikshank wishfully stated that the experiment in privatization had continued long enough to conclude that it had failed. Franz Goldmann portrayed labor's attitude as one of bare tolerance for the "makeshift solutions" that would occupy the interim prior to the enactment of satisfactory reform.[38]

Organized labor and a handful of allies never formally abandoned their defense of national health insurance throughout the fifties. Although they also judged private programs by the comprehensiveness of their benefits and other standards, the steadfast defenders of federal provision continued to uphold universality as the primary criterion for health policy. In 1952 Cruikshank told the President's Commission that "organized labor is united in demanding a system of national health insurance for the benefit of everyone." Of the sixteen members of this blue-ribbon commission, only three—Elizabeth Magee of the National Consumers League, Albert Hayes of the International Association of Machinists, and Walter Reuther—recommended such a course of action to the president. In contrast, the majority of the commissioners suggested only that "present prepayment plans be expanded to provide as much health service to as many people as they can." Similarly, of the thirty-four members of the Commission on Financing of Hospital Care, only the two labor representatives held out for federal insurance. CIO research director Stanley Ruttenberg couched his dissent from the bland recommendations of the overwhelming majority in terms of a "matter of right," a style of rhetoric seldom heard after 1950. With so many interested parties willing to watch the voluntarist experiment run its course, there was hardly any inclination at this juncture to resurrect any crusade for all-inclusive provision. The Committee for the Nation's Health, a bastion of universalism, did not survive Michael Davis's retirement in 1956. By that time, advocacy of universal public protection had diminished to a whisper. Leftist groups like the Physicians Forum had to divert their energies to defending themselves against raging McCarthyism. Prominent radical Henry Sigerist fled the witchhunt for exile in Switzerland. Absorbed in the complexities of contractual benefits, many unions paid only lip service to the cause.[39]

A few diehards criticized the new private health regime. Applying the standard of universal protection became a straightforward exercise as fairly reliable statistics accumulated on the extent of private coverage. In 1958, Wilbur Cohen, who had relocated to the University of Michigan with the advent of the Eisenhower administration, reminded union benefits experts: "Our objective is the coverage of all of the population with a broad scope of services." Cohen assessed the recent announcement that 72 percent of the population had obtained insurance: "This is a significant measure of progress. However, there is still twenty-eight percent of the population not yet covered under any form of health insurance." For Michael Davis, the deficiencies that rendered privatism "gravely insufficient" began with "the millions of persons yet unreached." The critics' skills extended beyond a mastery of subtraction. Supporters of federal intervention used fresh evidence indicating that existing insurance indemnified a small fraction of total health costs to attack the lack of breadth and depth of private benefits. The Eisenhower team sent I. S. Falk packing, as they had Cohen. In his new capacity as a consultant to the United Steelworkers, he estimated that employee benefits typically insured less than one-third of health expenses. At least one skeptic carried the critique one big step further. As early as 1954, Franz Goldmann blasted the private system for failing to demonstrate any evidence of improving health status among the insured.[40]

## Glimpses of the Uninsured

Despite the advance of privatization and the complacent tendency to ignore the excluded, health insecurity did not disappear. As time passed, the buoyant mood of expectancy began to fade. Extensive experience gradually exposed the limits of the private welfare state as well as its circumscribed potential for further growth. Both defenders and opponents of voluntarism studied the uninsured, a group that could not be dismissed by reference to bad consumer judgment or defective personal character. The task of elucidating the plight of the unprotected became more difficult in the placid postwar interval because, unlike during the turbulent depression years, the needy themselves were once again generally silent.[41]

The uninsured occasionally received scrutiny in high places even during the halcyon days of voluntarism. The Senate brought in a group of consultants led by Dean Clark, an administrator at Massachusetts General Hospital, to study the state of privatization at the beginning of the 1950s. Clark's nonpartisan team pointed to a lack of group affiliation, particularly participation in an employment relationship, as the common denominator among the approximately 75 million Americans without insurance. Beyond noting this general characteristic, the report helpfully named the types of people less likely to have insurance. These included the elderly, low-wage workers and other poor people, the disabled, the unemployed, the self-employed, employees in small organizations, African Americans, and residents of rural areas. Subsequent investigations filled in important information about each of these overlapping subgroups.[42]

The self-employed and employees in small establishments constituted a sizable share of the uninsured. In 1958, approximately 60 percent of uninsured workers in the state of New York worked for firms employing fewer than twenty people. Most of these vulnerable workers were concentrated in retail trade, transportation, and services. Less than half of the domestic servants in the state had health benefits. Twenty-nine percent of New York's self-employed had not obtained hospital insurance. Given the wide prevalence of family farms in rural areas, it was common to treat the problem of the rural uninsured as a facet of the larger problem of the self-employed. In the mid-1950s, most rural families lacked health insurance. Insurers understandably tended to shy away from smaller groups and isolated individuals as risky and time-consuming accounts. Nonetheless, many in these categories were considered promising prospects for inclusion into the private system by means of individual and family insurance policies. Self-employed farmers and their families could pursue this option as well. A further source of optimism with regard to independent operators and workers in small business was the increasing willingness of insurers to write policies for small groups. In 1954, one insurance executive predicted the imminent development of a movement to extend coverage to employee groups with as few as ten members. Three years later, HIAA research director J. F. Follmann Jr. announced that several insurers were selling policies to businesses with no more than four employees. He also reported fresh successes in reaching into rural areas but conceded that "the number of the rural population insured today is not known." A concurrent study found farm labor to be the nation's least insured occupation, with fewer than one in three protected.[43]

All but the most uncritical boosters of private insurance acknowledged obstacles to the complete inclusion of persons working on their own or in small enterprises. Some residents of remote, sparsely settled areas never gained a viable option for purchasing health insurance. Due to their inevitable administrative inefficiency, individual policies were always more expensive; of course, there was no employer to share the cost. For marginally profitable small operations, health insurance was sometimes prohibitively expensive. Still, insurers maintained guarded optimism about eventually reaching the vast majority of this relatively attractive and self-supporting population.[44]

The unemployed were another significant subgroup of uninsured Americans. As with almost all other components of welfare capitalism, employee benefits came with the job and generally ended when employment ended. This connection had proven fatal to the preceding version of corporate welfarism, which had ignominiously disintegrated in the Great Depression. However, the long postwar boom, a quarter century during which the annual unemployment rate never exceeded 7 percent, made this prospect less daunting. Nonetheless, even "full employment" left sizable numbers of people out of work. The business cycle became more moderate, but did not disappear. In the recession year of 1958, for example, the official jobless count reached 4.6 million. A study of applicants for unemployment insurance in New York that year discovered that less than half had health protection. Laid-off workers from apparel manufacturing and wholesale and retail trade were the least likely to have insurance. Some looked to the government to take care of the health needs of this group, much as it did their income-maintenance needs. But as with the self-employed and small businesses, extending coverage to the unemployed was seen primarily as a challenge manageable within private arrangements. By the mid-1950s, union negotiators were pressing for the continuation of coverage for those laid off. Common provisions kept furloughed union workers under their employer's umbrella for periods of a year or more. Sophisticated management in nonunion settings emulated this practice.[45]

Retired workers and other elderly men and women were another major category within the uninsured population. The rapidly growing aging population was a diffuse group largely disconnected from the workforce. One of the cardinal characteristics of the aged, of course, was inferior health status. The elderly were both afflicted with far more than their share of expensive chronic conditions and highly susceptible to ruinous acute diseases like pneumonia. In some measure as a consequence of their many maladies, a substantial fraction of older Americans were not affluent. These attributes made the elderly unattractive prospective customers of the insurance industry. Blatant age discrimination prevailed. A national study conducted in 1951 found that "most insurance carriers, including Blue Cross and Blue Shield, will not enroll for the first time any person who has reached the age of sixty or sixty-five." The resulting pattern of insecurity was not pleasant to behold. In 1952, insurers estimated that roughly one-quarter of those sixty-five and older had any private health coverage.[46]

Both profit and nonprofit insurers made a systematic, if somewhat ambivalent, attempt to enroll the elderly after 1950. They took on the elderly as a major test of the legitimacy of voluntarism. AMA President Louis Bauer argued that it was imperative to extend private protection to older citizens "if we are to preserve our American system of medicine." Indeed, covering a diffuse aggregation of individuals, the vast majority of whom had retired from the workforce, posed quite a challenge for a system founded on the employment relationship. In the mid-1950s, the industrial unions began to win demands that pensioners receive the same health benefits as active employees. Once again, breakthroughs at huge companies like General Motors spread rapidly across the less competitive sectors of the economy. On the other hand, this approach made virtually no headway among small employers in nonunion settings. Many insurers loosened discriminatory eligibility rules and sold individual policies to those over sixty-five. These measures brought immediate progress. By 1959, the HIAA considered it "reasonable to believe that the problem of financing health care costs of future older persons will be substantially eliminated through the proved and time-tested voluntary mechanisms presently in operation." In 1962, more than 9 million elderly Americans— slightly more than half of the population over sixty-five—had private coverage. Insurance industry leaders at that time made the valid observation that the recent rate of growth among the aged surpassed that for those younger than sixty-five, conveniently overlooking the slowing rate of enrollment in the latter. However, this progress still left unprotected more than 7 million older citizens, women and men who tended to be sicker and less well off than their insured cohorts.[47]

No such solicitude infused the relationship between the architects of voluntarism and Americans of color. Insurance carriers generally ignored the uninsured nonwhite masses. Besides its revelations about other facets of insecurity, the New York survey of the unemployed offered a rare glimpse of the situation of racial and ethnic minorities. The passing mention that African Americans and immigrants from Puerto Rico were more likely to be uninsured than other jobless New Yorkers was at least a minimal acknowledgment of disparity. The Clark report made no direct inquiry into the extent of protection in the African-American population; instead it inferred this from the lower rates of insurance in southern states with high concentrations of black residents. It attributed the infrequency of insurance in the South to "relatively fewer available medical personnel and facilities, economic status, educational levels, and other problems." Such skittishness about addressing racial segregation in employment and accommodation in health facilities was entirely the norm, as was skittishness about racial discrimination in the delivery of health care and the marketing of insurance. Despite the overall aversion to describing and explaining racism, some salient facts did emerge. For example, it came to light that only 46 percent of the nation's nonwhite population had any health insurance as late as 1963. Voluntarists seemed unwilling even to propose remedies for this thorny problem. Both labor representatives on the Commission on Financing of Hospital Care took their colleagues to task for failing to face the implications of racial discrimination. In 1961, the Health Information Foundation, a research organization supported by the pharmaceutical industry, reported that nonwhites constituted a disproportionately large share of the uninsured but offered no constructive remedial recommendation that explicitly addressed that disparity.[48]

Destitute or nearly destitute victims of various misfortunes were commonly lumped together. The profoundly disabled, those with drug and alcohol addictions, and others who either received public welfare or resided in public institutions made up a sizable segment of the uninsured population. In 1952, more than 5 million Americans received public relief, and countless others in this category subsisted with the help of private charity. Insurers considered this aggregation of indigents simply untouchable. Even the most reactionary opponents of government action expected public agencies to cope with the medical exigencies of the most poverty-stricken citizens. The HIAA's Follmann traced this tradition to the Elizabethan poor laws. Public provision in the middle of the twentieth century still centered on the direct delivery of elementary services in state, county, and municipal hospitals and other health-care facilities. Welfare medicine at the state and community level received fresh validation and, more important, financial support from the federal government through the Social Security amendments of 1950 and the Kerr-Mills Act of 1960. The consensus favoring government responsibility for uninsurable problem cases reinforced the view that only quadriplegics, schizophrenics, and those in the most dire straits deserved a modicum of government assistance. Conversely, all those who were not hopelessly unproductive could find jobs and thereby obtain insurance.[49]

Low-income workers and their families constituted the largest share of uninsured Americans in the postwar years. (Needless to say, the undifferentiated low-income classification took in many people from aforementioned groups.) In 1958, fully three-quarters of the nation's uninsured were members of working families. Whereas only 14 percent of the nation's insured at that time had annual family incomes below $3,500, 51 percent of the uninsured had incomes below that level. The same competitive forces that depressed wages precluded health benefits. Firms that relied heavily on easily replaceable unskilled labor had little incentive to introduce benefits. Accordingly, one third of unskilled nonagricultural workers remained uninsured in 1957. Firms trying to survive in industries with a plethora of small and medium-sized competitors often determined that the risk of adding a costly, complicated insurance plan outweighed the potential benefit in employee loyalty and productivity. In one such low-wage industry, cotton-textile manufacturing, more than a third of the workers lacked health insurance in the 1950s. Establishments capable of offering only bare-bones programs commonly assumed little or none of the expense of insuring employees' families, effectively leaving them unprotected. Almost 90 percent of the uninsured simply had no possibility of receiving insurance through their jobs. As a result, with individual insurance policies generally unaffordable to the working poor, tens of millions of working Americans had no viable means of achieving health security during the prosperous postwar years. The rebirth of welfare capitalism and the threat of unionism that often lay behind it did not compel a large share of employers to add health insurance to their compensation packages.[50]

This shortcoming stood as a powerful indictment of the voluntarist order. Employers, insurers, and other stakeholders in the system knew that they had to try to extend private insurance across the entire working population. Both the President's Commission on the Health Needs of the Nation and the Commission on Financing of Hospital Care highlighted this challenge. The *New England Journal of Medicine* interpreted the Truman commission findings in a way that left no room for evasion: "The report brings more clearly into the open than some proponents of the existing prepayment plans have been quite able to acknowledge the problem of low-income groups and the necessity for preparing to meet what may reasonably be considered as their basic needs." (The journal's uncritical reliance on the construct of need shows that the AMA had failed to excise it from the vocabulary of medical participants in policy discussion.) Beyond bearing witness to this shortcoming, neither commission offered much creative guidance for protecting the low-income population, in essence preferring to let the experiment in privatization run its course. Similarly, a 1956 congressional proposal for federal aid to help poorer Americans purchase voluntary insurance received much the same apathetic response that the Eisenhower reinsurance plan had. Instead, guardians of the status quo made the same assurances of increased underwriting flexibility and intensified marketing that they had used in addressing the intertwined difficulties of reaching small businesses, the self-employed, and rural areas. On occasion, the insurance industry added an analysis of the individual maladjustments or other deficiencies that kept the working poor from grasping that they could afford to purchase insurance on their own. There is no record of any corresponding psychological explanation of employers' inability to grasp that they could afford to offer employee health benefits.[51]

A large uninsured population persisted long after the inception of the voluntarist campaign in the 1940s. In the mid-1960s, more than 40 million people still had no health insurance. As time passed, it became inescapably clear that lack of insurance still meant lack of access to care. There was no seamless safety net to catch those who did not obtain private insurance. Although the combination of state welfare, community charity, and provider generosity enabled some to receive otherwise unaffordable care, this patchwork failed to accommodate many sick and injured citizens. The obligation to deliver free services imposed on hospitals by the Hill-Burton Act of 1946 sometimes remained nearly unknown in the community, making it meaningless to the uninsured throughout this period. When the President's Commission on the Health Needs of the Nation came to Philadelphia in 1952, CIO leader Harry Block informed the commissioners that "people are being turned away from our hospitals all the time, and one can only guess the number of others who do not even not even apply for admission because they have learned it is futile to do so." Block waved aside private insurance as "simply inadequate to provide a solution to the problem of bringing medical care to all of our citizens." Ten years later, Michael Harrington's exploration of life among the scarcely visible poor rediscovered the cycle of poverty, lack of care, and illness. "In every subculture of the other America," Harrington reported, "sickness and disease are the most important agencies of continuing misery." The vast majority of those deprived suffered in silence.[52]

For all its imperfections, the voluntarist approach did make great strides in the twenty years after World War II. By 1965, approximately three quarters of the working population enjoyed employment-based hospital and surgical benefits. As Jennifer Klein and other historians have documented, a substantial share of the nation's employers not only created new benefits but made employee security more of a priority. In the context of resurgent corporate paternalism, access to essential medical services improved markedly for most Americans. Health insecurity became the exception rather than the rule.[53]

Insuring most of the working class paid the voluntarists an enormous political dividend—demobilization of the natural core constituency for a universal public insurance plan. However far from universal, private measures reached far enough to preempt any sweeping state intervention into healthcare financing. These changes effectively placated the working and middle classes, two groups that overlapped considerably during this affluent era. One moment in June 1958 captured the futility of pursuing thoroughgoing universalism during this period. At the National Conference on Labor Health Services in Washington, Martha Eliot, professor of maternal and child health at the Harvard School of Public Health, tried to redirect the attention of union officials to unfinished business. Eliot reminded the conferees of the broad perspective and daring stance taken by union leaders at the National Health Conference (which she had helped to plan, while working at the Children's Bureau) twenty years earlier. She implored her audience "to take a long and a hard look once again at what needs to be done on a nationwide basis to fill the gaps that exist in the provision of services and facilities to meet the medical care needs of all the people of our country." This earnest plea did not move organized labor to reconsider its priorities, and no other strong social force stepped forward to fill the void. Those left out of the private system were, as usual, poorly positioned to make access to health care a major national concern. In these circumstances, the issue of universalistic reform virtually disappeared.[54]

# CHAPTER SIX

# As Much a Birthright as Education

Just as our National Government has moved to provide equal opportunity in areas such as education, employment and voting, so we must now work to expand the opportunity for all citizens to obtain a decent standard of medical care. We must do all we can to remove all racial, economic, social or geographic barriers which now prevent any of our citizens from obtaining adequate health protection.

—RICHARD NIXON, 1971

Do we believe that all people should be able to get needed medical care of dependable quality? . . . Do we all agree? On the surface, yes. But it is doubtful that we have developed, in our minds or in our plans, the consequences of these answers.

—GEORGE PICKETT, 1978

The idea of national health insurance came back from oblivion in the 1960s. Political leaders, most vested interests, and the general public recognized that a large share of the elderly and the poor would not gain private health protection. The establishment of the Medicare and Medicaid programs in 1965 remedied this deficiency for those over sixty-five and for a fraction of the very poorest Americans. To some activists, Medicare and Medicaid demonstrated the value of an incremental strategy that could culminate in national health insurance for all. To others, the fresh inroads of the central government into health-care financing reopened the possibility of immediate universal reform. Momentum for change soon reached the point that some form of all-inclusive health provision seemed not only inevitable but imminent.

Yet the universalist consensus proved to be fragile. Virtual unanimity of opinion in favor of unimpeded access to health care did not translate into any real right. Failure to grasp the opportunity presented in the early 1970s resulted from factors other than the obstruction of opposing interests. One of the important factors, heretofore underappreciated by historians—although, ironically, recognized at the time—was the lack of commitment to this issue.

A close examination of the policy discussion at this crucial moment reveals re-peated warnings that the nation would not have reform merely by achieving unanimity of opinion. It would take more than just lip service—universal health security would require great political will, strenuous effort, and con-siderable flexibility. None of these elements ever came about. Instead, policy intellectuals created a morass of new complications and diversions to com-pound the difficulties associated with the resumption of longstanding ideo-logical disputes. The ideal of universalism did not provide a rallying cry capa-ble of mobilizing a mass constituency for reform. Its proponents also failed to make it the preeminent principle driving policy formation. Instead, as health-care cost containment came to dominate the debate, fears of scarcity eclipsed the ideal of inclusion. By end of the 1970s, the cause of universal health secu-rity was not only politically dead but intellectually exhausted as well.

## Protection for the Residue

Even the voluntarist regime that dominated health affairs in the middle of the twentieth century conceded that the state should address social problems that were intractable to a market solution. In what Richard Titmuss called the "residual welfare model of social policy," governmental intervention served as a last resort for the needy and was associated with the marginal, "unproduc-tive" elements of society. Both the aged and the most impoverished became appropriate candidates for public protection after it became clear that neither employers nor the insurance industry wanted much to do with them.[1]

The Social Security amendments of 1965 extended health security to these two major segments of the uninsured. Under Title XVIII, the Medicare pro-gram granted federal insurance against hospital expenses and the option of additional coverage against medical and surgical expenses to virtually every-one starting at the age of sixty-five. Indeed, the program successfully enrolled almost all men and women in this open-ended age bracket as soon as it went into effect in 1966. Medicare thus became a system of universal protection for a sizable and growing share of the citizenry. As an integral part of a social insurance system based on contributory financing, Medicare gave its benefi-ciaries the respectable status of rightful claimants to deserved care.[2]

On the other hand, Medicaid made no pretense of conferring a right. Nor did Title XIX of the Social Security Act seek universal coverage for its target population, the medically needy. Largely an afterthought in the process of devising and revising a health plan for older Americans, Medicaid took a half-hearted step toward the nationalization of welfare medicine. Unlike the strictly federal initiative for the elderly, Medicaid was a joint undertaking of the federal government and the fifty states. Under fairly loose guidance from Washington, individual states were free to design insurance plans for impoverished residents. According to Robert Stevens and Rosemary Stevens, in their definitive dissection of the enactment and implementation of this legislation, "Perhaps the murkiest language of Title XIX was that which specified eligibility standards." Not surprisingly, some states sharply restricted Medicaid eligibility, especially where many potential recipients were not white. A number of states balked at participating in the program—Arizona held out until 1982. Nonetheless, taken together, the 1965 initiatives represented a huge advance in extending insurance protection to particularly needy citizens excluded from employment-based arrangements. Medicare and Medicaid served well over 40 million people by the early 1970s.[3]

Perhaps the only important common denominator of these two very different programs was their categorical nature. To some influential policy architects, this shared characteristic pointed to the viability of continuing along the path of incremental reform. In light of the fact that the central hospital-insurance component of Medicare had been invented at the end of the 1940s and had been regularly proposed since the early 1950s, another lesson of these developments seemed to be the virtue of patience. Partisans of universalism in the mid-1960s had good reason to believe that an incremental strategy would gradually bring about all-encompassing health security. Many in the policy world understood that the originators of Medicare intended it as a first step toward universal health insurance. The American Medical Association certainly saw it that way. In 1963, AMA president Edward Annis published a cautionary tale entitled "Government Health Care: First the Aged, Then Everyone." The momentum for federal expansionism embodied in Lyndon Johnson's drive for a Great Society stirred hopes that a step-by-step approach might not even require all that much patience. A series of limited reforms might flow in quick succession to the ultimate goal of health protection for all.[4]

## Kiddie Care

Flush with success from the Medicare campaign, liberal incrementalists quickly turned from the old to the very young. On April 8, 1966, while signing a bill that allowed more time for those over sixty-five to enroll in Medicare, Lyndon Johnson broached a maternalistic idea suggested to him by Wilbur Cohen. "I have been wondering for some time now," Johnson said, "why we shouldn't bring our compassion and our concern to bear not just on people over sixty-five but upon our young children under six." He did not elaborate on his intentions. Instead, he connected this venture to both the nation's founding purpose and his own legacy: "I want to be remembered as one who spent his whole life trying to get more people . . . to have medicine and have attention, nursing, hospital and doctors' care when they need it, and to have their children have a chance to go to school and carry out really what the Declaration of Independence says, 'All men are created equal.' But they are not equal if they don't have a chance . . . for a doctor to take care of their teeth or their eyes when they are little."[5]

Shortly thereafter, Eveline Burns, professor of social work at Columbia, pressed the issue by contrasting the nation's commitment to the well-being of the elderly with its treatment of its youngest and most vulnerable citizens. "Children, unless crippled or retarded or suffering specific handicaps, have been given no priority," she charged, "although one would think that a rational society would give them the highest preference." Burns proposed to redress this imbalance: "If we are really committed to the idea that health services should be available as a human right based on health needs alone, perhaps we should raise our sights and move toward a free health service for at least some sections of the population. Children suggest themselves as the obvious target for such a service." She defended this call for socialization of health care by pointing out that contributory social insurance could never reach all Americans and that the potential of Medicaid was cramped in states where racial discrimination and biases against unmarried mothers raised high barriers to access. Burns made clear that protection for all children constituted but one phase in the evolution of a campaign for similar protection for all members of society. In this regard, she departed from the traditional maternalist position, which made separate demands on behalf of mothers and children and took pains to differentiate their special situation from that of the rest of society.[6]

The Johnson administration did not immediately follow through on the idea of extending additional protection to children. Further amendments to the Social Security Act in 1967 expanded preexisting programs under Title V to make maternity care and other services more widely available. In January 1968 the president announced a plan to make maternal and infant services universally accessible through Medicare. In his State of the Union address, he asked Congress for a "child health program to provide, over the next five years, for families unable to afford it—access to health services from prenatal care of the mother through the child's first year." On April 26, 1968, Wilbur Cohen, in his capacity as secretary-designate of the Department of Health, Education, and Welfare, urged the Senate to act. Cohen had come up with not only the idea for this program but also its name, Kiddie Care. Earlier that month *Time* had called him the "salami slicer" for his willingness to advance his agenda one thin slice at a time. "You will find that comprehensive prenatal care has to be available to every mother before she delivers her child," this canny incrementalist advised lawmakers. "At the present time there are probably 500,000 to 750,000 women every year who deliver babies who have not had comprehensive prenatal care." Cohen stressed the human-capital dimension of maternal and child health, arguing that such programs represented the "best investment" for society. Speaking two weeks later, Eveline Burns reiterated her call for health care for all children, not just infants. Burns grounded her position in "the national interest in having a healthy and productive labor force."[7]

Lyndon Johnson himself couched insurance for mothers and babies in terms grander than those of productivity. To be sure, his address to the National Medical Association on August 14, 1968, declared this program "the best investment we can make in our future." But Johnson also stated that his administration looked upon insuring this small segment of the population as another installment in a drive for universal protection and presented that ultimate goal as a new right of citizenship. Straining to outdo Roosevelt's famous Four Freedoms, Johnson enumerated five new freedoms for his audience of two thousand African-American physicians. These included the right of "every American to as healthy a life as modern medicine can provide." His statement that "one day the healing hand of Medicare must reach out to every child in America" suggested that social insurance for all minors might be the next step in the incremental process after fetal and infant protection. However, with a war raging in Vietnam and conflict of all sorts erupting at home, the Kiddie Care proposal fell by the wayside in the waning days of the lame-duck Johnson administration.[8]

Richard Nixon's election to the presidency extinguished any prospects for the children's initiative. Nonetheless, on his way out in December 1968, Wilbur Cohen put his successors on notice regarding the need to act on this proposition. For good measure, the outgoing federal health executive called for universal access for Americans of all ages by the national bicentennial in 1976. Although it reappeared occasionally over the course of the following decade, the moment of enthusiasm for Kiddie Care had passed. In addition to the opposition of conservatives, who saw it as another step on the road to socialized medicine, the plan also drew only lukewarm support from many progressives, who saw it as too timid a step.[9]

## Medicare for All

The Social Security amendments of 1965 inspired progressives to consider more than incremental nibbling. The late 1960s were no time for half-measures. The bold (if only symbolic) policy declaration in favor of universality contained in 1966 health-planning legislation added fuel to the fire. The shifting stance of the nation's most influential newspaper signaled broadening horizons. While Medicare was making its way through Congress, the *New York Times* praised a gubernatorial committee's recommendation of requiring hospital insurance for all workers and their families in the state of New York. Less than a year later, however, the newspaper criticized the subsequent bill put forward by Governor Nelson Rockefeller embodying this very recommendation. Apparently caught up in the enthusiasm arising from the enactment of Medicare, the *Times* was now attacking partial arrangements and calling for hospital insurance for all residents of the state. Shortly thereafter, the paper commented that the American public was ready for President Johnson's universalistic aims in health policy. (A national survey soon found that a majority of Americans favored extending Medicare coverage to the entire population. This poll also discovered that about 40 percent of the population postponed necessary care due to financial considerations.) On May 1, 1966, the newspaper pushed Congress to "begin thinking seriously about the desirability of providing comprehensive health insurance for all Americans."[10]

Insurance for all the elderly also caused a stir in other liberal quarters. In January 1967, Americans for Democratic Action endorsed universal health insurance under Social Security. I. S. Falk understood that Medicare might well catalyze far-reaching change. However, recognition that further progress depended on successful implementation of the new legislation tempered his optimism. Falk promoted universal public insurance in 1966 by offering a "lesser of two evils" scenario: "Good performance will invite extension of the social insurance to broader groups or to all; bad performance or failure is more likely to invite development toward a national health service than toward a return to voluntary health insurance." While holding out hope that the insurance industry would still find a way to reach a large share of the insured, economist Anne Somers acknowledged the pressure to universalize Medicare in a 1968 overview of the policy scene.[11]

## From Civil Rights to Health Rights

The renewed campaign for universal health security drew upon sources other than the Medicare breakthrough. The electrifying success of the African-American civil rights movement fostered a renaissance of creative thinking about the full meaning of American citizenship. As James Patterson observed, "More than any other development of the early 1960s, the civil rights revolution spurred the idealism, egalitarianism, and rights-consciousness that galvanized many other groups and challenged social relations in the United States." The proliferation of contentious rights-seeking movements among racial and ethnic minority groups, students, women, and others served to amplify nascent concerns for equality in health care.[12]

In one instance, the black freedom struggle made a direct, programmatic contribution to reviving the cause of universal health security. In 1966, the A. Philip Randolph Institute, a new research and advocacy organization named for the longtime African-American leader of the Brotherhood of Sleeping Car Porters and run by his protégé Bayard Rustin, contested the Johnson administration's War on Poverty. Working with a coalition of labor, religious, academic, and civil rights activists, the institute produced a Freedom Budget. The coalition put forward a comprehensive social democratic agenda that centered on full employment. Among the seven basic objectives of this visionary document was "to provide, for all Americans, modern medical care . . . at costs within their means." The plan for reallocating national resources to meet this objective included "a nationwide, universal system of health insurance," and the group urged resumption of the long-dormant campaign for its establishment. In line with integrationist doctrine, the Freedom Budget sought the same protections for all citizens and eschewed any special pleading on behalf of African Americans. Its authors insisted that "the only reason why the Negro will benefit relatively more than others . . . is not because he is a Negro, but rather because he is at the bottom of the heap." Although it attracted little interest from political leaders, the Freedom Budget did help to return universal health insurance to the national policy agenda.[13]

Beyond the willingness of several labor officials to endorse the Freedom Budget, one unionist provided real leadership on the health question. Martha Eliot had challenged the labor movement in 1958 to "become again the bold spokesman for the people's health and the great advocate of more and better medical care for all who are in need of such care." Ten years later, Walter Reuther, president of the United Auto Workers, took up her challenge. Reuther's abiding social democratic dreams had not been fulfilled by the negotiation of a private welfare state for his million members and their families. On November 14, 1968, he brought his frustrations and ambitions to the annual meeting of the American Public Health Association in Detroit. Familiarity with western European developments in health care left him impatient with American complacency. The UAW leader observed that "if the rate of infant mortality in the United States last year had been comparable to the rate in Sweden, 50,000 fewer babies would have died in America." He also noted that nonwhite infants suffered a death rate almost 60 percent higher than white infants. "No amount of clever Madison Avenue public relations," Reuther mordantly commented, "can hide the ugly facts about the failure of our nation's health care system. He went on to blast "a disorganized, disjointed, antiquated, obsolete nonsystem" that left 30 million citizens uninsured.[14]

Walter Reuther had more than criticism on his mind. He announced the formation of the Committee of One Hundred for National Health Insurance, which soon renamed itself the Committee for National Health Insurance (CNHI). He expressed confidence "that we have in America the ingenuity and the social inventiveness to create a system of national health insurance that will be uniquely American." In his view, "comprehensive high quality health care must be made available to every citizen as a matter of right." The CNHI was the leading advocate of universal health care throughout the subsequent decade. After Reuther's death in a plane crash in 1970, his successor as UAW president, Leonard Woodcock, became chair of the committee.[15]

The CNHI's foremost guiding principle was the universal right to care, "with equal opportunity of access to the available services throughout the country." This commitment spoke directly to the long legacy of racial discrimination, especially in the South, and to abiding concerns about class discrimination in health care as well. It also echoed a broader theme of equal opportunity, a central concern of domestic policy at that time. The Economic

Opportunity Act of 1964, the Civil Rights Act of 1964, and other manifestations of federal activism advanced egalitarianism on many fronts. In this context, reformers naturally stressed that equal opportunity to enjoy the American way of life critically depended upon access to health care. Eveline Burns contended that the nation faced "a crucial test of our conviction that all people should have the assurance of an equal opportunity to obtain a high quality of comprehensive health care under self-respecting conditions." Even I. S. Falk, who communicated almost entirely in dry bureaucratic jargon, called for "equal opportunity for access to . . . [health] services by all persons."[16]

Rights claims commonly warranted equal opportunity to health care. That the recent effort to justify Medicare by emphasizing the "exceptional" needs of the elderly had undercut universalistic assertions apparently deterred nobody. Hospital administrator Peter Rogatz enumerated the ways in which urban hospitals failed to meet the many needs of the ailing poor. Implying that needs alone validated entitlements, Rogatz concluded that "first-class health care is the right of every citizen to enjoy and the duty of every community to provide." Wilbur Cohen maintained that planning legislation passed in 1966 had already established a broad right. "The American people . . . have declared through their Congress that each individual has the right to the best health care with equal opportunity to that care regardless of age, sex, color, or any other factor except medical need," Cohen contended. "All those concerned with delivering health care have an awesome responsibility and obligation, for we are still a long way from fulfilling that right."[17]

Political leaders espoused the right to health care, but did little to clarify its underpinnings. On April 22, 1968, Senator Abraham Ribicoff opened a round of hearings on health reform with a set of questions intended to frame the discussion. His first question presumed an entitlement: "Do all Americans, who should receive full and complete health care as a basic right and at a reasonable cost, actually receive this?" The Connecticut senator's statement allowed his witnesses to proceed from that premise. New York Governor Nelson Rockefeller, then contemplating a campaign for the Republican presidential nomination, told Ribicoff's subcommittee that because access to hospital services had become indispensable to full participation in "the opportunities of American life," he regarded universal access as a "basic human right." Senator Eugene McCarthy, running for the Democratic nomination, advocated "a new set of citizens' rights," which included the health protections granted in many other nations.[18]

Politicians were trying to keep up with prevailing attitudes, not to advance them. Reporting on the changing climate of public opinion in 1967, Harry Becker observed that market-based concepts of access were "being replaced with the idea that all people have the right to the best in health care without regard to their economic status." The following year, the National Opinion Research Center revealed that 87 percent of Americans viewed health care as the right of all citizens. Subsequent surveys discovered similar majorities holding this belief.[19]

Organized medicine formally embraced the majority view. The American Medical Association had pledged itself to the goal of universal health care in 1921, but had not posited an entitlement to care. In 1969, the AMA House of Delegates resolved that "it is a basic right of every citizen to have available to him adequate health care." The delegates decided that "the medical profession, using all means at its disposal, should endeavor to make good medical care available to each person." When the Committee for National Health Insurance met with the AMA in early 1970 to search (in vain) for a way to avert a confrontation in the legislative arena, it stressed the two groups' mutual adherence to universality. A rights-based perspective came easily for the National Medical Association. In 1971, outgoing president Wiley Armstrong promised that "the NMA will cooperate with whatever level of government necessary to achieve the goal that every American has the right to have accessibility to quality medical care regardless of his socio-economic standing."[20]

Many other interested parties took this position. In 1968, Olcott Smith, chairman of the board of Aetna Life and Casualty, then the nation's largest underwriter of group health insurance, told a Senate committee that "all Americans, regardless of income level or place of residence, expect and, in my opinion, are entitled to quality medical care. Quality medical care has become as much a birthright as education or pure drinking water." Smith characterized access to quality care as "one of those inalienable rights that you cannot find in the Constitution, but which I think you can find in the demands of society today." He estimated that failure to provide this entitlement resulted in thirteen thousand avoidable deaths a year in New York City alone. The American Public Health Association's policy statement of November 12, 1969, cited the ongoing quest for equal opportunity. The association also alluded to the nation's fundamental purposes: "Egalitarian principles and concepts of the rights of man are the high ideals upon which the United States was founded and which have shaped our political and social institutions. Health is no less a human aspiration than liberty and the pursuit of happiness. It should receive as firm a guarantee." A committee of the American Hospital Association concluded in 1970 that health care was "an inherent legal right" of all citizens.[21]

Some participants in the policy conversation refused to adopt the rights idiom. Perhaps most tellingly, President Nixon's health message to Congress of February 18, 1971, mentioned no rights in its promise of universal provision. By the same token, Aetna's Olcott Smith did not speak for all insurance carriers. The Health Insurance Association of America kept a healthy distance from these notions of entitlement. To be sure, the insurers' group proposed an agenda for the nation that acknowledged the centrality of the access question: "Achieving access to quality health care for all would be a fitting commemoration of our nation's bicentennial—truly in the spirit of the American dream of life, liberty, and the pursuit of happiness." Despite its willingness to quote the Declaration of Independence, the HIAA studiously avoided basing any rights assertions on it. Some physicians dissented from the AMA's pro-entitlement position. Former AMA president Edward Annis, a member of the U.S. Chamber of Commerce's board of directors, rallied doctors against social insurance. Annis derided as "absurd" the notion of a right to health care. Granting such a right would place the nation only one step away from "a revolutionary system bordering on Communism."[22]

These exceptions notwithstanding, the late 1960s and early 1970s witnessed the high tide of rights consciousness with respect to health care. Russell Roth of the AMA approvingly noted the "growing belief that medical care is an absolute right." In this exhilarating context, the CNHI could properly appeal to Congress to live up to "the oft-expressed declaration that good health care is the right of every man, woman, and child who lives in this land." Indicative of the temper of the times was the fact that neither the recalcitrant president nor the insurance interests explicitly denied the moral and quasi-constitutional contentions of their ideological opponents. The loose and cursory nature of most of the briefs for this entitlement was a further indication of the strength of rights consciousness at that moment. Universal health care had become an article of faith for all but a few.[23]

## Universal Universalism

By the end of the 1960s, health care for all Americans for all appearances was an idea whose time had finally come. In contrast to the immensity of other challenges like overcoming racism and ending the war in Vietnam, paying for medical care looked like a tractable problem for such an affluent nation. Indeed, the frequency of comments about the prevailing unanimity of opinion suggests a consensus about the universalist position. In 1970, the HIAA acknowledged the "general agreement today that every citizen should have access to quality health care." Discussion shifted from enunciating high principles to crafting feasible plans to realize them.[24]

The aura of inevitability compelled the major players to come up with remedies. In 1969, hospital executive J. Martin Stone alerted his colleagues to the mounting enthusiasm for national health insurance brought on by the promotional activities of Reuther, Rockefeller, and others. Stone urged hospital leaders to pursue a "positive and imaginative" alternative to the extreme possibilities on the horizon. The American Hospital Association quickly launched a study of the feasibility of universal health insurance.[25]

Such hasty conversions caused some skepticism. As befitted an organization that had revived this issue, the Committee for National Health Insurance continued to try to steer the discussion. At a coming-out conference in October 1969, the CNHI posed the question as one of true dedication, not merely pious declaration. Walter Reuther put the matter squarely before the policymakers: "We went to the moon because President Jack Kennedy made a commitment to the nation, and we allocated the resources necessary to carry out that commitment. We . . . will not deal effectively with the many problems at home until America reorders its priorities and until we all make a comparable commitment in terms of the national will and the allocation of our national resources." Endeavoring to build such a commitment by playing on feelings of embarrassment, the blunt union leader contended that no other industrialized nation in the world tolerated such disparities in access to care as existed in the United States.[26]

The CNHI used its 1969 conference to outline and refine its own formulation of universal provision. This plan would guarantee access to all U.S. residents through a seamlessly unitary federal insurance program, eliminating categorical programs like Medicare and Medicaid. The CNHI proposition became the basis for Senator Edward Kennedy's proposed Health Security Act. Introducing his bill in 1970, Kennedy stated that it would "enable our Nation to make the right to health care not merely a principle or a social goal, but a living and functioning reality."[27]

The Kennedy proposal was but one of a flood of measures. By early 1972, Congress had about forty bills under consideration. The alternatives came in two broad types. The more modest sought to build upon the existing system. The AMA, the AHA, and the Nixon administration favored measures that emphasized the use of tax credits to stimulate the purchase of private health insurance. Liberals chose instead to make the federal government the nation's health insurance carrier. Senator Jacob Javits of New York sponsored a series of bills to extend Medicare to citizens of all ages. Despite the myriad variations on such factors as scope of benefits, financing mechanisms, and delivery of services, leading legislative proposals all promised to reach some approximation of universal health security.[28]

In the ensuing debate, universality was but one criterion by which critics evaluated the propositions. Nonetheless, both the frequency and the intensity of criticism on this score signaled the importance of this consideration. Union leaders from AFL-CIO president George Meany on down assailed all bills that failed to take in the entire population. The AFL-CIO estimated that the original version of the Nixon plan, which combined tax credits with a new means-tested insurance program for the poor, would leave about 20 percent of the population without coverage. Both the NMA and the APHA questioned the adequacy of the AMA plan.[29]

In 1972, Princeton health economists Anne Somers and Herman Somers systematically assessed the pending reform proposals. Somers and Somers made unmistakably clear that certain approaches were doomed to fail a strict test of inclusiveness: "Universality cannot be achieved by voluntarism, even when supported by incentives. Publicly imposed means tests are destructive to universality and, when accompanied by a separate program for means test eligibles, almost always lead to a double standard and a 'two-class' quality of care." They predicted that the tax-incentive programs advocated by the AMA and the HIAA would leave millions out in the cold.[30]

## Radical Visions of Equality

The most fervent universalists lodged criticisms that went beyond the incomplete population coverage of some legislative measures. The disappointing shallowness and even emptiness of the rights rhetoric gave rise to more thoroughgoing, if not always more rigorous, critiques over the course of the 1970s. Some of this egalitarian rethinking came in response to the loose talk of politicians. Some of it came from doubts about the adequacy of the major reform schemes.[31]

A few dissident egalitarians criticized national health insurance. In June 1970, Yale health-policy scholar George Silver noted the general failure to scrutinize the appropriateness of social insurance as a policy instrument. In his view, universal coverage under national insurance would not, by itself, ensure access to some of those most in need. Silver contended that none of the current proposals went far enough to reorganize services in order to guarantee that care actually reached the poor, be they members of racial minorities concentrated in major cities or whites scattered in rural areas like Appalachia. He wanted an open discussion to enlighten the public: "Those who carry on the debate speak constantly as though what they were discussing was a national health *service*, and that is what the American people will think they have obtained when a national health *insurance* bill is passed." The former senior official of the Johnson administration suggested that national insurance incorporate such structural reforms as group medical practice and community control of hospital budgets.[32]

George Silver soon relinquished his faint hope for fundamental change through social insurance. Influenced by Eveline Burns, he began to argue for a federal takeover of the delivery of health services. In an editorial in the *American Journal of Public Health* in October 1970, Silver cited the failure of Medicare to improve substantially the distribution of services to the elderly. In his view, real universal protection required stronger state intervention: "We need a national health *service*, guaranteeing to all people equal access to modern medical care and a system designed to see to it that people have this access." Silver opposed interminable deliberation: "A definite time should be set—two years at most—at the end of which every American should be guaranteed the availability of modern medical care."[33]

Proponents of socialized services were motivated by more than doubts about insurance. Recent developments had inspired dreams of a fundamentally different system of care. By the 1970s, American health progressives in pursuit of profound change looked less to well-established but stodgy models like the British National Health Service than to ongoing domestic experiments. In 1964, the Economic Opportunity Act created the Neighborhood Health Center Program as an integral part of the War on Poverty. The program not only supported the operation of health facilities in underserved neighborhoods but also granted community members unprecedented powers to shape the assessment and satisfaction of medical needs. By 1971, about one hundred centers were functioning, many with evident success. Outreach to those in need and encouragement of patient participation in the planning of services demonstrated a concrete commitment to expanding access. The Nixon administration's promotion of privately and professionally controlled health maintenance organizations certainly paled in comparison to these experiments in participatory democracy. The 1973 HMO legislation brought many changes, to be sure, but it did very little to facilitate access to care for those with limited means or no insurance. The contrast between the two forms of restructuring was not lost on proponents of radical change.[34]

Thus inspired by democratic ventures in community self-help, proposals to socialize medicine from the bottom up appeared on the fringes of the policy conversation. As political scientist Alice Sardell has observed, "The advocates of the neighborhood health center program in its formative years believed that these projects would . . . serve as a model for the reorganization of health care services for the entire U.S. population." In 1971, the Medical Committee for Human Rights (MCHR), a physicians' group formed seven years earlier to support the black freedom struggle in Mississippi, demanded "a neighborhood-based, community-worker controlled, progressively financed, nondiscriminatory system which abolishes the profit motive from health care." As an alternative to what he termed "the hoax of national health insurance," MCHR activist Thomas Bodenheimer looked to a socialized system in which community health centers would constitute the basic institutional building blocks. These insurgents raised profound issues about what a commitment to universalism entailed.[35]

The MCHR activists helped bring about the introduction of a series of national health service bills by Representative Ronald Dellums of California, beginning in the mid-1970s. Dellums defended his advocacy of this impossible proposition in this way: "It is essential for a progressive to advocate from the left and to offer a principled alternative for debate and vote, and to work to shift the center of that debate." In the "insurance versus service" debate that arose within the APHA, Milton Roemer and Solomon Axelrod maintained that the thoroughly capitalistic United States was not ready to move to a nationalized service. In their assessment, "It would be regrettable if the advocacy of an immediate National Health Service, aside from its naivete, should lend strength to the many conservative forces opposing social security financing of health care for other reasons. History has too many stories of progress obstructed by divisiveness among the proponents of social change."[36]

Like mainstream politicians, the radical activists presumed a right to health care and, accordingly, felt little obligation to defend the proposition. A number of philosophers associated with the nascent field of medical ethics stepped forward to do the heavy lifting. As a warmup exercise, the ethicists disposed of the notion of a right to health, a utopian idea that found its way into the 1972 Democratic party platform. Georgetown University's Leon Kass maintained that health was "a state of being, not something that can be given" by the government. Kass argued that personal behavior, not state intervention, determined health status more than anything else. Daniel Callahan of the Institute of Society, Ethics and the Life Sciences, dismissed the right to health as unrealizable. "That kind of claim," Callahan tartly commented, "could only be entered against God Himself, or nature, or the evolutionary process." Even those most devoted to social equality recognized unavoidable limits on an absolute right to health. Callahan's colleague Robert Veatch drew on political philosopher John Rawls's leveling tenet that a just society strove to minimize the disadvantages suffered by its most unfortunate members. Veatch asserted that fundamental humanitarian values like freedom from suffering and maintenance of human dignity should govern society's allocation of health care resources. "Everyone," he contended, "has a claim to the amount of health care needed to provide a level of health equal to other persons' health." However, he qualified this proposition with the acknowledgment that for individuals with certain irreversible conditions like quadraplegia, the standard of truly equal health was unattainable.[37]

Philosophical work focused on the more feasible question of a right to health care. Gene Outka made need, not ability to pay, the primary criterion for access to care. Outka rejected Ayn Rand's view of the needy as weak, parasitical failures. Similarly, Daniel Callahan defined needs as "the minimal requirements for a satisfactory life" and maintained that under this definition they could be meaningfully distinguished from mere desires, which were "those things human beings want and demand as requirements for what they would consider an optimal life." Based on this distinction, Callahan defended a circumscribed right to care to meet elemental needs like survival through such actions as nonexperimental life-saving surgery. Veatch held that legitimate needs for health services varied so widely as to make health care uniquely unfit for market methods of allocation. University of Georgia philosophy professor William Blackstone weighed the satisfaction of health needs on a utilitarian scale: "The money taken from the rich means much less (in terms of producing their happiness) than it does to those whose most basic needs are unfulfilled." Blackstone attempted to place access to health services on a legal foundation by arguing that the United States had accepted Article 25 of the Universal Declaration of Human Rights, which set forth such a right. However, he had to concede that this acceptance did not establish a right "in a strict sense." Social economist Louis Buckley retraced the application of Roman Catholic natural law doctrine to health care. His review of doctrinal interpretation left Buckley "unable to locate any Catholic writer who has denied the existence of a right to health care."[38]

Most of the ethicists who explored this topic expressed sympathy for the cause of universal health insurance, at least in principle. Veatch assessed the major bills before Congress from the perspective of his avowed egalitarianism. Blackstone praised the CNHI proposal as an appropriate embodiment of the right to health care. Leon Kass's individualism, however, led to concerns that national health insurance might have perverse effects. If social insurance discouraged individual responsibility for activities like smoking, it might, in his view, actually diminish the nation's health.[39]

## Protecting the Protected

The intrepid health-rights advocates did relatively little to reshape the national debate. Instead, as political leaders and their advisors confronted the inevitable complexities of so vast an undertaking as universal health protection, a host of obstacles and constraints, new and old, loomed ever larger. More than any other factor, concentration on containing costs undercut efforts to help the uninsured. The rising level of expenditures on medical care had long caused concern among policy experts. Overall spending on health services had grown faster than the general rate of inflation since the 1950s, driven largely by heightened demand induced by private insurance. Medicare and Medicaid accelerated the pace of inflation. In no year during the interval 1966 through 1980 did health expenditures grow by less than 10 percent. The share of the gross domestic product devoted to health grew from 5 percent in 1960 to 9 percent in 1980. Thus, by the end of the 1970s, the typical American household worked more than one month a year to pay, directly or indirectly, for its health care. To make matters worse, by the late 1970s, the escalation of medical costs was occurring while the nation was dealing with alarming general inflation rates. Within the Carter administration, advocates of universal health security found themselves bogged down in a battle with economic advisors obsessed with rising prices. In this context it was quite understandable that controlling expenditures eclipsed expanding access as the nation's top health-policy priority.[40]

The increasing jeopardy of the previously secure middle class propelled this reorientation. All but the most generous employment-based health benefits imposed significant limits on the depth and breadth of coverage. Middle-class Americans with homes and other valuable assets to lose found themselves revisited by old fears. In 1973, the nation witnessed the spectacle of the former president's brother, Sam Houston Johnson, driven into insolvency by medical debts. Johnson hoped that his predicament would send a message to Washington: "It is embarrassing to me to take bankruptcy, but it will be worth it if it points out to Congress that many millions of Americans are forced into bankruptcy by medical costs they simply cannot meet." With exceedingly expensive procedures like organ transplantation becoming available but only half the costs covered by private insurance, insecurity now loomed over the vast majority of Americans. The prevalence of daunting chronic conditions like heart disease, diabetes, and cancer exacerbated these feelings of insecurity. Even though their jeopardy paled in comparison with that of the uninsured, the worried well-off had more political leverage. Widespread insecurity fostered interest in protection against frightening, if still rare, financial catastrophes. From the early 1970s on, Congress seriously examined a series of bills sponsored principally by Senator Russell Long to create a public safety net to supplement the private safety net. Governor Ronald Reagan announced his intention to develop catastrophic insurance for all Californians in January 1972. Legislative plans devoted to averting catastrophes drew attention away from proposals for basic protection. During hearings before the House Ways and Means Committee in 1974, one frustrated humanitarian attacked legislators' solicitude for the uneasy middle class. "The real crisis," maintained James McDaniel of the United Presbyterian Church, "is that our system has functioned for years while denying to millions of our fellow citizens anything approaching decent health care. The real crisis is that we have been willing to accept the fact that millions of Americans live in poor health and have limited or no access to health services." But the millions of needy citizens to whom McDaniel alluded to no significant extent made their voices heard. Their silence made it impossible for the handful of morally engaged participants in the discussion to redirect it by themselves.[41]

Another major response to the perceived crisis in health-care costs was deeper exploration of the role of market forces in effecting reform. Treating patients as consumers was not a novel idea in the post-1970 policy arena, but the invention of systematic plans to place cost-conscious consumption at the top of the agenda was quite a departure. Early on, the Nixon administration solicited proposals to introduce more competition into the health market-place and to make consumers more price-conscious. Academic economists and interest groups like the National Association of Manufacturers strove to provide plans. Although Martin Feldstein and Alain Enthoven, leading pro-ponents of the emerging competitive theory, averred their dedication to universality, their big concerns lay elsewhere. A fixation on disciplining the insured was eminently understandable at a time when a large majority of Americans enjoyed health insurance, much of it in forms that insulated them from the consequences of consumption patterns. Just as clearly, the new school of thought implicitly neglected the uninsured. No one adopted the ethic of competition primarily because they saw it as the best way to guaran-tee health services for all.[42]

One newly prominent band of critics went beyond a relative disregard for the plight of the uninsured. Led by the charismatic sophist Ivan Illich, these intellectuals challenged the value of health care and asserted the primacy of lifestyle in determining physical well-being. Oblivious to the situation of those cut off from elementary health services, public-policy scholar Aaron Wildavsky offered the generality that "more available medical care does not equal better health." From this truism, Wildavsky leapt to a fashionably avant-garde con-clusion: "If medical care does not equal health, access to medical care is irrel-evant to health." He advised against smoking, drinking, and skipping break-fast. (None of these men reported canceling his insurance policy or refusing life-saving services.) Whatever its value in deflating American culture's ro-mantic attitude toward the powers of medical science and technology, this strain of nihilism mocked the plight of the millions without ready access to care. Certainly, nihilist arguments provided ammunition for conservative economists crusading against the evil of inflation. On April 5, 1978, James McIntyre, director of the Office of Management and Budget, fallaciously ad-vised President Carter of an "expert consensus that no [national health insur-ance] plan will significantly improve the nation's health status." To be sure, the nihilist view was less than hegemonic in the Carter administration. When the president asked a group of his advisors whether a universal insurance plan covering more than catastrophes would affect the public's health, Hale Champion, Undersecretary of Health, Education and Welfare, reportedly replied, "For poor people, migrant workers and the like, yes."[43]

## From Foregone Conclusion to Forgone Opportunity

Perversely enough, revelations and reminders about the complications of and obstacles to reform did not lead to a substantial scaling back of progressive plans. Moreover, neither the rise of a new paradigm on the right nor the growing political strength of conservative business interests chastened the progressive side. Instead, the immensity of the challenge brought out a strain of rigidity in the dedicated universalists in the Committee for National Health Insurance. Leaders at successful labor organizations like the UAW could easily maintain a stance of ideological purity: all their members already had excellent health protection so they had nothing immediately at stake. Dogmatists like Falk had invested decades in defending a particular approach to social insurance. Rather than refocus to find a way to pay for basic services for all members of society, too many advocates of social justice in health affairs clung to seductive notions of wholesale transformation of health care and complete equality of access to all services. Voices of moderation went largely unheard. Amid mounting concern over costs and other competing considerations, compromise was essential. Yet at crucial junctures, key progressive advocates refused to alter their plans in order to make the goal of universal health care more likely in the long run.[44]

Throughout the 1970s, as the probability of transformative reform shrank into insignificance, the option of an incremental strategy remained available. The two most promising dimensions along which the gradualist method might have proceeded were population coverage or range of benefits. On both of these parameters, the CNHI staunchly opposed compromise. Because the committee held an authoritative position among liberals on this issue and because its lobbying arm, the Health Security Action Council, had enlisted dozens of progressive organizations to support its stance, this intransigence effectively blocked those seeking to accommodate to political reality. In a formative decision reached in 1970, a joint working group of AFL-CIO and CNHI technicians declared it "undesirable to 'stage' [i.e., introduce in stages] benefits or population." Subsequently, whenever accumulated defeats made limited reforms look more appealing to pragmatists like Wilbur Cohen and

Ted Kennedy, the hardline contingent raised objections. By 1974, the leaders of the committee understood that their approach had no chance but still could not agree upon a scaled-back alternative. Senator Kennedy broke ranks and joined Representative Wilbur Mills in sponsoring legislation that used such objectionable devices as mandated private insurance, copayment provisions, and a deductible of $1,000 per year—that is, one high enough to render it almost an anti-catastrophe measure. The CNHI stubbornly withheld its support, even though it knew that the Kennedy-Mills legislation would bring nearly universal protection and could potentially be improved upon in the future. In all probability, the leaders of the committee also understood that the American public very much favored a universal system built around mandatory employment-based benefits over a wholly federal program. The opposition of the CNHI proved fatal. Paul Starr considered this "the last moment in the 1970s when any such program had a serious chance of adoption."[45]

With respect to the specific alternative of restricting the share of the population to be covered initially, Wilbur Cohen and others attempted to revive federal insurance for children as the next step on the road to universal provision. In 1977, Theodore Marmor, then at the University of Chicago, suggested starting with "a comprehensive plan for preschool children and pregnant women," coupled with universal insurance against catastrophically high expenses. The following year, Lisbeth Schorr of the Children's Defense Fund advocated insuring all children and all mothers first. Other formulations sought gradual inclusion of various groups in stages until the entire population had come under the protective umbrella. With its Technical Committee, chaired by I. S. Falk, mounting a staunch defense, the CNHI repeatedly rejected this type of tactical retreat from immediate universal coverage. Besides the veteran infighter Falk, most of the union leaders who tended to dominate debate within the CNHI Executive Committee also held fast to the "everybody now or nobody at all" stand.[46]

Devotion to comprehensive benefits under social insurance had been a matter of liberal orthodoxy since the 1940s. This position paid insufficient attention to the spiraling cost of care. Proceeding from the understanding that hospital-centered benefits produced excessive hospitalization and surgery, progressives devised a long menu of services to be covered, with no assurances that adding outpatient services and preventive procedures would serve to reduce costs and with every assurance that adding custodial care and mental health benefits would increase the overall cost of the package. From the late 1960s on, I. S. Falk repeatedly criticized Medicare for its failure to insure "comprehensive preventive, diagnostic, therapeutic or rehabilitative services." As grudging supporters of health reform, Jimmy Carter and his advisors early on signaled their preference for phasing in benefits. On October 24, 1976, Falk told the Carter presidential campaign that such an approach amounted to "an invitation to disaster." When an acrimonious falling out occurred in 1978, the CNHI-Kennedy camp made the limited benefits proposed by their White House adversaries a major object of contention. Adhering to the standard of absolute equality inherent in a uniform package of comprehensive benefits, the CNHI found it "inconceivable that responsible people could sanction the idea that one American is entitled to better medical care than another with less ability to pay." With the nation's interest in this issue much diminished and the opposition revitalized, it was the wrong moment for utopianism.[47]

Of course, it was also the wrong moment for the Carter administration to give the most fervent supporters of reform further reason to believe that it sought to break its promise to fight for national health insurance. Doubts had surrounded the president's commitment to this issue ever since he pledged his support to universal health security in a perfunctory statement made in April 1976 in response to union pressure. The administration's delays in developing a concrete plan caused consternation. In April 1978, White House staff member Peter Bourne noted that Carter had "not made a speech on health since he assumed office." Certainly, there was a striking contrast between this administration's willingness to speak out on behalf of human rights abroad and its unwillingness to posit any right to health care for Americans. On May 8, 1978, Joseph Califano informed the World Health Assembly in Geneva that "President Carter holds to a simple belief that is also a central tenet of the World Health Organization: that a decent standard of health is a fundamental human right, for the world's poor no less than for the rich." Whereas thirty years earlier, Thomas Parran had immediately brought the World Health Organization's declaration of a global human right to health care into domestic political discourse as a standard for U.S. performance, Califano's pledge to the WHO seemed to have no bearing whatsoever on the White House's approach to the domestic issue of health-care financing. In fact, the Carter administration brought no rights contentions, new or old, into the national conversation on health reform. In mid-1978, as at other critical moments during his tenure, the president chose to heed economic policy advisors obsessed with inflation, not social policy advisors determined to make good on the campaign pledges made two years earlier. At the same time, the administration continued to profess its adherence to both universality and comprehensiveness, even while bowing to the greater imperative to avoid anything inflationary. Refusal to choose among these conflicting principles guaranteed inaction and, in turn, sharp feelings of betrayal from the Ted Kennedy camp.[48]

This predicament was not inevitable. By the mid-1970s, numerous respected experts were urging compromise. Hoping to salvage universal health insurance, these analysts understood that a growing public desire for limits on both government expansion and the soaring cost of health care doomed any scheme to pay for comprehensive services. In 1977, Daniel Callahan defended a restricted entitlement by citing the precedent of universal public education that extended only through high school. Fellow ethicist Joseph Boyle Jr. found it "reasonable . . . to suppose that a minimally decent level of health care is what the right to health care guarantees." In much the same vein, Columbia economist Eli Ginzberg tried to redirect attention to guaranteeing access to those services that saved lives and alleviated pain. A series of discussions among policy scholars in 1977 searched for a useful definition of adequate care. Distilling this conversation, Gerald Rosenthal and Daniel Fox suggested setting "standards for services at a level less than the best but adequate to maintain our notions of a decent society." Concerned that the prevailing rights discourse took inadequate account of limited resources in its construction of ideal standards of health care, Rosenthal and Fox argued that "the important conflict is not between minimum and ideal standards. Rather, it is between *any* standards and the present open-ended situation." They compared their approach to that of setting a minimum wage. Indeed, in a sense, this tendency hearkened back to the original Fabian strategy of encouraging state intervention to set modest standards of social protection. Political theorist Amy Gutmann proposed treating equal access as a guideline rather than a hard-and-fast rule. Gutmann concluded her critique of pure egalitarianism with a sober piece of advice for her colleagues: "Philosophers ought to resist basing their political recommendations solely upon a model of the best of all imaginable worlds."[49]

There was no shortage of ways to implement this approach. Jacob Javits had been advocating expansion of Medicare to take in all Americans since 1968. In adopting Medicare's limited coverage of hospital and doctor services, Javits's bills sought to forge a core entitlement to basic benefits. Whereas nobody could legitimately claim that this alternative would not entail additional costs to society, it was clearly a much more circumscribed program than that offered by the more liberal reformers. Nonetheless, Medicare-based proposals languished. In June 1979, a second alternative belatedly emerged from the White House. The initial phase of the Carter plan called for an all-inclusive entitlement to protection against catastrophically expensive illnesses and injuries. It saw this component of its plan "establishing the foundation of universality in health care coverage." The Carter plan also resurrected Kiddie Care, in modest form, by promising prenatal, obstetrical, and infant-care services for all babies and mothers, regardless of income. In announcing the administration's bill, HEW Secretary Joseph Califano stated, "There's no more chance of passing Kennedy's plan than there is of putting an elephant through a keyhole." The dogmatists in the CNHI rejected this measure. However, Nelson Cruikshank, retired from the AFL-CIO but still active in the leadership of its National Council of Senior Citizens, registered a notable dissent. From the vantage point of his extensive experience, Cruikshank argued for accepting the Carter measure as a valuable, if imperfect, first step. "We have had to literally nickel and dime ourselves into social legislation down through the years," he contended. "But once the outlines were on the books, we were able to build from there." He also attacked the all-or-nothing mentality among reformers that had long impeded social progress. At this point, however, the Carter and Kennedy camps were too bitterly divided to make a deal for the sake of the uninsured.[50]

For all its bright promise, universal health care did not result from the many plans that arose after the passage of Medicare. Broad support for the ideal of universality proved insufficient to reconcile conflicting approaches and overcome underlying ambivalence. Indeed, the consensus on a right to care, whether basic or comprehensive, turned out to be a fragile and evanescent one when put to the test. Rights assertions did little to deepen the superficial attraction of universal care. Few proponents of universalism were willing to confront American society with the necessity to spend large amounts of money to ensure that perhaps as many as 40 million of their fellow citizens would gain protection. Beyond the impediment raised by those who approved of universal health security only if it cost little or nothing stood other difficulties. The dark side of zealous commitment to the cause, irrespective of expense, was an inability to compromise on grandiose visions of transforming health care.

Much as they had during the 1950s, the uninsured receded into the background over the course of the 1970s. Their increasing marginality did not reflect decreasing numbers. Lack of insurance remained a common hazard for the working poor and other unfortunate groups. During the recessionary mid-1970s, a fresh cohort of researchers set out to count and describe the uninsured. In 1975, Leda Judd of the National Urban Coalition estimated that more than 40 million Americans lacked health insurance. For those under sixty-five, Judd found 44 percent of nonwhites, 30 percent of divorced women, and 26 percent of service workers unprotected. Karen Davis of the Brookings Institution helped to fill in the unhappy picture by observing that disproportionate numbers of low-wage workers, southerners, farmers, African Americans, and the disabled were without coverage. Davis noted that fully 75 percent of poor children had no hospital insurance. Critics aligned with the resurgent women's movement illuminated the extent to which the soaring divorce rate was cutting women off from their husband's employment-based benefits. Beyond the plight of the divorced, feminists brought attention to barriers to access for women who were separated, widowed, nonwhite, or poor. However, the sympathetic attention that the uninsured received from a small number of engaged intellectuals and other advocates of social justice did not do much to alter the tenor or direction of the policy discussion.[51]

By the end of the 1970s, another attempt to achieve universal health care had failed miserably. The short-lived rights revolution swept in neither incremental nor transformative change. Progressives had deployed their well-worn repertoire of humanitarian, rights, and productivist arguments in a different configuration, but with the same result. The contrast with the experience of the civil rights movement could hardly be starker. Claiming rights in the black freedom struggle helped to mobilize large numbers of African Americans to take highly committed, often life-endangering, action and galvanized white sympathizers into significant supporting work. Despite a universalist consensus, the language of health rights generated no mass activism. Just as the private welfare state had undercut the possibility for large-scale mobilization of the working class, the passage of Medicare and Medicaid drew much of the activist energy of the very poor and the elderly away from the cause of universal health care and into advocacy on behalf of their own special interests, especially as those interests were threatened by cutbacks.[52] Nonetheless, the public-private patchwork continued to exclude tens of millions of Americans, mainly in the ranks of the working poor, who might well have been receptive to such rhetoric if it had reached them. The paucity of effective channels of communication to the uninsured meant that this emancipatory message stayed largely within the confines of elite policy and political networks. Moreover, foreshadowings of a wholesale assault on social entitlements were already evident.

# Alone among the Developed Nations

> In a world where most industrialized countries concentrate their resources
> in one health insurance system that provides universal or nearly univer-
> sal coverage to their populations, the United States presents an altogether
> different picture. Its array of uncoordinated private and public programs
> underscores society's profound ambivalence about whether medical care
> for all is a social good, of which the costs should be borne by society.
>
> —JOHN IGLEHART, 1992

> Health care reform is necessary. The public recognizes that the United
> States stands alone among the developed nations in failing to ensure
> access to health care for all its citizens.
>
> —NICOLE LURIE, STEVEN MILES,
> AND DAVID HAUGEN, 1993

After 1980, the context of health policymaking in the United States changed profoundly. New currents of of globalization engendered a fresh receptivity to the possibility that this nation might be able to learn something of value from foreign experience. When the health status of citizens of many other nations surpassed that of American citizens, it became more difficult to ignore foreign patterns of delivering and financing health care. With the drive to restrain costs dominating the policy agenda in the United States, the ability of other advanced nations to cover their entire population at a significantly smaller share of their gross domestic product became a source of particular curiosity.[1]

In these much-altered circumstances, proponents of universal health in-surance attempted to use invidious international comparisons to reshape dis-cussion of the plight of those without ready access to care. To be sure, advo-cates of ameliorative change in the late twentieth century continued to rely upon and refashion familiar arguments based on rights, efficiencies, and hu-manitarianism. But clearly, the important innovative rationale for reform that came to the fore during the 1980s and 1990s was pragmatic: this nation could learn from other nations' success in achieving universal access. (American champions of state insurance during the second decade of the twentieth century sought to follow the precedents set in western Europe, but their touchstones were far from universal.) Universalists in the United States hoped that the wealth of foreign experience would reduce apprehension about the immensity of the challenge of reform.

## Privations of Privatism

Intensified global economic competition combined with escalating medical costs to undermine the private welfare state. A "race to the bottom" strategy caused countless American employers to curtail health benefits. Whereas some firms, especially those in the manufacturing sector, faced a genuine crisis, others used the pretext of globalization and the associated weakening of organized labor to reduce their commitment to employee health security. Even those American employers most insulated from foreign competition suffered from ever-increasing health-care costs, which translated directly into higher premium rates for employee insurance. Per capita expenditures on health services in the United States grew from $1,637 in 1984 to a staggering $4,631 in 2000. Many businesses discontinued longstanding benefit programs. One leading consultant group estimated that for every one percent increase in health costs, 300,000 people lost their insurance coverage. New businesses often excluded health insurance from their compensation plans. Many companies offered benefits only to a dwindling corps of full-time "core" staff. Many shifted so much of the premium payments to staff that many workers could not afford to participate in the insurance program. Abandonment or hollowing-out of employee protection extended from marginal enterprises all the way up to the Fortune 500. By the end of the century, a series of unsettling changes had installed an anti-paternalistic style of management, under which a much smaller share of the American workforce expected to attain health security (or any other form of security, for that matter) through the employment relationship. In 2003, less than half the nation's private-sector workers had employment-based health coverage.[2]

The goal of universal health care became ever more distant over the decades following the Carter administration. Since 1980, the number of uninsured Americans—the vast majority of whom are members of working families and a disproportionate share of whom are members of disadvantaged minorities—has risen almost without interruption. The revelation that the ranks of the uninsured swelled from 33 million in 1983, a year of severe recession, to 37 million in 1986, a year of buoyant recovery, underscored both the immensity of the problem and the degree to which this problem afflicted the employed as well as the unemployed. With so many other nations protecting all their citizens, the worsening situation stood out in stark relief. Economist Uwe Reinhardt did not mince words when he appraised the unique limitations of the American system for a congressional panel in 1986: "Canada, France, Germany, Italy—every other country in the civilized world—provides its citizens with the dignity of accessing health care without having to beg for it." In subsequent years, the architects of managed care did virtually nothing to bring a modicum of security to the working poor and others lacking health benefits. By the mid-1990s, the number of uninsured exceeded 40 million. In 2002, almost 44 million Americans had no health insurance.[3]

Awareness of the superior state of physical well-being enjoyed by citizens of many other nations helped to stimulate more rigorous inquiry into the unmet needs of the uninsured. Researchers investigated insurance status to see whether lack of coverage meant deprivation of services. In 1983, Karen Davis and Diane Rowland punctured the hardy illusion that the uninsured somehow managed to obtain all the care they needed. Davis and Rowland reported that those without insurance or cash "are turned away from hospitals even in emergency situations" and that insured Americans received 90 percent more hospital care than their uninsured fellow citizens, even though the latter tended to be sicker. They also noted that postponed care inflicted emotional strain and sometimes led to life-threatening crises. In its 1990 position paper supporting universal access, the American College of Physicians expressed its disappointment that for financial reasons hospitals refused to help at least a million people a year. A national survey in 1999 found that approximately half of all uninsured adults went without needed care during the previous year. Although quantitative analysis had become the norm in the burgeoning academic field of health services research, dramatic anecdotal reports continued to appear involving outright refusal to treat the uninsured or peremptory dumping after minimal treatment.[4]

Investigators assessed not only the amount of care received by uninsured Americans but also their level of well-being. They discovered that babies born into uninsured families had significantly higher rates of various immediate adverse outcomes, including death. They confirmed a long-suspected pattern: the uninsured waited until they were sicker to seek hospitalization; they received less care upon admission; as a result, they stood a higher risk of dying in the hospital. In 1993, the Institute of Medicine of the National Academy of Sciences concluded that inadequate care given to low-income uninsured individuals had "a profound impact on their health and well-being." By the beginning of the twenty-first century, numerous studies had shown that a lack of insurance contributed to elevated mortality and morbidity for cancer and other dreaded disorders. Moreover, two recent estimates have put the overall excess mortality due to lack of health insurance at roughly 18,000 deaths per year.[5]

## The Uninsured Can Wait Forever

Increased worldwide economic competition promoted harsh public policies for America's most unfortunate citizens. The tidal wave of competition inundating the health-care sector itself made market-oriented solutions irresistible to many designing and making health policy. Cost containment became the unquestioned priority in the political environment of the late twentieth century. Expanding access to care for the working class was very much on the back burner of the neo-Darwinist agenda. In the playground of health politics during the second Gilded Age, business was "the fat kid on the seesaw," as Linda Bergthold put it. Conversely, the ailing labor movement lost the capability to lead a strong countervailing progressive coalition.[6]

Health reformers relied less on rights rhetoric after 1980. The backlash against federal entitlements made extraconstitutional claims to health rights unattractive to all but the most intrepid universalists. Nonetheless, some medical ethicists joined a handful of progressive stalwarts in pressing the case for a moral, if not strictly legal, right to providing needed care despite the inhospitable political environment. But bioethicists hardly presented a monolithic front. A presidential commission on the ethics of access chose to cast its 1983 report in terms of societal obligations, not individual rights. The logic of rights invoked abroad did not easily translate into the distinctive idiom of American political culture. American reformers seldom stressed the point that European and Canadian health-care entitlements constituted social rights. Nancy Fraser and Linda Gordon found it "telling . . . that people in the United States rarely speak of 'social citizenship.'" Ongoing attempts to place health care within the framework of global human rights failed to gain traction.[7]

Doubts about the effectiveness of rights-based advocacy were evident even when it appeared to be on the verge of a renaissance. By far the most well-known assertion of a right to health services occurred in 1991 during the campaign to fill a vacated Senate seat in Pennsylvania. Before seizing on the health issue, Democratic candidate Harris Wofford trailed opponent Richard Thornburgh by more than forty points. Then the underdog began to emphasize this message: "If criminals have the right to a lawyer, I think working Americans should have the right to a doctor." Wofford won the election and resurrected universal health insurance as a national issue. However, Wofford's colleague Jay Rockefeller counseled the Clinton presidential campaign in August 1992 to avoid the "dead-end approach" of staking out a new right at a time when too few voters wanted to help pay for more generous social rights. The Clinton team heeded Rockefeller's advice.[8]

By the time Bill Clinton assumed the presidency in 1993, the plight of the uninsured had become a major national concern. As early as 1986, Willis Goldbeck of the Washington Business Group on Health projected a dismal scenario in which there would soon be 50 million uninsured. Emily Friedman's 1991 overview of the situation in the *Journal of the American Medical Association* appeared under the urgent title, "The Uninsured: From Dilemma to Crisis." "We claim that other nations ration care because the insured must wait sometimes," wrote Friedman. "In our nation, the uninsured can wait forever." There was a consensus that something had to be done for the expanding uninsured population, but nothing close to a consensus on the proper course of action. One contingent of reformers supported a Canadian-inspired proposal for national health insurance, under which the federal government would become the single payer of health-care bills. Although some advocates unquestionably favored the single-payer option primarily because it promised to curb rising costs, others were drawn mainly to its unequivocal universalism. However, skepticism about this approach left the door open to other alternatives, such as those based on mandated employee benefits, expansion of Medicare, or encouragement of market forces.[9]

Bill Clinton accepted the competitive paradigm. Both he and his wife Hillary Rodham Clinton, who chaired the White House health task force in 1993, spurned the Canadian model as infeasible in a society distrustful of government and in which the insurance industry and other conservative interests wielded great influence. Instead, the Clintons sought to reorganize the delivery and financing of health services by "managed competition." This centrist approach aimed to balance the operation of the marketplace and the intervention of the state. (A thorough historical review of this exceedingly complex initiative would be premature at this point. Existing accounts of the Clintons' attempt at reform have already criticized many of its errors of policy design and political execution.) In terms of the quest for all-inclusive health protection, what stands out is the Clinton administration's dedication to universality.[10]

From the outset, the administration made universal provision a crucial objective. The experts advising the presidential task force in 1993 demonstrated a thoroughgoing commitment to this objective. The working group on ethics offered a vision of a morally just health system that rested squarely on the principle of universality. The ethicists revisited the Great Society axiom that access to health care was a precondition for equality of opportunity. Proceeding from the assumption that achieving universal access would involve much more than issuing plastic cards to all Americans, the working group on the special problems of the poor searched for ways to surmount real-world obstacles to needed care.[11]

President Clinton's address to Congress on September 22, 1993, delineated the main features of his forthcoming plan. The speech reflected the shifting terms of social-policy discourse in a regressive time. The president invoked the Founding Fathers' pursuit of life, liberty, and the pursuit of happiness not as the foundation for health rights but only as the source of that most nebulous entity, the American dream. Clinton held that security stood foremost among his guiding principles: "At long last, after decades of false starts, we must make this our most urgent priority, giving every American health security, health care that can never be taken away." For the next several months, the president and his advisors emphasized not the extension of security to the exposed working poor but rather the guarantee of continued protection for a middle class worried about losing the benefits they already possessed. A month later, the final report of the White House task force, describing and explaining its proposal in more detail, carried an unqualified endorsement of universality. C. Everett Koop, a former surgeon general, set the tone for the chapter of the report spelling out the ideals underlying the proposed Health Security Act: "Some things, like universal access, are not negotiable. And that's exactly the way it should be."[12]

Universality remained a beacon for the Clinton administration throughout the ensuing no-holds-barred fight over its plan. In January 1994, the *New York*

*Times* observed that Clinton had "voiced a general willingness to negotiate on nearly all elements of his proposal except the guarantee of universal health insurance coverage." During the last stages of the battle several months later, after scuttling its incomprehensible managed-competition scheme in hopes of a compromise solution, the White House might well have contemplated abandoning universal provision. Nonetheless, the Clintons persevered in a last-ditch effort to salvage inclusive reform. On June 20, 1994, Hillary Clinton advised a group of core supporters to set aside other concerns and concentrate on universal access. A month later, the president finally conceded that he could tolerate legislation that approximated universal protection by taking in 95 percent of the population. This willingness to compromise accomplished nothing. It did, however, serve to illuminate the disingenuousness of some expressions of devotion to universality made by other participants in this exercise.[13]

The incrementalist approach returned to prominence in the aftermath of this debacle. Amid a variety of targeted proposals to build upon the existing system of public and private provision, the most important efforts focused on the vulnerable young. The plight of ten million uninsured children stirred state and then national lawmakers to take ameliorative action. Federal legislation in 1997 encouraged states to extend coverage to low-income children and adolescents either through existing Medicaid plans or through the new State Children's Health Insurance Program. This initiative has achieved only modest gains. In 2002, there were still about eight million uninsured young people in America.[14]

At the beginning of the twenty-first century, the goal of universal health care remains elusive. Future attempts to guarantee care for all Americans will have to confront powerful interests. Obviously, an understanding of the history of the ideal of universal access does not contribute very much, by itself, to surmounting this formidable opposition. However, if reformers embrace a more participatory strategy, an awareness of the universalist tradition may be of significant value. The failure of several reform campaigns relying heavily on elite expertise suggests the imperative need to build a mass movement among the uninsured to reframe the policy debate and the political contest. Needless to say, organizing such a movement among a diffuse and shifting aggregation of disadvantaged individuals will be, under any circumstances, an exceedingly difficult undertaking. However, the success of other unlikely movements offers a glimmer of hope. If breathless coal miners, AIDS victims, and profoundly disabled Americans can build effective mass movements, why can't the uninsured? Large-scale mobilization in pursuit of universal health care by groups like Jobs with Justice since the early 1990s is encouraging in this regard, as is the proliferation of new grassroots health-reform organizations. Taken together, these efforts suggest the potential for a robustly democratic approach. With more than 40 million Americans currently uninsured, there is certainly no shortage of prospective activists. The experience of previous initiatives from below shows the importance of fundamental legitimating principles around which activists can rally. Universality, defined simply as health security for all, may well serve as such a rallying principle for the tens of millions without any protection. After a century of failure to win reform from the top down, maybe it is time for a new strategy.[15]

Even a militant mass movement of the working poor will need allies motivated by a sense of moral purpose. The historical record shows the importance of cross-class coalitions in achieving social reform. This study has shown that doctors have done much more in the policy arena than denounce socialized medicine. Consider Rosemary Stevens's suggestion that renovation of the medical profession's tradition of delivering charity care might "lead to strong political positions on universal health insurance, or some other means of providing reasonable access to services for the whole population." With members of racial and ethnic minorities comprising almost half the uninsured, minority-rights advocates who challenge the inequity of the current state of affairs may find themselves with additional support from concerned scholars and other experts. Others who retain strong humanitarian values could also become more conscientiously engaged with the moral dimensions of health reform. Progressive faith-based organizations, children's advocates, and feminist groups are well positioned to offer both a distinctive critique of the inequities in the prevailing system and compelling arguments for the fairness of universalism.[16]

It is impossible to predict how the conversation on universal health protection will evolve. Nonetheless, it is entirely possible that emerging problems will make insured Americans less resistant to lower-class demands. The rise of new infectious diseases and the resurgence of old ones may turn the uninsured into a greater source of fear for both the insured population in general and those managing industries prone to disruption by outbreaks of fearsome contagious disorders in particular. Ethicist Larry Churchill has noticed that an elevated risk of communicable disease can force a rethinking of individual interest: "The new TB epidemic, superimposed over the AIDS epidemic, is just one indication that, at least in health care, we cannot isolate our self-interest and make trade-offs against the needs of others. The needs of others are not distant objects of my philanthropy but part of my own security." If our society becomes even more unequal, masters and mistresses may want to take steps to avoid acquiring a lethal condition from their uninsured servants. Typhoid Mary, the notorious cook, could well return as SARS Maria, a notorious nanny. The overrepresentation of recent immigrants from the Third World and others of color in both the service occupations and the ranks of the uninsured could also help to stir an anxious white elite to support corrective action. Perhaps researchers will estimate how many Americans suffer illness or death due to diseases transmitted to them by uninsured persons. Economists could calculate what this toll in morbidity and mortality costs the nation in dollars and cents. Such a line of reasoning might sway a society weary of rights claims and unmoved by humanitarian appeals. As historian David Rothman observed in 1993, "Americans do not like to think of themselves as callous and cruel, and yet in their readiness to . . . withhold this most elemental social service, they have been so." Maybe it is time to speak to the callous and cruel in a language they understand.[17]

Future attempts to achieve universal health care will have to overcome the defeatism that surrounds the issue. A fuller awareness of the ingenuity, tenacity, and accomplishments of previous generations of reformers should encourage those who take up this historic challenge. The efforts of champions like C.-E. A. Winslow, Michael Davis, and Martha Eliot, who stayed with this cause for the long haul despite countless setbacks, should be particularly encouraging. A further reminder that past defeats sometimes involved opportunities missed due to dogmatism and misplaced optimism can perhaps prevent the recurrence of those errors. In a battle in which the stakes are life and death, the perfect should never again become the enemy of the good. A century of frustrated universalism should temper the transformative temptation but not extinguish the dreams of those pursuing one of the essential elements of a humane society.[18]

# Acknowledgments

I am happy to acknowledge some of the formative influences that brought me to the subject of this book. During my tenure at the Textile Workers' Health Plan three decades ago, I worked closely with the plan's founding administrator, Dorothy Garfein, who never wavered in her determination to find ways to make good health care accessible to more of the working poor. At the Institute for Health Policy Studies at the University of California at San Francisco, where I spent three years as a Pew Fellow in the early 1980s, I learned a great deal from Phil Lee and his ingenious crew about both the possibilities and the difficulties of crafting a more humane policy. In much the same vein, the sagacious George Silver has spent twenty years trying to teach me how to mix idealism and realism. My late father-in-law, Paul Spear, devoted virtually his entire career to public medicine, committing his considerable skills to the service of some of the nation's poorest citizens and noncitizens in a truly inspiring and unassuming way. It is a real pleasure to have a chance to express my admiration for all these tireless partisans of health security for all. By articulating and, more important, by acting on strong egalitarian convictions, they gave me my bearings for this journey.

Without the help of many able archivists and librarians, I would not have gotten very far with this project. I very much appreciate the efforts of the staff at the Wisconsin Historical Society, the Yale University Library, the National Archives, the Library of Congress, the Jimmy Carter Library, the Catherwood Library and the Olin Library at Cornell University, the Butler Library at Columbia University, the American Philosophical Society Library, the American College of Physicians–American Society of Internal Medicine Archives, the George Meany Memorial Archives, the Reuther Library at Wayne State University, the New York Academy of Medicine, the Paterno Library and the Pattee Library at the Pennsylvania State University, the Lane Medical Library at Stanford University, the Hagley Museum and Library, the Archives Service Center at the University of Pittsburgh, the American Catholic History Research

Center at the Catholic University of America, the Georgetown University Library, and the Moorland-Spingarn Research Center at Howard University. At the risk of overlooking other worthy individuals, I want to thank Peter Gottlieb, Richard Strassberg, Lee Sayrs, and Megan Phillips for their extraordinary helpfulness.

Penn State has supported this venture since its inception. The Department of Labor Studies and Industrial Relations, the Department of History, and the College of the Liberal Arts have provided financial support and other resources. I have been fortunate to work with a series of talented and diligent research assistants—Mark Longfellow, Hai Yi, April Deng, Janet Schaeffer, Kanika Suri, and Suzanna Martin. I have also been the beneficiary of a great deal of patient clerical assistance, for which I am most grateful. Numerous colleagues have given this project their moral support. I thank Ron Filippelli, Mark Wardell, Paul Clark, Gregg Roeber, and especially Nan Woodruff and Dan Letwin for this encouragement.

Since its first incarnation as a sketchy conference paper in 1991, many colleagues have graciously refused to take refuge in the abundance of good excuses for not reading my work. I have benefited from the comments by these readers of various drafts of various portions of the book: Edward Berkowitz, David Brody, Theodore Brown, Dan Cornford, Liz Fee, Gil Gall, Gary Gerstle, Jim Gregory, Beatrix Hoffman, Philip Jenkins, Michael Kazin, the late Stuart Kaufman, Jennifer Klein, Daniel Leab, Mark Leff, Dan Letwin, Nelson Lichtenstein, Jeff Manza, David McBride, Daniel Rodgers, George Silver, Kitty Sklar, and David Thelen. I am most deeply indebted to those hardy readers who took on the full-length manuscript: Daniel Fox, Ron Numbers, Jackie Wehmueller, Martin Schneider, and an anonymous colleague.

The members of my immediate family get their thanks last, yet another indication of their long-suffering plight. My wife, Margaret Spear, has supported this marathon undertaking in countless ways. Her approach to the practice of medicine constantly reminds me that caring is the essence of health care and that everyone deserves decent care. She is also a terrific editor. Words cannot express my gratitude for her loving commitment all along the way. I am delighted to dedicate this book to my daughters, Katherine and Elizabeth. As I worked on a subject that too often seemed like a hopeless quest, I have had the advantage of these two great sources of hope for the future in the midst of my life.

# Notes

| | |
|---|---|
| AALL | American Association for Labor Legislation |
| AFL | American Federation of Labor |
| *AHR* | *American Historical Review* |
| *AJPH* | *American Journal of Public Health* |
| *ALLR* | *American Labor Legislation Review* |
| AMA | American Medical Association |
| APHA | American Public Health Association |
| CNHI | Committee for National Health Insurance |
| CNH | Committee for the Nation's Health |
| CCMC | Committee on the Cost(s) of Medical Care* |
| CIO | Congress of Industrial Organizations |
| *JAH* | *Journal of American History* |
| *JAMA* | *Journal of the American Medical Association* |
| *JNMA* | *Journal of the National Medical Association* |
| *NEJM* | *New England Journal of Medicine* |
| *NYT* | *New York Times* |

## Preface

Epigraphs: Harry S. Truman, "Special Message to the Congress Recommending a Comprehensive Health Program," Nov. 19, 1945, in *Public Papers of the Presidents of the United States: Harry S. Truman, 1945* (Washington: GPO, 1961), 475; George W. Bush, "The State of the Union Address," *Congressional Record* 149 (2003): H212.

1. *NYT*, Feb. 28, 2002, A16 (quotations); Jack Hadley, "Sicker and Poorer—The Consequences of Being Uninsured: A Review of the Research on the Relationship between Health Insurance, Medical Care Use, Health, Work, and Income," *Medical Care Research and Review* 60: suppl. (2003): 3S-75S, esp. 62S; Institute of Medicine, *Care without Coverage: Too Little, Too Late* (Washington: National Academies Press, 2002), passim, esp. 161–65; Peter Franks, Carolyn Clancy, and Marthe Gold, "Health Insurance and Mortality: Evidence from a National Cohort," *JAMA* 270 (1993): 737–41; John Ayanian et al., "Unmet Health Needs of Uninsured Adults in the United States," ibid. 284 (2000): 2061–69; Richard Roetzheim et al., "Effects of Health Insurance and Race on Breast Carcinoma Treatments and Outcomes," *Cancer* 89 (2000): 2202–13; John

---

*Group changed name from "Cost" to "Costs" in 1930.

Ayanian et al., "The Relation between Health Insurance Coverage and Clinical Outcomes among Women with Breast Cancer," *NEJM* 329 (1993): 326–31; David W. Baker et al., "Lack of Insurance and Decline in Overall Health in Late Middle Age," ibid. 345 (2001): 1106–12; Paul Sorlie et al., "Mortality in the Uninsured Compared with That in Persons with Public and Private Health Insurance," *Archives of Internal Medicine* 154 (1994): 2409–16; Natalie Freeman, Dona Schneider, and Patricia McGarvey, "The Relationship of Health Insurance to the Diagnosis and Management of Asthma and Respiratory Problems in Children in a Predominantly Hispanic Urban Community," *AJPH* 93 (2003): 1316–20; John Ayanian et al., "Undiagnosed Hypertension and Hypercholesterolemia among Uninsured and Insured Adults in the Third National Health and Nutrition Examination Survey," ibid., 2051–54. For recent estimates of the uninsured, see U.S. Congressional Budget Office, *How Many People Lack Health Insurance and for How Long?* ([Washington]: Congressional Budget Office, 2003); *NYT*, May 13, 2003, A20; Kim Krisberg, "Uninsurance Rates Signaling Health Crisis," *Nation's Health*, Dec. 2002–Jan. 2003, 14; "US Uninsured Now Number 43.6 Million," ibid., Nov. 2003, 6. On bankruptcies attributable to illness and injury, see Melissa Jacoby, Teresa Sullivan, and Elizabeth Warren, "Rethinking the Debates over Health Care Financing: Evidence from the Bankruptcy Courts," *New York University Law Review* 76 (2001): 375–418.

2. The most helpful overviews are Paul Starr, *The Social Transformation of American Medicine* (New York: Basic Books, 1982); Daniel M. Fox, *Health Policies, Health Politics: The British and American Experience, 1911–1965* (Princeton: Princeton University Press, 1986); David Rothman, *Beginnings Count: The Technological Imperative in American Health Care* (New York: Oxford University Press, 1997); Colin Gordon, *Dead on Arrival: The Politics of Health Care in Twentieth-Century America* (Princeton: Princeton University Press, 2003); Jaap Kooijman, *. . . And the Pursuit of National Health: The Incremental Strategy toward National Health Insurance in the the United States of America* (Amsterdam: Rodopi, 1999); Rosemary Stevens, *In Sickness and in Wealth: American Hospitals in the Twentieth Century* (New York: Basic Books, 1989); Ronald Numbers, ed., *Compulsory Health Insurance: The Continuing American Debate* (Westport, Conn.: Greenwood Press, 1982). Among the most valuable monographs on specific reform campaigns are Ronald Numbers, *Almost Persuaded: American Physicians and Compulsory Health Insurance, 1912–1920* (Baltimore: Johns Hopkins University Press, 1978); Beatrix Hoffman, *The Wages of Sickness: The Politics of Health Insurance in Progressive America* (Chapel Hill: University of North Carolina Press, 2001); Daniel Hirshfield, *The Lost Reform: The Campaign for Compulsory Health Insurance in the United States from 1932 to 1943* (Cambridge: Harvard University Press, 1970); Monte Poen, *Harry S. Truman versus the Medical Lobby: The Genesis of Medicare* (Columbia: University of Missouri Press, 1979); Theodore Marmor, *The Politics of Medicare*, 2d ed. (New York: Aldine de Gruyter, 2000); Theda Skocpol, *Boomerang: Clinton's Health Security Effort and the Turn against Government in U.S. Politics* (New York: W. W. Norton, 1996); Jacob Hacker, *The Road to Nowhere: The Genesis of President Clinton's Plan for Health Security* (Princeton: Princeton University Press, 1997).

CHAPTER ONE: A Fertile and Lively Cause of Poverty

1. Paul Starr, *The Social Transformation of American Medicine* (New York: Basic Books, 1982), 60–117, 155–56; Kenneth Ludmerer, *Learning to Heal: The Development of*

*American Medical Education* (New York: Basic Books, 1985), 3–71; Charles Rosenberg, *The Care of Strangers: The Rise of America's Hospital System* (New York: Basic Books, 1987), 212–28.

2. Sandra Opdycke, *No One Was Turned Away: The Role of Public Hospitals in New York City since 1900* (New York: Oxford University Press, 1999), 4, 10; Harry Dowling, *City Hospitals: The Undercare of the Underprivileged* (Cambridge: Harvard University Press, 1982), 25–44; Rosenberg, *Care of Strangers*, 97–261; Charles Rosenberg, "Social Class and Medical Care in Nineteenth-Century America: The Rise and Fall of the Dispensary," *Journal of the History of Medicine and Allied Sciences* 29 (1974): 32–54.

3. Rosenberg, "Class and Care," 34, 38; Rosenberg, *Care of Strangers*, 238–42; George Rosen, *Fees and Fee Bills: Some Economic Aspects of Medical Practice in Nineteenth-Century America* (Baltimore: Johns Hopkins Press, 1946), 52ff; John Duffy, *From Humors to Medical Science: A History of American Medicine*, 2d ed. (Urbana: University of Illinois Press, 1993), 214–16; Starr, *Social Transformation*, 204–9.

4. Samuel Gompers, *Seventy Years of Life and Labor: An Autobiography*, 2 vols. (New York: E. P. Dutton, 1925), 1: 156–57; David Rosner, "Health Care for the 'Truly Needy': Nineteenth-Century Origins of the Concept," *Milbank Memorial Fund Quarterly* 60 (1982): 355–85, esp. 365–67, 376–80; David Rosner, *A Once Charitable Enterprise: Hospitals and Health Care in Brooklyn and New York, 1885–1915* (Cambridge: Cambridge University Press, 1982), 23, 57; Rosenberg, "Class and Care," 51–52.

5. Starr, *Social Transformation*, 138 (quotation), 134–44; Rosenberg, *Care of Strangers*, 142–65; Duffy, *Humors to Science*, 167–202; Bert Hansen, "America's First Medical Breakthrough: How Popular Excitement about a French Rabies Cure in 1885 Raised New Expectations for Medical Progress," *AHR* 103 (1998): 373–418; Bert Hansen, "New Images of a New Medicine: Visual Evidence for the Widespread Popularity of Therapeutic Discoveries in America after 1885," *Bulletin of the History of Medicine* 73 (1999): 629–78.

6. Martin Bulmer, Kevin Bales, and Kathryn Kish Sklar, eds., *The Social Survey in Historical Perspective, 1880–1940* (Cambridge: Cambridge University Press, 1991); Theda Skocpol, *Protecting Soldiers and Mothers: The Political Origins of Social Policy in the United States* (Cambridge: Belknap Press of Harvard University Press, 1992), 161–71; Kathryn Kish Sklar, *Florence Kelley and the Nation's Work: The Rise of Women's Political Culture, 1830–1900* (New Haven: Yale University Press, 1995), passim, esp. 277–79; Dorothy Ross, *The Origins of American Social Science* (Cambridge: Cambridge University Press, 1991), 143–59; Mary Furner, *Advocacy and Objectivity: A Crisis in the Professionalization of American Social Science, 1865–1905* (Lexington: University Press of Kentucky, 1975), passim, esp. 265–73; Alice O'Connor, *Poverty Knowledge: Social Science, Social Policy, and the Poor in Twentieth-Century U.S. History* (Princeton: Princeton University Press, 2001), 25–44.

7. Robert Hunter, *Poverty* (New York: Macmillan, 1904), 148 (quotation), 143 (quotation), 144 (quotation), 2.

8. Ibid., 148 (quotation), 146–49.

9. Ibid., 12 (quotation), 181 (quotation), 338–39 (quotation), 11–13, 338–40.

10. Louis More, *Wage Earners' Budgets: A Study of Standards and Cost of Living in New York City* (New York: Henry Holt, 1907), 144 (quotation), 115–16, 150; Edward Devine, *Misery and Its Causes* (New York: Macmillan, 1909), 54 (quotation), 108 (quotation), 53–112; Margaret Byington, *Homestead: The Households of a Mill Town* (1910;

Pittsburgh: University of Pittsburgh Press, 1974), 87 (quotation), 82–96, 182. On the larger project of which Byington's work formed a part, see Steven R. Cohen, "The Pittsburgh Survey and the Social Survey Movement: A Sociological Road Not Taken," in *Social Survey in Perspective*, ed. Bulmer, Bales, and Sklar, 245–68.

11. Lawrence Glickman, *A Living Wage: American Workers and the Making of Consumer Society* (Ithaca: Cornell University Press, 1997), 55–91. Recent studies of the health implications of low wages and economic inequality include R. G. Wilkinson, "Income Distribution and Life Expectancy," *British Medical Journal* 304 (1992): 165–68; George A. Kaplan et al., "Inequality in Income and Mortality in the United States: Analysis of Mortality and Potential Pathways," ibid., 312 (1996): 999–1003; Bruce Kennedy et al., "Income Distribution and Mortality: Cross Sectional Ecological Study of the Robin Hood Index in the United States," ibid., 1004–7; Norman Daniels, Bruce Kennedy, and Ichiro Kawachi, *Is Inequality Bad for Our Health?* (Boston: Beacon Press, 2000).

12. Richard Ely, "Introduction," in John A. Ryan, *A Living Wage: Its Ethical and Economic Aspects* (New York: Macmillan, 1906), xii (quotation), xi–xiii; Glickman, *Living Wage*, 134–35. For the inspiration, see Pope Leo XIII, *Rerum Novarum*, in National Conference of Catholic Bishops, comp., *Contemporary Catholic Social Teaching* (Washington: United States Catholic Conference, 1991), 15–43; Aaron Abell, "The Reception of Leo XIII's Labor Encyclical in America, 1891–1919," *Review of Politics* 7 (1945): 464–95. On Protestantism and Progressivism, see Robert Crunden, *Ministers of Reform: The Progressives' Achievement in American Civilization, 1889–1920* (New York: Basic Books, 1982); Ross, *Origins of American Social Science*, chaps. 9–10; Linda Gordon, "Social Insurance and Public Assistance: The Influence of Gender in Welfare Thought in the United States, 1890–1935," *AHR* 97 (1992): 23. On the antecedents of Progressive Catholicism, see Robert D. Cross, *The Emergence of Liberal Catholicism in America* (Cambridge: Harvard University Press, 1958).

13. Ryan, *Living Wage*, 64 (quotation), 67 (quotation), 326 (quotation), 312 (quotation), 43–80, 324–26.

14. Ibid., 127 (Smart quotation), 132 (quotation), 328 (quotation), 107–8 (quotation), 110–36; William J. White, "The Facts Considered," *Charities and the Commons*, Nov. 17, 1906, 321–22; William J. White, review of *A Living Wage*, ibid., Dec. 15, 1906, 471–72; John A. Ryan, *Social Doctrine in Action: A Personal History* (New York: Harper and Brothers, 1941), 80–82. Alice Kessler-Harris has trenchantly observed that defenders of a living wage for female workers during the Progressive Era believed that it should be less generous than the living wage for men. See Alice Kessler-Harris, *A Woman's Wage: Historical Meanings and Social Consequences* (Lexington: University Press of Kentucky, 1990), 8–12. For an argument (helpfully pointed out to me by Eileen Boris) that a living wage was thought to be instrumental to a right to a healthy childhood free from premature labor, see Florence Kelley, *Some Ethical Gains through Legislation* (New York: Macmillan, 1905), 5, 66, 69.

15. Samuel Gompers, "Wages and Health," *American Federationist*, Aug. 1914, 642–44; Glickman, *Living Wage*, 62ff.

16. James Kloppenberg, *Uncertain Victory: Social Democracy and Progressivism in European and American Thought, 1870–1920* (New York: Oxford University Press, 1986); Daniel Rodgers, *Atlantic Crossings: Social Politics in a Progressive Age* (Cambridge: Belknap Press of Harvard University Press, 1998), esp. 209–66; David A. Moss, *Socializing Security: Progressive-Era Economists and the Origins of American Social Policy*

(Cambridge: Harvard University Press, 1996); Beatrix Hoffman, *The Wages of Sickness: The Politics of Health Insurance in Progressive America* (Chapel Hill: University of North Carolina Press, 2001), 24–56.

17. Moss, *Socializing Security*, 4–6.

18. John Commons and Arthur Altmeyer, "The Health Insurance Movement in the United States," in Ohio, Health and Old Age Insurance Commission, *Health, Health Insurance, Old Age Pensions: Report, Recommendations, Dissenting Opinions* (Columbus: F. J. Heer, 1919), 291; Starr, *Social Transformation*, 237–38; Hoffman, *Wages of Sickness*, 27–29.

19. [AALL], "Necessary Standards for Sickness Insurance," June 13, 1914 (quotation), *American Association for Labor Legislation Papers, 1905–1945*, microfilm ed., 71 reels (Glen Rock, N.J.: Microfilming Corporation of America, 1973), reel 11; [Joseph] Chamberlain and [Isaac] Rubinow, "Necessary Standards of Sickness Insurance," June 1914, ibid., reel 62; Joseph Chamberlain, "Compulsory Health Insurance and Its Organization," Sept. 14, 1916, ibid.; I. M. Rubinow, "Health Insurance in Its Relation to Public Health," *JAMA* 67 (1916): 1011–12; Commons and Altmeyer, "Health Insurance Movement," 287–88, 297–99. For an estimate that the workers' compensation laws of the 1910s covered about a quarter of the workforce, see Morton Keller, *Regulating a New Society: Public Policy and Social Change in America, 1900–1933* (Cambridge: Harvard University Press, 1994), 201. On Progressives and efficiency, see James A. Smith, *The Idea Brokers: Think Tanks and the Rise of the New Policy Elite* (New York: Free Press, 1991), 46–67; Samuel Haber, *Efficiency and Uplift: Scientific Management in the Progressive Era* (Chicago: University of Chicago Press, 1964). For a highly tortuous defense of social insurance based on an especially expansive notion of efficiency, see Louis Brandeis, "Workingmen's Insurance—The Road to Social Efficiency," *Proceedings of the National Conference of Charities and Correction, Thirty-Eighth Annual Session, 1911* (Fort Wayne, Ind.: Fort Wayne Printing, 1911), 156–62. For emphasis on male wage-earners, see William Willoughby, *Workingmen's Insurance* (New York: T. Y. Crowell, 1898); Lee Frankel and Miles Dawson, *Workingmen's Insurance in Europe* (New York: Charities Publication Committee, 1910); Hoffman, *Wages of Sickness*, 29–31. On gender inequality in U.S. social provision, see, among others, Gordon, "Social Insurance and Public Assistance," 19–54; Linda Gordon, *Pitied But Not Entitled: Single Mothers and the History of Welfare* (Cambridge: Harvard University Press, 1995); Barbara Nelson, "The Origins of the Two-Channel Welfare State: Workmen's Compensation and Mothers' Aid," in *Women, the State, and Welfare*, ed. Linda Gordon (Madison: University of Wisconsin Press, 1990), 123–51; Ann Shola Orloff, "Gender in Early U.S. Social Policy," *Journal of Policy History* 3 (1991): 249–81; Skocpol, *Protecting Soldiers and Mothers*.

20. I. M. Rubinow, "Medical Services under Health Insurance," in U.S. Bureau of Labor Statistics, *Proceedings of the Conference on Social Insurance*, Bulletin 212 (Washington: GPO, 1917), 686 (quotation), 685–86; I. M. Rubinow, *Standards of Health Insurance* (New York: Henry Holt, 1916), 22; Olga Halsey to Josephine Baker, Jan. 27, 1916, *AALL Papers*, reel 16.

21. Lee Frankel, "Some Fundamental Considerations in Health Insurance," in BLS, *Conference on Social Insurance*, 212 (quotation; italics in original); AALL, *The Gist of the Health Insurance Bill* (New York: AALL, [1916]); John Andrews to Social Insurance Committee, Nov. 3, 1916, *AALL Papers*, reel 17. For loose use of the term "universal" by the AALL, see "Recent American Opinion in Favor of Health Insurance," *ALLR* 6

(1916): 348–49; John Andrews, "Proposed Legislation for Health Insurance," in BLS, *Conference on Social Insurance*, 554, 557.

22. Rubinow, *Standards of Health Insurance*, 30 (quotation), 91 (quotation), 29–39, 90–93; Olga Halsey to John Andrews, Nov. 3, 1914, *AALL Papers*, reel 13; John Andrews to Olga Halsey, Nov. 7, 1914, ibid.; Halsey to Eden Delphey, Feb. 5, 1916, ibid., reel 16; Louis Harris, "Discussion," in BLS, *Conference on Social Insurance*, 715. On Halsey and her important contributions, see Hoffman, *Wages of Sickness*, passim, esp. 39–41. For an overview of Rubinow's activism, see J. Lee Kreader, "Isaac Max Rubinow: Pioneering Specialist in Social Insurance," *Social Service Review* 50 (1976): 402–25. On the problematic notion of "dependency" and its relation to the family-wage ideal, see Nancy Fraser and Linda Gordon, "A Genealogy of *Dependency*: Tracing a Keyword of the U.S. Welfare State," *Signs* 19 (1994): 309–36, esp. 314–19.

23. S. S. Goldwater, "Why I Favor the Mills Bill," Mar. 1917, *AALL Papers*, reel 62; Editorial, "Social Insurance in California," *JAMA* 65 (1915): 1560 (quotation); B. S. Warren, "Sickness Insurance: A Preventive of Charity Practice," ibid., 2059 (quotation), 2056–59; Hoffman, *Wages of Sickness*, 30.

24. Ronald Numbers, *Almost Persuaded: American Physicians and Compulsory Health Insurance, 1912–1920* (Baltimore: Johns Hopkins University Press, 1978), 37ff; Hoffman, *Wages of Sickness*, 45ff.

25. Samuel Gompers, "Statement," in U.S. House of Representatives, Committee on Labor, *Commission to Study Social Insurance and Unemployment: Hearings . . . on H. J. Res. 159*, 64th Cong., 1st sess., 1916 (Washington: GPO, 1918), 130 (quotation), 129–30; Samuel Gompers, "Labor versus Its Barnacles," *American Federationist*, Apr. 1916, 271 (quotation), 268–74; Frederick Hoffman to Irving Fisher, Dec. 11, 1916 (quotation), *AALL Papers*, reel 17; Samuel Gompers to William Gorgas, Apr. 8 and Apr. 12, 1916, in AFL, *Letterpress Copybooks of Samuel Gompers and William Green, Presidents, 1883–1925*, microfilm ed., 343 reels (Washington: Library of Congress, 1967), reel 206; Samuel Gompers, "Not Even Compulsory Benevolence Will Do," *American Federationist*, Jan. 1917, 47–48. For estimates of union membership, see Leo Troy, *Trade Union Membership, 1897–1962* (New York: National Bureau of Economic Research, 1965), 2.

26. D. R. Kennedy, "General Discussion [at AALL annual meeting]," *ALLR* 7 (1917): 62 (quotation); Samuel Gompers, *Seventy Years of Life and Labor: An Autobiography*, 2 vols. (New York: E. P. Dutton, 1925), 1: 42, 144–45, 167; Samuel Gompers, "The Next Step toward Emancipation," *American Federationist*, Dec. 1899, 248–49; James B. Kennedy, *Beneficiary Features of American Trade Unions* (Baltimore: Johns Hopkins Press, 1908), 7–83; Olga Halsey, "What's Wrong with the Bill," [spring 1917], *AALL Papers*, reel 62; Frederick Hoffman to John Andrews, Jan. 13, 1915, ibid., reel 13; Frederick Hoffman, "Systems of Wage-Earners' Insurance," *ALLR* 3 (1913): 227–28; T. Leigh Thompson, "The Un-American Doctrine of Compulsory Health Insurance," *Economic World*, Mar. 4, 1916, 315; David Beito, *From Mutual Aid to the Welfare State: Fraternal Societies and Social Services, 1890–1967* (Chapel Hill: University of North Carolina Press, 2000), 152.

27. B. S. Warren and Edgar Sydenstricker, "The Relation of Wages to the Public Health," *AJPH* 8 (1918): 887 (quotation); Irving Fisher, "The Need for Health Insurance," *ALLR* 7 (1917): 9–23 passim, esp. 23; U.S., Commission on Industrial Relations, *Industrial Relations: Final Report and Testimony*, 11 vols. (Washington: GPO, 1916), 1: 68, 124–27. On the Commission on Industrial Relations, its context, and its recommendations, see Julie Greene, "Negotiating the State: Frank Walsh and the Transfor-

mation of Labor's Political Culture in Progressive America," in *Organized Labor and American Politics, 1894–1994: The Labor-Liberal Alliance*, ed. Kevin Boyle (Albany: State University of New York Press, 1998), 71–102, esp. 78–81; Leon Fink, *Progressive Intellectuals and the Dilemmas of Democratic Commitment* (Cambridge: Harvard University Press, 1997), 80–113.

28. Administrative Committee of the National Catholic War Council, *Program of Social Reconstruction*, in *Justice in the Marketplace: Collected Statements of the Vatican and the United States Catholic Bishops on Economic Policy, 1891–1984*, ed. David Byers (Washington: United States Catholic Conference, 1985), 374 (quotation), 377 (quotations), 372–78, 382–83; John A. Ryan, *Social Reconstruction* (New York: Macmillan, 1920), 203 (quotation), 10–21, 81–99, 202–3, 208–9; Francis Broderick, *Right Reverend New Dealer: John A. Ryan* (New York: Macmillan, 1963), 105 (quotation), 104–8; William Kerby, *The Social Mission of Charity: A Study of Points of View in Catholic Charities* (New York: Macmillan, 1921), 61–71; Edward Hanna to Bishop [Peter] Muldoon, [Apr. 1919?], National Catholic War Council Records, box 5, folder 14, American Catholic History Research Center and University Archives, Catholic University of America, Washington; John A. Ryan, "The Workingman's Needs," [Nov. 1922?], John A. Ryan Papers, box 63, folder 9, ibid.; John A. Ryan, "The Teaching of the Catholic Church," *Annals of the American Academy of Political and Social Science* 103 (1922): 76–80, esp. 76; Joseph McShane, *"Sufficiently Radical": Catholicism, Progressivism, and the Bishops' Program of 1919* (Washington: Catholic University of America Press, 1986); Dorothy M. Brown and Elizabeth McKeown, *The Poor Belong to Us: Catholic Charities and American Welfare* (Cambridge: Harvard University Press, 1997), 63–64. On gendered wage policy, see Martha May, "The Historical Problem of the Family Wage: The Ford Motor Company and the Five Dollar Day," *Feminist Studies* 8 (1982): 399–424; Kessler-Harris, *Woman's Wage*, 1–56.

29. Fisher, "Need for Insurance," 14 (quotation), 13–14; Edgar Sydenstricker, "Existing Agencies for Health Insurance in the United States," in BLS, *Conference on Social Insurance*, 471 (quotation), 430–75 passim, esp. 431–32, 470–71, 475; Pauline Newman, "What Will Health Insurance Mean to the Insured?" *American Journal of Nursing* 17 (1917): 943 (quotation), 942–45; Rubinow, *Standards*, 21–22; "Prominent Labor Organizations Already on Record for Health Insurance," *ALLR* 8 (1918): 319. On Pauline Newman's career, see Ann Schofield, *"To Do and to Be": Portraits of Four Women Activists, 1893–1986* (Boston: Northeastern University Press, 1997), 82–112. On the ILGWU health program, see Gus Tyler, *Look for the Union Label: A History of the International Ladies' Garment Workers' Union* (Armonk, N.Y.: M. E. Sharpe, 1995), 125–33; Daniel E. Bender, "Inspecting Workers: Medical Examination, Labor Organizing, and the Evidence of Sexual Difference," *Radical History Review* 80 (2001): 51–75, esp. 62–68. On the insurance debate within organized labor, see Alan Derickson, " 'Take Health from the List of Luxuries': Labor and the Right to Health Care, 1915–1949," *Labor History* 41 (2000): 173–77.

30. Grant Hamilton, "Proposed Legislation for Health Insurance," in BLS, *Conference on Social Insurance*, 563 (quotation), 564 (quotation); Gompers, "Compulsory Benevolence," 48 (quotation); Committee on Social Insurance, AFL, "Report," in AFL Executive Council, "Minutes of Meetings," Feb. 25, 1920, Appendix, 9, AFL Executive Council Minutes [Collection], George Meany Memorial Archives, Silver Spring, Md.; National Industrial Conference Board, *Sickness Insurance or Sickness Prevention?*

(Boston: National Industrial Conference Board, 1918), 14 (quotation), 22; Olga Halsey, "Objections against Health Insurance Urged by Dr. Hoffman," 1917, *AALL Papers*, reel 62; Hoffman, *Wages of Sickness*, 58–60. For a reformer who saw no point in denying that state health insurance was class legislation, see I. M. Rubinow, "Sickness Insurance," *ALLR* 3 (1913): 162.

31. John Andrews to Willard Fisher, Mar. 17, 1916, *AALL Papers*, reel 16; Frederick L. Hoffman to John Andrews, Oct. 21, 1914, ibid., reel 14; Moss, *Socializing Security*, 142–43; Michael T. Bennett, "The Movement for Compulsory Health Insurance in Illinois, 1912–1920," *Illinois Historical Journal* 89 (1996): 236. On the general pattern of governmental investigation, see Mary Furner, "Knowing Capitalism: Public Investigation and the Labor Question in the Long Progressive Era," in *The State and Economic Knowledge: The American and British Experiences*, ed. Mary Furner and Barry Supple (Cambridge: Cambridge University Press, 1990), 241–86; Dietrich Rueschemeyer and Theda Skocpol, eds., *States, Social Knowledge, and the Origins of Modern Social Policies* (Princeton: Princeton University Press, 1996). On the misplaced optimism of reformers and their historians, see Daniel M. Fox, "The Decline of Historicism: The Case of Compulsory Health Insurance," *Bulletin of the History of Medicine* 57 (1983): 596–609.

32. "Scope and Methods of Investigations," *ALLR* 8 (1918): 142–46; John Andrews to Ira Cross, June 2, 1915, *AALL Papers*, reel 14; [Isaac Rubinow] to Barbara Nachtrieb, Mar. 27, 1916, Isaac Rubinow Papers, box 2, folder 31, Kheel Center for Labor-Management Documentation and Archives, Catherwood Library, Cornell University, Ithaca.

33. California, Social Insurance Commission, *Report, 1917* (Sacramento: State Printing Office, 1917), 9 (quotation), 10 (quotation), 28 (quotation), 9–10, 27–29; John Andrews to Ira Cross, June 2, 1915, *AALL Papers*, reel 14; [Isaac Rubinow] to Barbara Nachtrieb, Mar. 27, 1916, Isaac Rubinow Papers, box 2, folder 31; Arthur Viseltear, "Compulsory Health Insurance in California, 1915–18," *Journal of the History of Medicine and Allied Sciences* 24 (1969): 154–56; Barbara Nachtrieb Armstrong, interview by Peter Corning, Dec. 19, 1965, transcript, 6, 20, Oral History Collection, Oral History Research Office, Butler Library, Columbia University, New York.

34. California Commission, *Report*, 33 (quotation), 53 (quotation), 30–53.

35. Ibid., 16 (quotation), 14, 84, 229, 232, 240.

36. Ibid., 39 (quotation), 45 (quotation), 15, 34–46, 116; *San Francisco Chronicle*, Nov. 22, 1916, 8.

37. California Commission, *Report*, 52 (quotation), 46–54; California Social Insurance Commission, *Do You Know This Girl?* (San Francisco: The Commission, [1918]).

38. California Commission, *Report*, 16 (quotation), 16–23, 287–89. Although the estimate of the covered population apparently indicated the absence of "dependent" coverage, the commission proposed language for a constitutional amendment that contradicted that position: "It is hereby declared to be the policy of the State of California to make special provision for the health and welfare of those classes of persons, and their dependents, whose incomes, in the determination of the legislature, are not sufficient to meet the hazards of sickness. The legislature may establish a health insurance system, applicable to any or all such persons." California Commission, *Report*, 17 (quotation), 17–18.

39. Ohio, Health and Old Age Insurance Commission, *Health, Health Insurance, Old Age Pensions: Report, Recommendations, Dissenting Opinions, 1919* (Columbus: F. J.

Heer, 1919), 156 (quotation), 159; Pennsylvania, Health Insurance Commission, *Report, 1919* (Harrisburg: J. L. L. Kuhn, 1919), 158; Illinois, Health Insurance Commission, *Report, 1919* (Springfield: Illinois State Journal, 1919), 108–48, esp. 108, 142; John Andrews, "Recent Developments in the United States in Favor of Health Insurance," [late 1919], *AALL Papers*, reel 63; Massachusetts, Special Commission on Social Insurance, *Report, 1917* (Boston: Wright and Potter, 1917), 18, 32, 175.

40. Massachusetts Commission, *Report*, 20 (quotation), 19–20; Pennsylvania Commission, *Report*, 6 (quotation), 4; Commons and Altmeyer, "Health Insurance Movement," 632; Frederick Davenport, "Address before United Meeting of Women's Conference of the State of New York and State Federation of Labor," Aug. 27, 1919, *AALL Papers*, reel 63.

41. [Olga Halsey], "Health Insurance," 4 (quotation), 1919, *AALL Papers*, reel 63; Pennsylvania Commission, *Report*, 107, 114–15; Ohio Commission, *Report*, 2, 59–60; Illinois Commission, *Report*, 18–22; Wisconsin, Special Committee on Social Insurance, *Report, 1919* (Madison: Democrat Printing, 1919), 12.

42. Massachusetts Commission, *Report*, 11 (quotation); [Halsey], "Health Insurance," 6, *AALL Papers*, reel 63; Gordon, "Insurance and Assistance," 30–31; Skocpol, *Protecting Soldiers and Mothers*, 182–83. On AALL faith in social science, see Moss, *Socializing Security*, 26–27, 36–38. For the many uses of government statistics, see William Alonso and Paul Starr, eds., *The Politics of Numbers* (New York: Russell Sage Foundation, 1987). For quantitative policy-related work by early female social investigators, see Ellen Fitzpatrick, *Endless Crusade: Women Social Scientists and Progressive Reform* (New York: Oxford University Press, 1990), passim, esp. 66–69, 87–91; Gordon, "Social Insurance and Public Assistance," 40–41.

43. John Lapp, "The Findings of Official Health Insurance Commissions," *ALLR* 10 (1920): 27–40; Numbers, *Almost Persuaded*, 64–109; Hoffman, *Wages of Sickness*, 55ff; Starr, *Social Transformation*, 252–57; Viseltear, "Insurance in California," 171–82.

44. *San Francisco Chronicle*, Nov. 22, 1916, 8 (Whitney quotation, Harris quotation), Nov. 21, 1916, 9 (Mullen quotation), Nov. 23, 1916, 2; C. D. Stuart to John Andrews, Nov. 10, 1918 (quotations), *AALL Papers*, reel 18; Charles Henderson, "The Right of the Worker to Social Protection," *Proceedings of the National Conference of Charities and Corrections at the 41st Annual Session, 1914* (Fort Wayne, Ind.: Fort Wayne Printing, 1914), 356–57 (quotation; italics in original).

45. Rufus Potts, "Statement," in House, *Commission*, 20 (quotation), 23–24, 29–31; Rufus Potts, *Addresses and Papers on Insurance* (Springfield, Ill.: Schnepp and Barnes, 1917), 11 (quotation), 19 (quotation), 21 (quotation), 15 (quotation), 7–21, 34, 83–97; Rufus Potts, "Extracts from Preliminary Report to the Social Insurance Committee of the National Convention of Insurance Commissioners," in House, *Commission*, 229–30; Rufus Potts, "Joint-Stock Company Health Insurance," in BLS, *Conference on Social Insurance*, 517–18; Bennett, "Movement in Illinois," 234–35.

46. James Warbasse, "The Socialization of Medicine," *JAMA* 63 (1914): 264 (quotation); Eden Delphey, "Discussion," in BLS, *Conference on Social Insurance*, 622 (quotation); John Lentz, "Fraternal Societies under Universal Health Insurance," *ALLR* 7 (1917): 79–81, 84. On the tendency to justify social protection by service to the common welfare, see Orloff, "Gender in Policy," 256–57. For an echo of Warbasse's argument, albeit in defense of a nonuniversal proposition, see S. S. Goldwater, "Why I Favor the Mills Health Insurance Bill," Mar. 1917, *AALL Papers*, reel 62. On a few occasions, AALL

leaders made rights arguments for their less-than-universal plan. See Miles Dawson, "What Will Health Insurance Do for the American Citizen?" Mar. 1917, ibid.

47. James T. Patterson, *America's Struggle against Poverty in the Twentieth Century* (Cambridge: Harvard University Press, 2000), 18 (quotation); Forrest Walker, "Compulsory Health Insurance: 'The Next Great Step in Social Legislation,'" *JAH* 56 (1969): 300, 304.

48. Martha Russell, "What Social Insurance Will Mean to Nurses," *American Journal of Nursing* 17 (1917): 388 (quotation), 389; Kerby, *Social Mission*, 4 (quotation), 56 (quotation), 1–4, 56–110, 120–22; William Kerby, "Address," in BLS, *Conference on Social Insurance*, 419–20. From much the same perspective as that of those seeking reform of curative services, Assistant Surgeon John Trask saw preventive governmental activities in terms of a mixture of rights and duties: "Health is the right of every man and ... the preservation of one's own health and that of his neighbor is a moral duty." See John Trask, "The Citizen and the Public Health," *Public Health Reports* 28 (1913): 2343 (quotation), 2339–45.

49. Donald B. Johnson, comp., *National Party Platforms*, rev. ed., 2 vols. (Urbana: University of Illinois Press, 1978), 1: 142, 166, 240.

CHAPTER TWO: One of the Most Radical Moves Ever Made

Epigraph: Roger I. Lee and Lewis W. Jones, *The Fundamentals of Good Medical Care: An Outline of the Fundamentals of Good Medical Care and an Estimate of the Service Required to Supply the Medical Needs of the United States* (Chicago: University of Chicago Press, 1933), 10.

1. Joel Howell, *Technology in the Hospital: Transforming Patient Care in the Early Twentieth Century* (Baltimore: Johns Hopkins University Press, 1995); Stanley Joel Reiser, *Medicine and the Reign of Technology* (Cambridge: Cambridge University Press, 1978), 144–231; Margarete Sandelowski, *Devices and Desires: Gender, Technology, and American Nursing* (Chapel Hill: University of North Carolina Press, 2000); Judith Walzer Leavitt, *Brought to Bed: Childbearing in America, 1750–1950* (New York: Oxford University Press, 1986), 171–95; Charles Rosenberg, *The Care of Strangers: The Rise of America's Hospital System* (New York: Basic Books, 1987), 142–336; Paul Starr, *The Social Transformation of American Medicine* (New York: Basic Books, 1982), 134–79.

2. Social Insurance Committee, AALL, "Standards of Sickness Insurance," Dec. 26, 1914 (quotation), *American Association for Labor Legislation Papers, 1905–1945*, microfilm ed., 71 reels (Glen Rock, N.J.: New York Times Microfilming Corporation of America, 1973), reel 62; Michael M. Davis, "Existing Conditions of Medical Practice, Forms of Service under Health Insurance, and Preventive Work," in U.S. Bureau of Labor Statistics, *Proceedings of the Conference on Social Insurance*, Bulletin 212 (Washington: GPO, 1917), 681 (quotation), 677–83; John Andrews, "Proposed Legislation for Health Insurance," in ibid., 555; [AALL], "Brief for Health Insurance," *ALLR* 6 (1916): 230–36; [AALL], "Health Insurance Standards," ibid., 238; John Andrews, "Industrial Hygiene and Health Insurance," *AJPH* 6 (1916): 960–62; I. M. Rubinow, *Standards of Health Insurance* (New York: Henry Holt, 1916), 68–69; Hornell Hart to John Andrews, June 7, 1918, *AALL Papers*, reel 18; John Andrews to Hornell Hart, July 2, 1918, ibid.; Roy Lubove, *The Struggle for Social Security, 1900–1935* (Pittsburgh: University of Pittsburgh Press, 1986), 70.

3. National Industrial Conference Board, *Sickness Insurance or Sickness Prevention?* (Boston: The Board, 1918), 22 (quotation), 24 (quotation), 14–19, 22–24; National Industrial Conference Board, *Is Compulsory Health Insurance Desirable?* (Boston: The Board, 1919), 11 (quotation), 10–12; Margaret Stecker, statement, Mar. 31, 1919, 11 and passim, National Industrial Conference Board Records, series V, box 9, folder: "Insurance, Health, 1917–22," Manuscripts and Archives Department, Hagley Museum and Library, Greenville, Del.; Margaret Stecker, "A Critical Analysis of the Standard Bill for Compulsory Health Insurance with Constructive Suggestions," [1919?], 14, 41–42, ibid.; "If Not Compulsory Insurance—What," *National Civic Federation Review*, June 5, 1919, 1, 2, 16–17; "Compulsory Sickness Insurance," ibid., Apr. 1, 1920, 6–8; Frederick Hoffman, "A Plan for More Effective Federal and State Health Administration," *AJPH* 9 (1919): 161–69, 275–83.

4. Sidney Webb to Miss [Olga] Halsey, Aug. 26, 1916 (quotation), *AALL Papers*, reel 17; [Hornell Hart], "The New Social Order in America: A Study Outline," [June 7, 1918?], 17 (quotation), 2, ibid., reel 18; John Commons and Arthur Altmeyer, "The Health Insurance Movement in the United States," in Ohio, Health and Old Age Insurance Commission, *Health, Health Insurance, Old Age Pensions: Report, Recommendations, Dissenting Opinions* (Columbus: F. J. Heer Printing, 1919), 297 (quotations); John Commons, "A Reconstruction Health Program," *Survey*, Sept. 6, 1919, 801 (quotation), 834; Alice Hamilton, "Health and Labor," ibid., Nov. 11, 1916, 137; Hornell Hart to John Andrews, June 7, 1918, *AALL Papers*, reel 18; John Andrews to Hornell Hart, July 2, 1918, ibid.; John F. Anderson, "Some Important Public Health Problems," *AJPH* 6 (1916): 1145–47. On Webb's plan for postwar reconstruction and its reception in the United States, see Daniel Rodgers, *Atlantic Crossings: Social Politics in a Progressive Age* (Cambridge: Belknap Press of Harvard University Press, 1998), 293–308.

5. Rupert Blue, "Some of the Larger Problems of the Medical Profession," *JAMA* 66 (1916): 1901 (quotation); B. S. Warren and Edgar Sydenstricker, "Health Insurance, the Medical Profession, and the Public Health, Including the Results of a Study of Sickness Expectancy," *Public Health Reports* 34 (1919): 787 (quotation), 789 (quotation), 786–89; B. S. Warren, "A Unified Health Service," ibid., 380 (quotation), 381 (quotations); "Conference of Health Authorities with the Public Health Service," *JAMA* 66 (1916): 1713–14. For a concise summary of the wide-ranging social and economic research agenda of the PHS in the 1910s, see Nancy Krieger and Elizabeth Fee, "Measuring Social Inequalities in Health in the United States: A Historical Review, 1900–1950," *International Journal Health Services* 26 (1996): 394–98. For the most policy-relevant study, see U.S. Public Health Service, *Health Insurance: Its Relation to the Public Health*, by B. S. Warren and Edgar Sydenstricker, Public Health Bulletin 76 (Washington: GPO, 1916). On the extraordinary scope envisioned for preventive medicine at this time, see Milton Rosenau, *Preventive Medicine and Hygiene* (New York: D. Appleton, 1914).

6. William H. Welch, "Foreword," in Arthur Newsholme, *Medicine and the State: The Relation between the Private and Official Practice of Medicine, with Special Reference to Public Health* (Baltimore: Williams & Wilkins, 1932), 8; Arthur Newsholme, *The Last Thirty Years in Public Health: Recollections and Reflections on My Official and Post-Official Life* (London: George Allen & Unwin, 1936), 253–54, 264–66; Elizabeth Fee, *Disease and Discovery: A History of the Johns Hopkins School of Hygiene and Public Health, 1916–1939* (Baltimore: Johns Hopkins University Press, 1987), 66–67, 79; John Eyler, *Sir*

*Arthur Newsholme and State Medicine, 1885–1935* (Cambridge: Cambridge University Press, 1997), 341–46.

7. Eyler, *Newsholme and State Medicine*, 343 (quotation), 354–55; Newsholme, *Last Thirty Years*, 248–50; Arthur Newsholme, *Public Health and Insurance: American Addresses* (Baltimore: Johns Hopkins Press, 1920), 73 (quotation), 71–102, esp. 83–86, 98.

8. Newsholme, *Public Health and Insurance*, 101 (quotation), 179 (quotation), 71 (Burton quotation), 77 (quotation), 71–102, 178–79.

9. Ibid., 43 (quotation), 101 (quotation), 71 (quotation), 42–102, 115, 187–88. On universalistic goals (and practical shortcomings in achieving these goals) in U.S. public health at that time, see John Trask, "The Citizen and the Public Health: The Individual's Relation to the Health of the Community," *Public Health Reports* 28 (1913): 2343; John Duffy, *The Sanitarians: A History of American Public Health* (Urbana: University of Illinois Press, 1990), 193–255; Werner Troesken, "Race, Disease, and the Provision of Water in American Cities, 1889–1921," *Journal of Economic History* 61 (2001): 750–76. For an attempt to use universalistic public-health activities to justify expanded access to medical care, see John Kingsbury, "Health Centers," Apr. 26, 1928, Milbank Memorial Fund Records, box 24, folder 13, Manuscripts and Archives, Yale University Library, New Haven.

10. Newsholme, *Public Health and Insurance*, 35 (quotation), 33–36, 66–70, 103–19, 190.

11. Judith Walzer Leavitt, *The Healthiest City: Milwaukee and the Politics of Health Reform* (Princeton: Princeton University Press, 1982), 4, 216; James Warbasse, "The Socialization of Medicine," *JAMA* 63 (1914): 264; Ralph Pumphrey, "Michael Davis and the Transformation of the Boston Dispensary, 1910–1920," *Bulletin of the History of Medicine* 49 (1975): 463–65; Frederic Almy, "Free Health," *Survey*, May 13, 1911, 270. By the time he returned to the United States for another round of lectures in 1926, Newsholme's harsh assessment of public insurance had mellowed somewhat. See Arthur Newsholme, *Health Problems in Organized Society: Studies in the Social Aspects of Public Health* (London: P. S. King and Son, 1927), 148, 154; Eyler, *Newsholme*, 357–58.

12. Hermann Biggs, "The New York Health Center Bill," Apr. 12, 1920, repr. in C.-E. A. Winslow, *The Life of Hermann M. Biggs, M.D., D.Sc., LL.D.: Physician and Statesman of the Public Health* (Philadelphia: Lea & Febiger, 1929), 402 (quotation), 402–5; Augustus Wadsworth, "The Development of the State Departments of Health in Relation to Health Insurance and Industrial Hygiene," *AJPH* 10 (1920): 56 (quotation), 55–56 (quotation), 53–58; Hermann Biggs, "Presidential Address," *Transactions of the Association of American Physicians* 35 (1920): 1–6; Hermann Biggs, "The State Board of Health," *New York State Journal of Medicine* 21 (1921): 6–7; Winslow, *Life of Biggs*, 346–55, 364; Milton Terris, "Hermann Biggs' Contribution to the Modern Concept of the Health Center," *Bulletin of the History of Medicine* 20 (1946): 387–412, esp. 394–95. On the 1921 version of the proposal, known as the Robinson-Moore Bill, see Terris, "Biggs' Contribution," 399. On the reactionary atmosphere of the 1920 session of the New York legislature, see Beatrix Hoffman, *The Wages of Sickness: The Politics of Health Insurance in Progressive America* (Chapel Hill: University of North Carolina Press, 2001), 163–80. On the passage in 1923 of a very modest plan to subsidize rural health services in New York, see Winslow, *Life of Biggs*, 368–69. On changing forms of organization, see Michael M. Davis, *Clinics, Hospitals and Health Centers* (New York: Harper and Brothers, 1927).

13. Gerald Morgan, "To Conserve the Human Resources of the State," *New Republic*, Mar. 23, 1921, 106 (quotation), 102–9; Gerald Morgan, *Public Relief of Sickness* (New York: Macmillan, 1922), 158–59 (quotation), 158–61. For another critique and remedy in this vein, see Glenn Frank, "Trailing the Robin Hoods of Medicine," *Century Magazine*, Oct. 1921, 953–60.

14. AMA House of Delegates, "Proceedings of the Boston Session," *JAMA* 76 (1921): 1756 (Medical Society of New Hampshire quotation), 1756–57; Terris, "Biggs' Contribution," 399–400; Morris Fishbein, *A History of the American Medical Association, 1847 to 1947* (Philadelphia: W. B. Saunders, 1947), 333.

15. Julia Lathrop, "Income and Infant Mortality," *AJPH* 9 (1919): 274 (quotation), 270–74; Kriste Lindenmeyer, *"A Right to Childhood": The U.S. Children's Bureau and Child Welfare, 1912–46* (Urbana: University of Illinois Press, 1997), 52–107; Richard Meckel, *Save the Babies: American Public Health Reform and the Prevention of Infant Mortality, 1850–1929* (Ann Arbor: University of Michigan Press, 1998), 200–219; Theda Skocpol, *Protecting Soldiers and Mothers: The Political Origins of Social Policy in the United States* (Cambridge: Belknap Press of Harvard University Press, 1992), 480–524; J. Stanley Lemons, "The Sheppard-Towner Act: Progressivism in the 1920s," *JAH* 55 (1969): 776–86; Ellen More, *Restoring the Balance: Women Physicians and the Profession of Medicine, 1850–1995* (Cambridge: Harvard University Press, 1999), 158, 162–63.

16. Katharine Tucker, "Response and President's Address," *American Journal of Nursing* 20 (1920): 785 (quotation); Josephine Goldmark, "Report on a Survey," in Committee for the Study of Nursing Education, *Nursing and Nursing Education in the United States: Report of the Committee for the Study of Nursing Education and Report of a Survey* (New York: Macmillan, 1923), 79 (quotations), 34–35, 82–93, 127–29; Elspeth Vaughan, "The Interdependence of Physicians and Public Health Nurses in Community Health Work," *Public Health Nurse* 16 (1924): 452; Haven Emerson, "Meeting the Demands for Community Health Work," ibid., 485–89; Anna Haines, "High Lights in Russian Public Health," *Public Health Nurse* 19 (1927): 56–60. On public health nursing and its relations with the medical profession, see Karen Buhler-Wilkerson, *False Dawn: The Rise and Decline of Public Health Nursing, 1900–1930* (New York: Garland Publishing, 1989); Karen Buhler-Wilkerson, "Bringing Care to the People: Lillian Wald's Legacy to Public Health Nursing," *AJPH* 83 (1993): 1778–86, esp. 1783; Barbara Melosh, *"The Physician's Hand": Work Culture and Conflict in American Nursing* (Philadelphia: Temple University Press, 1982), 113–43.

17. Frank Billings, "The Future of Private Medical Practice," *JAMA* 76 (1921): 349–54. On Billings's importance in the AMA, see Fishbein, *History of AMA*, 224.

18. Billings, "Future of Practice," 352 (quotations), 353 (quotation), 352–54.

19. House of Delegates, "Boston Session," 1757 (anonymous circular quotation), 1758, 1761–62.

20. Victor Vaughan, "Rural Health Centers as Aids to General Practitioners," *JAMA* 76 (1921): 985 (quotation), 983–86. On Vaughan's career, see John Duffy, *The Sanitarians: A History of American Public Health* (Urbana: University of Illinois Press, 1990), 152, 198, 199, 222, 251.

21. House of Delegates, "Boston Session," 1671 (Council on Medical Education and Hospitals quotation), 1672 (quotation), 1673 (quotation), 1671–78.

22. House of Delegates, "Boston Session," 1672 (Council on Medical Education and Hospitals quotation), 1672–73. On the tensions between specialists and generalists, see

Rosemary Stevens, *American Medicine and the Public Interest* (New Haven: Yale University Press, 1971), 146–56.

23. House of Delegates, "Boston Session," 1754.

24. Ray Lyman Wilbur, "Human Welfare and Modern Medicine," *JAMA* 80 (1923): 1890 (quotation), 1892 (quotation), 1889 (quotation), 1889–93; Ray Lyman Wilbur, "Address of President Ray Lyman Wilbur," *JAMA* 82 (1924): 1968 (quotation), 1968–69.

25. Ray Lyman Wilbur, "The Lag in the Health Program," in Wilbur, *The March of Medicine: Selected Addresses and Articles on Medical Topics, 1913–1937* (Stanford: Stanford University Press, 1938), 130 (quotation), 133–34 (quotation), 122–34.

26. [C.-E. A. Winslow] to Arthur Newsholme, Jan. 24, 1920 (quotation), C.-E. A. Winslow Papers, box 21, folder 529, Manuscripts and Archives, Yale University Library, New Haven; C.-E. A. Winslow, "The Untilled Fields of Public Health," *Modern Medicine* 2 (1920): 189 (quotation), 183–91; Newsholme, *Public Health and Insurance*, 157. For many insights into Winslow's thought and action, see Arthur Viseltear, "C.-E. A. Winslow: His Era and His Contribution to Medical Care," in *Healing and History: Essays for George Rosen*, ed. Charles Rosenberg (New York: Science History Publications, 1979), 205–28; Viseltear, "Compulsory Health Insurance," 25–54.

27. [C.-E. A. Winslow] to John B. Andrews, Jan. 16, 1923, Winslow Papers, box 1, folder 16; [C.-E. A. Winslow] to Arthur Newsholme, Nov. 21, 1922, ibid., box 21, folder 529; Arthur Newsholme to C.-E. A. Winslow, June 25, 1923, ibid.

28. C.-E. A. Winslow, *The Evolution and Significance of the Modern Public Health Campaign* (New Haven: Yale University Press, 1923), 63 (quotation), 49–65; Winslow, *Life of Biggs*, passim; Viseltear, "Winslow," 208–9.

29. C.-E. A. Winslow, "Public Health at the Crossroads," *AJPH* 16 (1926): 1076–85; Roemer, "Force for Change," 339–41. By one estimate, approximately 80 percent of APHA members were physicians in the early twentieth century. See Allan Brandt and Martha Gardner, "Antagonism and Accommodation: Interpreting the Relationship between Public Health and Medicine in the United States during the Twentieth Century," *AJPH* 90 (2000): 709–10.

30. Winslow, "Crossroads," 1084 (quotation), 1083 (quotation).

31. Ibid., 1082 (Meeker quotation), 1084 (quotation). For an instance of the negative response that Winslow anticipated, see Morris Fishbein, "Socialized Medicine," *NEJM* 199 (1928): 472–73.

32. C. F. Wilinsky, "The Health Center," *AJPH* 17 (1927): 679 (quotation), 677–82; John Duffy, "The American Medical Profession and Public Health: From Support to Ambivalence," *Bulletin of the History of Medicine* 53 (1979): 20–21.

33. Fox, *Health Policies*, 46 (quotation); Jonathan Engel, *Doctors and Reformers: Discussion and Debate over Health Policy, 1925–1950* (Columbia: University of South Carolina Press, 2002), 16–27; Douglas R. Parks, "Expert Inquiry and Health Care Reform in New Era America: Herbert Hoover, Ray Lyman Wilbur, and the Travails of the Disinterested Experts" (Ph.D. diss., University of Iowa, 1994), 243; Viseltear, "Winslow," 214–15; Ray Lyman Wilbur, *The Memoirs of Ray Lyman Wilbur*, ed. Edgar E. Robinson and Paul C. Edwards (Stanford: Stanford University Press, 1960), 308. For a list of the members of the committee as of October 31, 1932, see CCMC, *Medical Care for the American People: The Final Report of the Committee on the Costs of Medical Care* (Chicago: University of Chicago Press, 1932), xi. On the changing role of foundations, see Daniel Fox, "Policy and Vulnerability: Foundations in Twentieth-Century Health

Affairs," *Minerva* 35 (1997): 311–19. On 1920s corporatism, see Ellis Hawley, "Herbert Hoover, the Commerce Secretariat, and the Vision of an 'Associative State,' 1921–1928," *JAH* 61 (1974): 116–40; Guy Alchon, *The Invisible Hand of Planning: Capitalism, Social Science, and the State in the 1920s* (Princeton: Princeton University Press, 1985).

34. Harry H. Moore, *American Medicine and the People's Health: An Outline with Statistical Data on the Organization of Medicine in the United States, with Special Reference to the Adjustment of Medical Service to Social and Economic Change* (New York: D. Appleton, 1927), 325 (quotation), 352 (quotation), 309–14, v–vii, 339; Milton Roemer, "I. S. Falk, the Committee on the Costs of Medical Care, and the Drive for National Health Insurance," *AJPH* 75 (1985): 841–48; Engel, *Doctors and Reformers*, 28–33; Harry Moore to C.-E. A. Winslow, Jan. 7, 1927, Winslow Papers, box 62, folder 744; [C.-E. A. Winslow] to Harry Moore, Oct. 29, 1927, ibid., folder 746; Executive Committee, CCMC, "Minutes," May 18, 1927, ibid., box 63, folder 774; Harry Moore to Ray Lyman Wilbur, Sept. 28, 1927, Ray Lyman Wilbur Papers, box 95, folder 2, Special Collections and Archives, Lane Medical Library, Stanford University, Palo Alto.

35. Editorial, "The Cost of Medical Care," *AJPH* 17 (1927): 723 (quotation); CCMC, *Five-Year Program of the Committee on the Cost of Medical Care* (Washington: CCMC, 1928), 6 (Wilbur quotation), 7 (Wilbur quotation), 25; Committee of Five, "Conference on the Economic Factors Affecting the Organization of Medicine," May 17, 1927, Wilbur Papers, box 95, folder 2; Parks, "Expert Inquiry," 249–54.

36. Ray Lyman Wilbur, "The Cost of Medical Care," *California and Western Medicine* 29 (1928): 1 (quotation), 2 (quotation).

37. Ray Lyman Wilbur, "Introduction," in CCMC, *Medical Care for the American People*, vi–ix; Committee of Five, "Researches Recommended," [early 1927?], Winslow Papers, box 61, folder 718. For a list of all its publications, see CCMC, *Medical Care for the American People*, unpaginated end matter.

38. Michael Davis, *Paying Your Sickness Bills* (Chicago: University of Chicago Press, 1931), 8 (quotation), passim, esp. 8–9, 181–98, 202–3 (Davis's book was not published under the direct auspices of the CCMC itself, but he drew heavily on its ongoing research); I. S. Falk, C. Rufus Rorem, and Martha D. Ring, *The Costs of Medical Care: A Summary of Investigations on the Economic Aspects of the Prevention and Care of Illness* (Chicago: University of Chicago Press, 1933), vi (quotation), passim, esp. v–vi, 70, 113–16, 148; CCMC, *Medical Care for the American People*, 19; Louis Reed, *The Ability to Pay for Medical Care* (Chicago: University of Chicago Press, 1933), passim, esp. 70–75; Leon Henderson, *The Use of Small Loans for Medical Expenses* (Washington: CCMC, 1930), 6–7; I. S. Falk, Margaret Klem, and Nathan Sinai, *The Incidence of Illness and the Receipt and Costs of Medical Care among Representative Families: Experiences in Twelve Consecutive Months during 1928–31* (Chicago: University of Chicago Press, 1933).

39. Executive Committee, CCMC, "Minutes of a Meeting," June 2, 1930, Wilbur Papers, box 93, folder 4; Reed, *Ability to Pay*, passim, esp. 21–26; Pierce Williams, *The Purchase of Medical Care through Fixed Periodic Payment* (New York: National Bureau of Economic Research, 1932); Parks, "Expert Inquiry," 249; Perkins, "Economic Organization," 1724. On the unpublished study of the Biggs centers, see Alden Mills, "The Biggs Health Center Plans," [Aug. 1932?], Winslow Papers, box 65, folder 848; Alden Mills to C.-E. A. Winslow, Aug. 20, 1932, ibid.; CCMC, *Medical Care for the American People*, unpaginated end matter. On developments abroad, see Megan J. Davies, "Competent Professionals and Modern Methods: State Medicine in British Columbia

during the 1930s," *Bulletin of the History of Medicine* 76 (2002): 56–83, esp. 59–62; Newsholme, *Medicine and the State.* For a dismissive reference to higher wages suggestive of the CCMC's lack of interest in the living wage, see Michael Davis, "Doctors' Bills and People's Billions," *JAMA* 94 (1930): 1014. For physicians' objections to spending on fur coats, bootleg liquor, patent medicines, and other questionable items, see George Follansbee, "A Doctor Diagnoses the Bills," *Survey,* Jan. 1, 1930, 376–77; Executive Committee, CCMC, "Minutes of a Meeting," Jan. 13, 1930, Wilbur Papers, box 93, folder 2.

40. CCMC, *Medical Care for the American People,* 10 (quotation); Jennifer Klein, *For All These Rights: Business, Labor, and the Shaping of America's Public-Private Welfare State* (Princeton: Princeton University Press, 2003), 122–25. On racial segregation and discrimination in health care in the early twentieth century, see W. Michael Byrd and Linda A. Clayton, *An American Dilemma,* vol. 2: *Race, Medicine, and Health Care in the United States, 1900–2000* (New York: Routledge, 2002), 35–131; David McBride, *Integrating the City of Medicine: Blacks in Philadelphia Health Care, 1910–1965* (Philadelphia: Temple University Press, 1989), 3–30; Thomas J. Ward Jr., *Black Physicians in the Jim Crow South, 1880–1960* (Fayetteville: University of Arkansas Press, 2003); Vanessa Northington Gamble, *Making a Place for Ourselves: The Black Hospital Movement, 1920–1945* (New York: Oxford University Press, 1995); Edward Beardsley, *A History of Neglect: Health Care for Blacks and Mill Workers in the Twentieth-Century South* (Knoxville: University of Tennessee Press, 1987), 11–41, 77–155; Darlene Clark Hine, *Black Women in White: Racial Conflict and Cooperation in the Nursing Profession, 1890–1950* (Bloomington: Indiana University Press, 1989), 3–62; James H. Jones, *Bad Blood: The Tuskegee Syphilis Experiment* (New York: Free Press, 1981).

41. Lee and Jones, *Fundamentals of Good Care,* 3 (quotation), 10 (quotation), 91–128; Falk, Rorem, and Ring, *Costs of Medical Care,* 135 (quotation), 7.

42. CCMC, *Medical Care for the American People,* passim, esp. v–xi, 121, 130, 201. The proponents of compulsory, albeit nonuniversal, insurance doubted that voluntary insurance would ever reach low-paid workers. See ibid., 131.

43. Editorial, "The Committee on the Costs of Medical Care," *JAMA* 99 (1932): 1951 (quotation), 1952 (quotation), 1950–52; Editorial, "The Report of the Committee on the Costs of Medical Care," ibid., 2035 (quotation), 2034–35; Editorial, "The Report of the Committee on the Costs of Medical Care," *NEJM* 207 (1932): 1059; Editorial, "Interpretations of the Work of the Committee on the Costs of Medical Care," ibid., 1162–63; Editorial, "Confronting the Peril of Thought," *American Journal of Nursing* 32 (1932): 1295; Forrest Walker, "Americanism versus Sovietism: A Study of the Reaction to the Committee on the Costs of Medical Care," *Bulletin of the History of Medicine* 53 (1979): 489–504; Engel, *Doctors and Reformers,* 41–52. For the ambivalence of the African-American medical community, see Editorial, "Committee on the Cost of Medical Care: Open Season in No Man's Land," *JNMA* 25 (1933): 18–19; John Kenney et al., "Reaction of the North Jersey Medical Society to the Report of the Committee on the Cost of Medical Care," ibid., 26 (1934): 10–13. For evidence that the conflict over insurance and group practice did not entirely obscure the CCMC's call for universalism, see Editorial, "The Final Report of the Committee on the Costs of Medical Care," *NEJM* 207 (1932): 1001; Haven Emerson, "Medical Care for All of Us," *Survey,* Dec. 1, 1932, 629–32; I. M. Rubinow, "The Medical Report," Dec. 30, 1932, Isaac Rubinow Papers, box 12, folder: "Manuscripts, Medical," Kheel Center for Labor-Management Documentation and Archives, Catherwood Library, Cornell University, Ithaca.

44. Ray Lyman Wilbur, "The Economics of Public Health and Medical Care," *Milbank Memorial Fund Quarterly* 10 (1932): 178 (quotation), 169–90; "An Analysis of the Task of the Committee on the Cost of Medical Care," [Oct. 28, 1929?], Wilbur Papers, box 93, folder 2; Executive Committee, CCMC, "Executive Committee Meeting," Oct. 28, 1929, ibid.; "A New Analysis of the Task of the Committee on the Cost of Medical Care: Revised Copy," Jan. 6, 1930, ibid.; "Status of the Committee's Work," June 1, 1931, ibid., folder 6; CCMC, "Final Report of the Committee on the Costs of Medical Care to Be Made Public on November 29th, Says Dr. Wilbur," May 24, 1932, ibid., box 94, folder 4; Haven Emerson, "Health—the Business of Each of Us," *Survey*, Jan. 1, 1930, 373. For studies that give little or no attention to the universalism of the CCMC, see Daniel Hirshfield, *The Lost Reform: The Campaign for Compulsory Health Insurance in the United States from 1932 to 1943* (Cambridge: Harvard University Press, 1970), 31–37; Starr, *Social Transformation*, 261–67; Fox, *Health Policies*, 45–51; Engel, *Doctors and Reformers*, 11–52; Barbara Bridgman Perkins, "Economic Organization of Medicine and the Committee on the Costs of Medical Care," *AJPH* 88 (1998): 1721–26. For an exception, see Rosemary Stevens, *In Sickness and in Wealth: American Hospitals in the Twentieth Century* (New York: Basic Books, 1989), 135, 154.

45. CCMC, *Medical Care for the American People*, x (Wilbur quotation), 41–42 (quotation), 195–96 (Hamilton quotation), 2–43, 118–19, 189–200.

46. Ibid., 168 (quotation), 151–83 passim, esp. 167.

47. CCMC, "Reports of Four Subcommittees," May 16, 1931, 24 (Roberts quotation), 26 (Schwitalla quotation), 24–28, Wilbur Papers, box 93, folder 6.

CHAPTER THREE: No Poor-Man's System

1. Franklin Roosevelt to Thomas Parran, Nov. 26, 1932 (quotation), Thomas Parran Papers, box 11, folder 94, Archives Service Center, University of Pittsburgh; Thomas Parran, address, Nov. 29, 1932, 5 (quotation), 5–6, ibid. Parran's measured support for universalism at this event contrasted with the unbridled enthusiasm of other participants who seemed oblivious to the depression. See Ray Lyman Wilbur, "The High Points in the Recommendations of the Committee on the Costs of Medical Care," *NEJM* 207 (1932): 1073–78; C.-E. A. Winslow, "The Recommendations of the Committee on the Costs of Medical Care," ibid., 1138–42; Lewellys Barker, "The Present and Future Significance of the Findings and Recommendations of the Committee on the Costs of Medical Care—from the Physician's Point of View," ibid., 1193–95.

2. John Kenneth Galbraith, *The Great Crash, 1929* (Boston: Houghton Mifflin, 1997); Robert McElvaine, *The Great Depression: America, 1929–1941* (New York: Times Books, 1993), 72–94; Irving Bernstein, *The Lean Years: A History of the American Worker, 1920–1933* (Boston: Houghton Mifflin, 1960), 251–513.

3. Kenneth Kusmer, *Down and Out, on the Road: The Homeless in American History* (New York: Oxford University Press, 2002), 193–220; Gerald Markowitz and David Rosner, eds., *"Slaves of the Depression": Workers' Letters about Life on the Job* (Ithaca: Cornell University Press, 1987); Bernstein, *Lean Years*, 293–333, 361–65; McElvaine, *Great Depression*, 170–95.

4. W. Michael Byrd and Linda A. Clayton, *An American Health Dilemma*, vol. 2: *Race, Medicine, and Health Care in the United States, 1900–2000* (New York: Routledge, 2002), 138–39; Bernstein, *Lean Years*, 364; Abraham Epstein, *The Case for Health Insurance*

(New York: American Association for Social Security, [1936]), 5; George Perrott and Selwyn Collins, "Sickness among the 'Depression Poor,'" *AJPH* 24 (1934): 101–7.

5. Margaret Klem, "Illness and the Receipt and Cost of Medical Care among California Families of Low and Moderate Incomes," *Western Hospital Review* 22 (1935): 5–8; E. T. Remmen, "Compulsory Health Insurance," ibid., 21 (1934): 6; T[hurston] S. W[elton], untitled editorial, *American Journal of Surgery* 15 (1932): 554–55.

6. Rosemary Stevens, *In Sickness and in Wealth: American Hospitals in the Twentieth Century* (New York: Basic Books, 1989), 142–49; Paul Benzoni, *Beyond the Mine: A Steelworker's Story* (Superior, Wis.: Savage Press, 1997), 65, 79; Paul Starr, *The Social Transformation of American Medicine* (New York: Basic Books, 1982), 270–71; U.S. Bureau of the Census, *Historical Statistics of the United States, Colonial Times to 1970*, 2 vols. (Washington: GPO, 1976), 1: 74.

7. Barbara Nachtrieb Armstrong, *Insuring the Essentials: Minimum Wage Plus Social Insurance: A Living Wage Program* (New York: Macmillan, 1932), xiii (quotation), xiv, 553–62.

8. Ibid., xiii (quotation), xiii–xvii, 4.

9. Ibid., 297 (quotations), 297–98, 374.

10. Ibid., 284 (quotation), 312–62, 374, 561, 673–83.

11. John Andrews to I. M. Rubinow, Nov. 16, 1932 (quotation), Isaac Rubinow Papers, box 1, folder 18, Kheel Center for Labor-Management Documentation and Archives, Catherwood Library, Cornell University, Ithaca; I. M. Rubinow, "The Medical Report," Dec. 30, 1932, 5 (quotation), 6–7, ibid., box 12, folder: "Manuscripts, Medical"; I. M. Rubinow to John Andrews, Dec. 13, 1932, box 1, folder 19; "Health Insurance," *ALLR* 22 (1932): 162.

12. Abraham Epstein, *Insecurity, a Challenge to America: A Study of Social Insurance in the United States and Abroad* (New York: Harrison Smith and Robert Haas, 1933), vii (quotations), 421 (quotation), 19 (quotation), vii–viii, 6–19; I. M. R[ubinow] to John Andrews, Nov. 8, 1925, Rubinow Papers, box 1, folder 17; David A. Moss, *Socializing Security: Progressive-Era Economists and the Origins of American Social Policy* (Cambridge: Harvard University Press, 1996), 161.

13. Epstein, *Insecurity*, 458 (quotations), 473 (quotation), 432–81, esp. 471–74.

14. I. M. Rubinow, *The Quest for Security* (New York: Henry Holt, 1934), iv (quotation), iii–iv, 207–14.

15. Ibid., 8 (quotation), iv (quotation), 8–18, 175, 205–6. On his preference that state health insurance cover only wage earners, see I. M. Rubinow, "Health Insurance," May 24, 1935, Rubinow Papers, box 12, folder: "Manuscripts, Health Insurance."

16. Alice Kessler-Harris, "In the Nation's Image: The Gendered Limits of Social Citizenship in the Depression Era," *JAH* 86 (1999): 1259 (quotation), 1251–79.

17. Clyde Kiser, *The Milbank Memorial Fund: Its Leaders and Its Work, 1905–1974* (New York: Milbank Memorial Fund, 1975), 22–55; Daniel M. Fox, *Health Policies, Health Politics: The British and American Experience, 1911–1965* (Princeton: Princeton University Press, 1986), 38–42.

18. Albert Milbank, "Socialized Individualism," *Milbank Memorial Fund Bulletin Quarterly* 11 (1933): 88–96.

19. Arthur Newsholme and John Kingsbury, *Red Medicine: Socialized Health in Soviet Russia* (Garden City, N. Y.: Doubleday, Doran, 1933), vii (quotation), passim, esp. 221, 268–70, 294. At one point, Newsholme felt compelled to remind his co-author that

the Soviet system was not one that any other nation could borrow. See Arthur Newsholme to John Kingsbury, Sept. 18, 1935, John Kingsbury Papers, pt. II, box 16, folder: "Newsholme, Arthur, 1935," Manuscript Division, Library of Congress, Washington; Beatrice Webb to Sir Arthur [Newsholme], May 16, 1932, ibid., box 68, folder: "Webb, Sidney and Beatrice"; Arthur Newsholme, *Medicine and the State: The Relation between the Private and Official Practice of Medicine, with Special Reference to Public Health* (Baltimore: Williams and Wilkins, 1932); John Eyler, *Sir Arthur Newsholme and State Medicine, 1885–1935* (Cambridge: Cambridge University Press, 1997), 360–73.

20. John Kingsbury, "A Health Plan for the Nation," *Survey*, Nov. 1933, 373 (quotations); John Kingsbury, "A Program for National Health Insurance," *ALLR* 23 (1933): 188 (quotation), 185–88; J[ohn] K[ingsbury] to Franklin Roosevelt, Jan. 24, 1934, Kingsbury Papers, pt. II, box 18, folder: "Roosevelt, Franklin D."; John Kingsbury to Mrs. Franklin D. Roosevelt, Apr. 19, 1933, Milbank Memorial Fund Records, box 24, folder 14, Manuscripts and Archives, Yale University Library, New Haven.

21. Edgar Sydenstricker, "Medical Practice and Public Needs," in American Academy of Political and Social Science, *The Medical Profession and the Public: Currents and Counter-Currents* (Philadelphia: American Academy of Political and Social Science, 1934), 25 (quotation), 28 (quotation), 29 (quotations), 30 (quotation), 21–30; I. S. Falk to Abraham Epstein, Jan. 11, 1934, American Association for Social Security Records, box 3, folder 3, Kheel Center for Labor-Management Documentation and Archives, Catherwood Library, Cornell University, Ithaca; AASS, "Minutes of the Regular Annual Meeting," Feb. 7, 1934, Rubinow Papers, box 1, folder 22.

22. Morris Fishbein, "The Doctor and the State," in American Academy, *Medical Profession*, 101 (quotation), 88–101; Thomas Parran, "Health Services of Tomorrow," in ibid., 79 (quotation), 75–79; William T. Foster, "Doctors, Patients, and the Community," in ibid., 103, 108, 111–12.

23. Parran, "Health Services of Tomorrow," 77 (Blackstone quotation; italics in original), 76 (quotations), 84–85. Parran proudly proclaimed this an important expression of his own credo. See Thomas Parran to Donald Armstrong, May 8, 1934, Parran Papers, box 32, folder 360.

24. E. T. Remmen, "Compulsory Health Insurance," *Western Hospital Review* 21 (1934): 5 (quotation), 5–6, 24–25; I. S. Falk, "Report to the Round Table on Medical Care," Mar. 14, 1934, 3 (quotations), I. S. Falk Papers, box 8, folder 130, Manuscripts and Archives, Yale University Library, New Haven.

25. Falk, "Report to the Round Table," 5–6, 10–12.

26. Ibid., A (quotation), passim, esp. A–A2; James A. Miller, "Report of Round-Table on Medical Care," in Milbank Memorial Fund, *Problems of Health Conservation: Proceedings of the Twelfth Annual Conference of the Advisory Council of the Milbank Memorial Fund* (New York: The Fund, 1934), 15–17, 23–24, 34.

27. Albert Milbank, "Greetings on Behalf of the Board of Directors," in ibid., 75 (quotation), 75–77; Henry Sigerist, "Trends toward Socialized Medicine," in ibid., 82 (quotation), 81–83; Harry Hopkins, "Health Planning in the Recovery Program," in ibid., 90–91 (quotation), 86–91; Kiser, *Milbank Memorial Fund*, 56.

28. John Kingsbury, "Is America Headed for State Medicine?" Apr. 13, 1934, 15 (quotation), 1, 13–15, Kingsbury Papers, pt. II, box 80, folder: "Is America Headed for State Medicine?"; J[ohn] K[ingsbury] to Arthur Newsholme, Mar. 17, 1934, ibid., box 16, folder: "Newholme, Arthur, 1934."

29. Kingsbury, "Is America," 11 (quotation), 12 (Newsholme quotation), 4–6.

30. Ibid., 8, 14, 21, 23–24.

31. John Kingsbury, "Adequate Health Service for All the People," in National Conference of Social Work, *Proceedings of the National Conference of Social Work at the Sixty-First Annual Session, 1934* (Chicago: University of Chicago Press, 1934), 315 (quotation), 320 (quotation), 304–24; AMA, House of Delegates, "Proceedings of the Cleveland Session," *JAMA* 102 (1934): 2200.

32. I. S. Falk, "Formulating an American Plan of Health Insurance," *ALLR* 24 (1934): 88 (quotation), 87–90

33. Michael M. Davis, "The American Approach to Health Insurance," *Milbank Memorial Fund Quarterly* 12 (1934): 215 (quotation), 203–17; Michael Davis to I. M. Rubinow, Apr. 5, 1934, Rubinow Papers, box 3, folder 2. For further criticism of exclusionary policies abroad, see Michael Davis, "Medical Service in Europe," [1934], ibid.

34. Edwin E. Witte, *The Development of the Social Security Act: A Memorandum on the History of the Committee on Economic Security and Drafting and Legislative History of the Social Security Act* (Madison: University of Wisconsin Press, 1963), 3–37, esp. 30–31; Daniel Hirshfield, *The Lost Reform: The Campaign for Compulsory Health Insurance in the United States from 1932 to 1943* (Cambridge: Harvard University Press, 1970), 44–45.

35. Edgar Sydenstricker and I. S. Falk to Mr. Witte, Aug. 28, 1934 (quotation), RG 47, Records of the Social Security Administration, Records of the Committee on Economic Security, box 35, folder: "Health Studies," Archives II, National Archives, College Park, Md.; Edgar Sydenstricker and I. S. Falk, "Economic Insecurity Arising out of Illness," sec. II-4, [Sept. 12, 1934?], ibid., box 5, folder: "Early Drafts." For the priorities of Roosevelt and Perkins, see Frances Perkins, *The Roosevelt I Knew* (New York: Viking Press, 1946), 278–301; Arthur Altmeyer, *The Formative Years of Social Security* (Madison: University of Wisconsin Press, 1966), 27.

36. Thomas Parran to Edgar Sydenstricker, Sept. 22, 1934 (quotation), Parran Papers, box 14, folder 191; Edgar Sydenstricker to Thomas Parran, Sept. 24, 1934 (quotation), ibid.; C. B. Cates to Parran, Sept. 21, 1934, ibid.; A[braham] E[pstein] to Edwin Witte, Sept. 25, 1934, AASS Records, box 6, folder 20; Abraham Epstein, "Social Security—Fiction or Fact?" *American Mercury*, Oct. 1934, 136–37. On Epstein's difficult personality, see Hirshfield, *Lost Reform*, 75–76.

37. Edwin Witte to Abraham Epstein, Sept. 28, 1934 (quotation), AASS Records, box 6, folder 20; Edgar Sydenstricker and I. S. Falk, Appendix D, 4 (quotation), 2 (quotation), 11–16, in Staff, CES, "Preliminary Report," Sept. 1934, Edwin Witte Papers, box 70, folder: "Staff Report," Archives Division, Wisconsin Historical Society, Madison; CES Staff, "Preliminary Report," 63–64, ibid.

38. Technical Board on Economic Security, "Preliminary Recommendations of the Technical Board to the Committee on Economic Security," [Oct. 1, 1934?] (quotation), RG 47, Records of the CES, box 1, folder: "Technical Board Reports"; Sydenstricker and Falk, Appendix D, 4 (quotation), in Staff, CES, "Preliminary Report," Sept. 1934, Witte Papers, box 70, folder: "Staff Report"; Witte, *Development*, 37–39; cf. Hirshfield, *Lost Reform*, 47.

39. National Conference on Economic Security, proceedings, Nov. 14, 1934, 247 (Stewart Roberts quotations), 217–19, 229, 232–33, 240, 243, Witte Papers, box 65, folder:

"Committee Activities"; Witte, *Development*, 41–44. For one AMA opponent who agreed that the CES felt no public demand for health security, see Abraham Epstein, *Insecurity, a Challenge to America: A Study of Social Insurance in the United States and Abroad*, 2d rev. ed. (New York: Random House, 1938), 692.

40. Edwin Witte, "Suggestions for a Long-Time and an Immediate Program for Economic Security," Nov. 15, 1934, passim, esp. 13–14, Witte Papers, box 65, folder: "Committee Activities"; Witte, *Development*, 47–56.

41. [Edgar] Sydenstricker and [I. S.] Falk, "A Statement of General Principles," [Nov. 15, 1934?] (quotation), RG 47, Records of the CES, box 35, folder: "Health Studies"; Edgar Sydenstricker, "Health in the New Deal," *Annals of the American Academy of Political and Social Science* 176 (1934): 131 (quotation), 131–37, esp. 134; Edgar Sydenstricker and I. S. Falk, "Preliminary Draft: Abstract of a Program for Social Insurance against Illness," [Nov. 15, 1934?], passim, esp. III-1–3; CES Staff, "Risks to Economic Security Arising out of Ill Health," Dec. 4, 1934, RG 47, Records of the CES, box 2, folder: "Health Reports"; Frances Perkins, "The Way of Security," *Survey Graphic*, Dec. 1934, 621–22; Perkins, *The Roosevelt I Knew*, 289.

42. U.S., Committee on Economic Security, *Report to the President of the Committee on Economic Security* (Washington: GPO, 1935), 41 (quotation), 6, 40–43; CES, "Minutes of Meetings," Dec. 4, 1934, Witte Papers, box 65, folder: "Committee Activities"; Advisory Council on Economic Security, CES, "Report," Dec. 18, 1934, 30, ibid.; Witte, *Development*, 181–82.

43. Barbara Nachtrieb Armstrong, "Reminiscences," interview by Peter Corning, Dec. 19, 1965, transcript, 153 (quotation), 206–7, Oral History Collection, Oral History Research Office, Butler Library, Columbia University, New York; Thomas Parran, "A Coordinated Plan to Achieve Health Security," [Jan. 29, 1935?], Parran Papers, box 14, folder 191; Medical Advisory Board [*sic*], CES, "Proceedings," Jan. 29 and Jan. 30, 1935, Witte Papers, box 68, folder: "Medical Advisory Board Proceedings"; CES, "Minutes of Meetings," Mar. 15, 1935, 21–22, ibid., box 65, folder: "Committee Activities"; Edgar Sydenstricker and I. S. Falk, "Report of the Committee on Economic Security to the President: Final Report on Risks to Economic Security Arising out of Illness," [June 15, 1935?], passim, esp. 37–38, ibid., box 67, folder: "Health in Relation to Economic Security"; Frances Perkins to the President, June 15, 1935, Arthur Altmeyer Papers, box 2, folder: "Health Insurance Report of 1935," Archives Division, Wisconsin Historical Society, Madison; Witte, *Development*, 135–45, 173–74, 185–89; Hirshfield, *Lost Reform*, 54–59. On the March 1935 decision of the California Medical Association to support legislation mandating insurance for all families making less than $3,000 per year, see Arthur Viseltear, "Compulsory Health Insurance in California, 1934–1935," *AJPH* 61 (1971): 2119–21. On the influence of federalism and other strong conservative factors in shaping the Social Security Act, see, among many others, James T. Patterson, *The New Deal and the States: Federalism in Transition* (Princeton: Princeton University Press, 1969); G. John Ikenberry and Theda Skocpol, "Expanding Social Benefits: The Role of Social Security," *Political Science Quarterly* 102 (1987): 389–416; Colin Gordon, *New Deals: Business, Labor, and Politics in America, 1920–1935* (New York: Cambridge University Press, 1994), 261–79; Linda Gordon, *Pitied but Not Entitled: Single Mothers and the History of Welfare, 1890–1935* (Cambridge: Harvard University Press, 1994), 253–306; Suzanne Mettler, *Dividing Citizens: Gender and Federalism in New Deal Public Policy* (Ithaca: Cornell University Press, 1998).

44. Fox, *Health Policies, Health Politics*, 81–82 (quotation), 79–83; James Rorty, *American Medicine Mobilizes* (New York: W. W. Norton, 1939), 116 (quotation), 116–30; Kiser, *Milbank Memorial Fund*, 59–63. On the Townsend movement and its influence, see Daniel J. Mitchell, "Townsend and Roosevelt: Lessons from the Struggle for Elderly Income Support," *Labor History* 42 (2001): 255–76; Altmeyer, *Formative Years*, 10, 13, 32; Edwin Amenta and Yvonne Zylan, "It Happened Here: Political Opportunity, the New Institutionalism, and the Townsend Movement," *American Sociological Review* 56 (1991): 250–65; Abraham Hoffman, *The Townsend Movement: A Political Analysis* (New York: Octagon Books, 1975). On other insurgencies at this time and their impact on social policy, see Gordon, *Pitied*, 209–51.

45. Sydenstricker and Falk, "Report to President," [June 15, 1934?] (quotation), Witte Papers, box 67, folder: "Health in Relation to Economic Security." On (white male) individualism and Americanism as important ingredients in New Deal social policy, see Kessler-Harris, "In the Nation's Image," 1251–72; Daniel Nelson, *Unemployment Insurance: The American Experience, 1915–1935* (Madison: University of Wisconsin Press, 1969), passim, esp. 30, 146–48; Ikenberry and Skocpol, "Expanding Social Benefits," 412–13. On jingoistic attacks on reform in the 1910s, see Beatrix Hoffman, *The Wages of Sickness: The Politics of Health Insurance in Progressive America* (Chapel Hill: University of North Carolina Press, 2001), 45–67, 163–80.

46. Stewart Roberts, "The Social Trends Underlying Health and Hospital Insurance," *NEJM* 212 (1935): 1124 (quotations), 1128 (quotation), 1129 (quotation), 1123–29; W. L. Bierring et al. to Edwin Witte, May 22, 1935, Altmeyer Papers, box 2, folder: "Health Insurance Report of 1935."

CHAPTER FOUR: American Democratic Medicine

1. On labor's impasse in the Progressive Era, see Solon DeLeon, "Year's Developments toward Health Insurance Legislation," *ALLR* 8 (1918): 316–18; AFL, *Report of Proceedings of the Thirty-Eighth Annual Convention, 1918* (Washington: Law Reporter Printing, 1918), 94, 282–83; AFL, *Report of Proceedings of the Fortieth Annual Convention, 1920* (Washington: Law Reporter Printing, 1920), 176, 387; AFL, *Report of Proceedings of the Forty-First Annual Convention, 1921* (Washington: Law Reporter Printing, 1921), 147–48, 310–11; Beatrix Hoffman, *The Wages of Sickness: The Politics of Health Insurance in Progressive America* (Chapel Hill: University of North Carolina Press, 2001), 115–36. On some of the meanings of the New Deal for workers, see Irving Bernstein, *A Caring Society: The New Deal, the Worker, and the Great Depression* (Boston: Houghton Mifflin, 1985); Lizabeth Cohen, *Making a New Deal: Industrial Workers in Chicago, 1919–1939* (Cambridge: Cambridge University Press, 1990), 251–89.

2. AFL, *Report of Proceedings of the Fifty-Fifth Annual Convention, 1935* (Washington: Judd and Detweiler, n.d.), 593 (quotation), 93 (quotation), 91–93, 269–70.

3. Harold Maslow, "Labor Leadership Needed for Health Insurance," *American Federationist*, Oct. 1937, 1071–73; Andrew Biemiller, "Medical Care for Wage Earning Groups," ibid., Oct. 1938, 1054–59. In California, a similar proposal in 1939 met the same fate. See Daniel J. Mitchell, "Earl Warren's California Health Insurance Plan: What Might Have Been," *Southern California Quarterly* 85 (2003): 210–11.

4. [William Green], "Health a Public Responsibility," *American Federationist*, July 1937, 703 (quotation), 702–3; [William Green], "Health for All," ibid., May 1938, 471

(quotation), 470–71; [William Green], "Toward Social Security," ibid., Feb. 1937, 130–31; [William Green], "National Health Survey," ibid., Feb. 1938, 130–31.

5. William Green, *Labor and Democracy* (Princeton: Princeton University Press, 1939), 26–38; Craig Phelan, *William Green: Biography of a Labor Leader* (Albany: SUNY Press, 1988), 20–21; United Mine Workers of America, *Proceedings of the Twenty-Seventh Consecutive and Fourth Biennial Convention, 1919*, 3 vols. (Indianapolis: Book-walter-Ball Printing, 1919), 2: 682–83; [William Green] to James Duncan, July 24, 1919, AFL, Office of the President, William Green Papers, RG-019, box 1, folder 7, George Meany Memorial Archives, Silver Spring, Md.; William Green to Daniel Tobin, June 2, 1920, ibid., folder 9. On social unionism, see Joseph Shister, "Unresolved Problems and New Paths for American Labor," *Industrial and Labor Relations Review* 9 (1956): 447–57; Jack Fiorito, "Unionism and Altruism," *Labor Studies Journal* 17 (1992): 19–34.

6. Edwin Witte, *The Development of the Social Security Act: A Memorandum on the History of the Committee on Economic Security and Drafting and Legislative History of the Social Security Act* (Madison: University of Wisconsin Press, 1963), 165–73; Bernstein, *Caring Society*, 58–59; John Duffy, *The Sanitarians: A History of American Public Health* (Urbana: University of Illinois Press, 1990), 258–61; Isidore Falk, "Reminiscences," interview by Peter Corning, Oct. 3, 1968, transcript, 55–56, Oral History Collection, Oral History Research Office, Butler Library, Columbia University, New York; I. S. Falk to C.-E. A. Winslow, Aug. 28, 1936, C.-E. A. Winslow Papers, box 10, folder 247, Manuscripts and Archives, Yale University Library, New Haven.

7. Edgar Sydenstricker, "The Changing Concept of Public Health," *Milbank Memorial Fund Quarterly* 13 (1935): 303 (quotations), 301–10.

8. Thomas Parran, "Health Security," *AJPH* 26 (1936): 333 (quotation), 329–35; Thomas Parran, "Trends in Public Health," *Annals of Internal Medicine* 12 (1938): 116 (quotations), 115 (quotation), 119 (quotation), 115–20.

9. Josephine Roche, "Medical Care as a Public Health Function," *AJPH* 27 (1937): 1221 (quotation), 1221–26; Editorial, "Public Health and Private Rights," *Christian Century*, Nov. 17, 1937, 1414–15; Michael Davis, *Public Medical Services: A Survey of Tax-Supported Medical Care in the United States* (Chicago: University of Chicago Press, 1937).

10. Grace Abbott, *From Relief to Social Security: The Development of the Public Welfare Services and Their Administration* (Chicago: University of Chicago Press, 1941), 295 (quotation), 297 (quotation), 290–97. On Abbott, see Lela Costin, *Two Sisters for Social Justice: A Biography of Grace and Edith Abbott* (Urbana: University of Illinois Press, 1983).

11. Henry Sigerist, *Socialized Medicine in the Soviet Union* (New York: W. W. Norton, 1937), 15, 17, 57, 59, 83–84, 86, 96–98, 278, 307–8; John F. Hutchinson, "Dances with Commissars: Sigerist on Soviet Medicine," in *Making Medical History: The Life and Times of Henry E. Sigerist*, ed. Elizabeth Fee and Theodore M. Brown (Baltimore: Johns Hopkins University Press, 1997), 229–58; Elizabeth Fee, "The Pleasures and Perils of Prophetic Advocacy: Socialized Medicine and the Politics of American Medical Reform," ibid., 197–228; John Andrews to Henry Sigerist, Dec. 11, 1937, *American Association for Labor Legislation Papers, 1905–1945*, microfilm ed., 71 reels (Glen Rock, N.J.: Microfilming Corporation of America, 1973), reel 57.

12. Henry Sigerist, "Socialized Medicine," *Yale Review* 27 (1938): 464 (quotation), 470 (quotation), 463–81.

13. Fee, "Pleasures and Perils," 210. For a most curious example of curiosity about state medicine, see J. Strom Thurmond to American Association for Social Security, July 18, 1939, American Association for Social Security Records, box 2, folder 42, Kheel Center for Labor-Management Documentation and Archives, Catherwood Library, Cornell University, Ithaca. For an analysis that focuses on AMA opposition to state insurance (but not state medicine), see Ronald Numbers, "The Specter of Socialized Medicine: American Physicians and Compulsory Health Insurance," in *Compulsory Health Insurance: The Continuing American Debate*, ed. Ronald Numbers (Westport, Conn.: Greenwood Press, 1982), 3–24.

14. U.S. Interdepartmental Committee to Coordinate Health and Welfare Activities, news release, Mar. 27, 1938 (quotation), Altmeyer Papers, box 3, folder: "National Health Conference"; Rollo Britten, "The National Health Survey: Receipt of Medical Services in Different Urban Populations and Groups," *Public Health Reports* 55 (1940): 2200 (quotation), 2220 (quotation), 2199–2224, esp. 2219–22; Rollo Britten, Selwyn Collins, and James Fitzgerald, "The National Health Survey: Some General Findings as to Disease, Accidents, and Impairments in Urban Areas," ibid., 444–70; U.S. Public Health Service, *The National Health Survey: 1935–1936: Illness and Medical Care in Relation to Economic Status* (Washington: The Service, 1938). A federal survey of household expenditures in 1917 had disclosed a similar racial disparity in spending on and, presumably, access to heath care. See Joel D. Howell and Catherine G. McLaughlin, "Race, Income, and the Purchase of Medical Care by Selected 1917 Working-Class Urban Families," *Journal of the History of Medicine and Allied Sciences* 47 (1992): 439–61. The National Health Survey notwithstanding, federal officials (in part because of their ongoing reliance on the whites-only CCMC studies) continued to ignore racial aspects of health-care access in the late 1930s. See George Perrott, "Health Problems of Low Income Families," *Health Officer* 2 (1938): 488–95; Joseph Mountin and Hazel O'Hara, "Differences in Opportunities for Health," *Public Health Reports* 53 (1938): 485–96.

15. U.S. Interdepartmental Committee to Coordinate Health and Welfare Activities, Technical Committee on Medical Care, "A National Health Program: Report of the Technical Committee on Medical Care," Feb. 14, 1938, in U.S. Interdepartmental Committee to Coordinate Health and Welfare Activities, *Proceedings of the National Health Conference* (Washington: GPO, 1938), 29 (quotation), 60 (quotation), 55 (quotation), 64 (quotation), 29–64.

16. Josephine Roche, "The Worker's Stake in a National Health Program," *ALLR* 28 (1938): 125 (quotation), 125–30; I. S. Falk, "The Committee on the Costs of Medical Care: Twenty-Five Years of Progress: Introductory Remarks," *AJPH* 48 (1958): 982 (quotation); Interdepartmental Committee, *National Health Conference*, 14–15; Michael M. Davis, *Medical Care for Tomorrow* (New York: Harper and Brothers, 1955), 278. For Falk's recollection of the conference as a "blowout" with the AMA, see Falk, "Reminiscences," 211.

17. Davis, *Medical Care for Tomorrow*, 278 (quotation). On the upsurge in unionism, see, among many others, Irving Bernstein, *Turbulent Years: A History of the American Worker, 1933–1941* (Boston: Houghton Mifflin, 1970); Robert Zieger, *The CIO, 1935–1955* (Chapel Hill: University of North Carolina Press, 1995), 22–140; Janet Irons, *Testing the New Deal: The General Textile Strike of 1934 in the American South* (Urbana: University of Illinois Press, 2000); Dana Frank, "Girl Strikers Occupy Chain Store, Win Big: The Detroit Woolworth's Strike of 1937," in Howard Zinn, Dana Frank, and Robin

D. G. Kelley, *Three Strikes: Miners, Musicians, Salesgirls, and the Fighting Spirit of Labor's Last Century* (Boston: Beacon Press, 2001), 57–118.

18. Interdepartmental Committee, *National Health Conference*, 84 (Greenberg quotations), 26–27, 84–85; Roche, "Worker's Stake," 127.

19. Interdepartmental Committee, *National Health Conference*, 122 (Stone quotation), 14 (Bellanca quotation), 106 (Pressman quotation), 13 (Green quotation), 12–15, 105–7, 120, 122–24.

20. Ibid., 1 (Roche quotation), 5 (Parran quotation), 94 (Silverman quoting Parran), 1–7, 93–95; Thomas Parran, "The Significance of the National Health Conference," July 19, 1938, Parran Papers, box 39, folder 492; People's National Health Committee, "The People's Fight for Health and Life," July 18, 1938, John Kingsbury Papers, pt. II, box 61, folder: "National Health Conference," Manuscript Division, Library of Congress, Washington.

21. Interdepartmental Committee, *National Health Conference*, 9 (Abell quotation), 11 (Kahn quotation), 87 (Wright quotations), 9–12, 16–18, 79, 154–56. On Wright's career, see P. Preston Reynolds, "Dr. Louis T. Wright and the NAACP: Pioneers in Hospital Racial Integration," *AJPH* 90 (2000): 883–92.

22. Interdepartmental Committee, *National Health Conference*, 19 (Cabot quotation), 146 (Baehr quotation), 149 (Winslow quotation), 19–21, 24, 70–71, 130–32, 134–37, 141–42, 146–47, 149–52.

23. Josephine Roche to the President, July 23, 1938 (quotation), Altmeyer Papers, box 3, folder: "National Health Conference"; Editorial, "National Health Conference," *NEJM* 219 (1938): 136–37; Editorial, "The National Health Problem," ibid., 209–10; Robert F. Wagner, "The National Health Bill," *ALLR* 29 (1939): 13–17; Hirshfield, *Lost Reform*, 138–39.

24. Wagner, "National Health Bill," 16 (quotations), 13–17.

25. Morris Fishbein, "American Medicine and the National Health Program," *NEJM* 220 (1939): 495–504; Editorial, "The Special Session of the American Medical Association," *American Journal of Surgery* 42 (1938): 287–88; Hirshfield, *Lost Reform*, 124–51; James Rorty, *American Medicine Mobilizes* (New York: W. W. Norton, 1939), 104, 320–23; Alan Brinkley, *The End of Reform: New Deal Liberalism in Recession and War* (New York: Vintage Books, 1996).

26. U.S. Senate, Committee on Education and Labor, *To Establish a National Health Program: Hearings . . . on S. 1620*, 76th Cong., 1st sess., 1939 (Washington: GPO, 1939), 882 (Polakov quotation), 205–13, 224–31, 876–88; Michael Davis to Thomas Parran, Mar. 24, 1939, Michael Davis Papers, box 71, folder: "Parran, Thomas," Historical Collections, New York Academy of Medicine, New York.

27. U.S. National Resources Planning Board, *National Resources Development: Report for 1942* (Washington: GPO, 1942), 1 (quotation), 3, 8–9, 15, 110, 112; Franklin D. Roosevelt, "Message to the Congress on the State of the Union," Jan. 11, 1944, in *Public Papers and Addresses of Franklin D. Roosevelt*, comp. Samuel Rosenman, 13 vols., vol. 13: *Victory and the Threshold of Peace* (New York: Harper and Brothers, 1950), 41 (quotations), 40–41. On the National Resources Planning Board, see Nelson Polsby, *Political Innovation in America: The Politics of Policy Initiation* (New Haven: Yale University Press, 1984), 105–6. On the promise of the Declaration of Independence, see Charles L. Black Jr., *A New Birth of Freedom: Human Rights, Named and Unnamed* (New York: Grosset/Putnam, 1997).

28. Arthur Altmeyer, *The Formative Years of Social Security* (Madison: University of Wisconsin Press, 1966), 74–151; U.S. Social Security Board, *Eighth Annual Report, Fiscal Year 1942–43* (Washington: GPO, 1943), 32–39; Great Britain, Interdepartmental Committee on Social Insurance and Allied Services, *Social Insurance and Allied Services: Report by Sir William Beveridge*, Cmd 6404 (London: HMSO, 1942); I. S. Falk, "Mobilizing for Health Security," in *War and Post-War Social Security: The Outlines of an Expanded Program*, ed. Wilbur J. Cohen (Washington: American Council on Public Affairs, 1942), 68–77; Wilbur J. Cohen, "Next Steps and Future Goals," in ibid., 31–42; Edwin Amenta and Theda Skocpol, "Redefining the New Deal: World War II and the Development of Social Provision in the United States," in *The Politics of Social Policy in the United States*, ed. Margaret Weir, Theda Skocpol, and Ann Shola Orloff (Princeton: Princeton University Press, 1988), 81–122; Jill Quadagno, *The Color of Welfare: How Racism Undermined the War on Poverty* (New York: Oxford University Press, 1995), 19–24, 157–58; Hirshfield, *Lost Reform*, 163–65; Monte Poen, *Harry S. Truman versus the Medical Lobby: The Genesis of Medicare* (Columbia: University of Missouri Press, 1979), 29–33.

29. *Congressional Record* 89 (1943): 5258–67, esp. 5261–62.

30. I. S. Falk, "Social Security for Everyone," Feb. 10, 1943, Falk Papers, box 79, folder 859; *Congressional Record* 89 (1943): 5262. On contributory funding as an article of faith, see J. Douglas Brown, *An American Philosophy of Social Security: Evolution and Issues* (Princeton: Princeton University Press, 1972), 17–23, 43–64; Colin Gordon, *Dead on Arrival: The Politics of Health Care in Twentieth-Century America* (Princeton: Princeton University Press, 2003), 92–100.

31. Poen, *Truman versus Medical Lobby*, 51–53; David McCullough, *Truman* (New York: Touchstone, 1993), 166–75; Starr, *Social Transformation*, 280–82; Douglas E. Ashford, *The Emergence of the Welfare States* (Oxford: Basil Blackwell, 1986), 240–99; Peter Baldwin, *The Politics of Social Solidarity: Class Bases of the European Welfare States, 1875–1975* (Cambridge: Cambridge University Press, 1990), 107–207; Raymond Richards, *Closing the Door to Destitution: The Shaping of the Social Security Acts of the United States and New Zealand* (University Park: Pennsylvania State University Press, 1994).

32. Health Program Conference, *Principles of a Nation-wide Health Program: Report of the Health Program Conference* (New York: Committee on Research in Medical Economics, 1944); Michael Davis to Robert Wagner, Apr. 27, 1945, Robert F. Wagner Papers, Legislative Files, box 265, folder 11, Special Collections Division, Georgetown University Library, Washington; Robert Wagner to Michael Davis, May 10, 1945, Davis Papers, box 72, folder: "Robert F. Wagner, Sr., 1944–46"; Michael Davis, "Report of the President to the Annual Meeting," May 9, 1947, ibid., box 54, folder: "Minutes of Annual Membership Meetings—from 1946"; Margaret I. Stein, "Meeting of the Health Program Steering Group," Feb. 15, 1946, Wilbur Cohen Papers, box 27, folder 3, Archives Division, Wisconsin Historical Society, Madison; Poen, *Truman versus Medical Lobby*, 83; Starr, *Social Transformation*, 280. The Committee for the Nation's Health was an offshoot of the Social Security Charter Committee, a lobbying group also created by Michael Davis. See Starr, *Social Transformation*, 280; [Wilbur Cohen], "Draft of Opening Remarks of Senator Wagner at Conference in His Office, February 5, 1944," Feb. 2, 1944, Cohen Papers, box 53, folder 4.

33. Edwin Witte, "American Post-War Social Security Proposals," *American Economic Review* 33 (1943): 832 (quotation), 835–36; Altmeyer, *Formative Years*, 146; Wilbur

Cohen to I. S. Falk, John Corson, and O. C. Pogge, Mar. 19, 1943, Falk Papers, box 59, folder 514; Philip Murray to Robert Wagner, May 15, 1943, ibid., box 60, folder 525; M[ichael] M. D[avis] to Thomas Parran, June 3, 1943, Davis Papers, box 71, folder: "Parran, Thomas"; Alan Derickson, "Health Security for All? Social Unionism and Universal Health Insurance, 1935–1958," *JAH* 80 (1994): 1340–43. For union influence on social policy more broadly, see Edward Berkowitz, "How to Think about the Welfare State," *Labor History* 32 (1991): 499–502; Seth Wigderson, "How the CIO Saved Social Security," ibid. 44 (2003): 483–507.

34. Interdepartmental Committee, *National Health Conference*, 22 (McCormack quotation), 21–23; Milton Roemer, "The American Public Health Association as a Force for Change in Medical Care," *Medical Care* 11 (1973): 339–41; John Duffy, "The American Medical Profession and Public Health: From Support to Ambivalence," *Bulletin of the History of Medicine* 53 (1979): 20–21.

35. C.-E. A. Winslow, "The Public Health Aspects of Medical Care," *AJPH* 29 (1939): 20 (quotation), 16 (quotation), 16–22; Edward Godfrey, "Health for Three-Thirds of the Nation," ibid., 1288 (quotations), 1283–91; Abel Wolman, "A Century in Arrears," ibid., 28 (1938): 1369–75; Thomas Parran, "The Health of the Nation," ibid., 1376, 1380; Senate, *To Establish*, 130–39. For a wide-ranging argument for prevention as a crucial component of universal health protection, see Thomas Parran, "The Right to Health— and How to Win It," June 20, 1939, Parran Papers, box 40, folder 523.

36. Social Security Board, *Report, 1942–43*, 24 (quotation); APHA, "Medical Care in a National Health Program: An Official Statement of the American Public Health Association Adopted October 4, 1944," *AJPH* 34 (1944): 1253 (quotation), 1252–56; Subcommittee on Medical Care, Committee on Administrative Practice, APHA, "Preliminary Report on a National Program on Medical Care," ibid., 984–88; Joseph W. Mountin, "Content and Administration of a Medical Care Program: A Brief of the Report on Medical Care in a National Health Program," ibid., 1217–22; I. S. Falk, "Some Notes on a National Health Service and a General Medical-Care Program," Mar. 31, 1944, Winslow Papers, box 10, folder 249; Arthur Viseltear, *Emergence of the Medical Care Section of the American Public Health Association, 1926–1948: A Chapter in the History of Medical Care in the United States* (Washington: APHA, 1972), 12–16; Roemer, "Force for Change," 341–44, 348; Thomas Parran to All Officers of the Public Health Service, Dec. 10, 1945, repr. in Editorial, "General Parran Addresses His Officers," *JAMA* 130 (1946): 84.

37. Raymond P. Alexander, "The Legal Aspects of Medical Economics," *JNMA* 28 (1936): 158 (quotation); Editorial, "Committee on the Cost of Medical Care: An Open Season in No Man's Land," ibid., 25 (1933): 18–19; "Dr. Fishbein Guest Speaker at National Medical Association Banquet, August 1933," ibid., 19–20; G. Hamilton Francis, "The Negro Doctor and the Threatened Socialization of Medicine," ibid., 20; Editorial, "Group Hospitalization," ibid., 28 (1936): 127–28.

38. Editorial, "A Plea for Independent Racial Thought and Action," *JNMA* 30 (1938): 121–22; C. A. Whittier et al., "The Report of the Committee on Medical Economics," ibid., 172–73; "Excerpts from [AMA] House of Delegates Proceedings of the Special Session," ibid., 173–79; Editorial, "The Federal Government and Organized Medicine in Closer Accord," ibid., 159; J[ohn] A. K[enney], "The Status of the Negro Doctor in the National Health Program," ibid. 31 (1939): 29–30; J[ohn] A. K[enney], "The Relationship between the NMA and the AMA and the Federal Government,"

ibid., 150–51; John Kenney to Robert Wagner, telegram, May 23, 1939, reprinted in ibid., 175–76; John Kenney, "The New York Meeting of the NMA," ibid., 221–22.

39. Senate, *To Establish*, 240 (Wright quotation), 237–43, 891–98; Charlie [Houston] to Walter White, Nov. 18, 1939 (quotation), National Association for the Advancement of Colored People Records, pt. I, series C, box 257, folder: "Congressional Action, Wagner Health Bill, May 26—Dec. 26, 1939," Manuscript Division, Library of Congress, Washington; Dona Cooper Hamilton and Charles V. Hamilton, *The Dual Agenda: Race and Social Welfare Policies of Civil Rights Organizations* (New York: Columbia University Press, 1997), 2 (quotation); Louis T. Wright to E. Worth Higgins, July 28, 1938, NAACP Records, pt. I, series C, box 306, folder: "Health and Hygiene, 1938"; W[alter] W[hite] to Fred Hoehler, Dec. 22, 1938, ibid.; Frances H. Williams to William Imes, Nov. 2, 1939, ibid., box 257, folder: "Congressional Action, Wagner Health Bill, May 26–Dec. 26, 1939"; Elmer H. Carter, "The AMA and the Negro," *Opportunity*, May 1939, 130–31. On the general political reorientation of the African-American community, see Harvard Sitkoff, *A New Deal for Blacks: The Emergence of Civil Rights as a National Issue: The Depression Decade* (New York: Oxford University Press, 1978); August Meier and John Bracey, "The NAACP as a Reform Movement, 1909–1965: 'To Reach the Conscience of America,'" *Journal of Southern History* 59 (1993): 15–21, 23; Beth Tompkins Bates, "A New Crowd Challenges the Agenda of the Old Guard in the NAACP, 1933–1941," *AHR* 102 (1997): 340–77.

40. Senate, *To Establish*, 894 (Davis quotation), 891–98; Louis T. Wright to Josephine Roche, July 30, 1938 (quotation), NAACP Records, pt. I, series C, box 306, folder: "Health and Hygiene, 1938"; T[hurgood] Marshall, "Suggested Amendments to S. 1620," Apr. 11, 1939, ibid., folder: "Health and Hygiene, 1939"; W[alter] W[hite] to Robert Wagner, Feb. 10, 1939, ibid., box 257, folder: "Congressional Action, Wagner Health Bill, Feb. 7–May 25, 1939"; Walter White, blank form letter, Dec. 4, 1939, ibid., folder: "Congressional Action, Wagner Health Bill, May 26–Dec. 26, 1939"; Thurgood Marshall to Philip Levy, Jan. 8, 1941, ibid., pt. II, series B, box 71, folder: "Federal Health Bill, 1941"; Reynolds, "Wright and NAACP," 888–89; Ruby Yearwood, "The Wagner-Murray-Dingell Bill," *Opportunity*, Jan. 1944, 9–11; Louis T. Wright to Ernst Boas, June 24, 1944, Ernst Boas Papers, series I, box: Mo-New York He, folder: "NAACP," American Philosophical Society Library, Philadelphia. For a sharp critique of the all-white CCMC as naively oblivious to racial realities, see John A. Kenney et al., "Reaction of the North Jersey Medical Society to the Report of the Committee on the Costs of Medical Care, June 14, 1933," *JNMA* 26 (1934): 12–13. On Montague Cobb, see E. H. Beardsley, "Good-bye to Jim Crow: The Desegregation of Southern Hospitals, 1945–70," *Bulletin of the History of Medicine* 60 (1986): 367–86. On the war as a catalyst to activism by African-American physicians, see Darlene Clark Hine, "Black Professionals and Race Consciousness: Origins of the Civil Rights Movement, 1890–1950," *JAH* 89 (2003): 1279–94.

41. Warren Draper, "A National Health Program," *NEJM* 220 (1939): 43–47; Falk, "Reminiscences," 63ff; Arthur Altmeyer, "Reminiscences," interview by Peter Corning, Sept. 14, 1966, transcript, passim, esp. 225–27, Oral History Collection, Oral History Research Office, Butler Library, Columbia University, New York; Wilbur Cohen to Robert Wagner, Mar. 23, 1946, Cohen Papers, box 27, folder 4; I. S. Falk to Wilbur Cohen, Jan. 11, 1943, Falk Papers, box 59, folder 514; [I. S. Falk], "Summary Notes

Recording Evolution of President Truman's Message to Congress on a National Health Program," Dec. 4, 1945, ibid., box 6, folder 111; Milton Roemer, "I. S. Falk, the Committee on the Costs of Medical Care, and the Drive for National Health Insurance," *AJPH* 75 (1985): 841, 847; Poen, *Truman versus Medical Lobby*, 33–35. On bureaucratic influence on social policy in this era, see Brian Balogh, "Securing Support: The Emergence of the Social Security Board as a Political Actor, 1935–1939," in *Federal Social Policy: The Historical Dimension*, ed. Donald Critchlow and Ellis W. Hawley (University Park: Pennsylvania State University Press, 1988), 55–78; Theodore Marmor and Philip Fellman, "Entrepreneurship in Public Management: Wilbur Cohen and Robert Ball," in *Leadership and Innovation: A Biographical Perspective on Entrepreneurs in Government*, ed. Jameson Doig and Erwin Hargrove (Baltimore: Johns Hopkins University Press, 1987), 246–81; Edward D. Berkowitz, *Mr. Social Security: The Life of Wilbur J. Cohen* (Lawrence: University Press of Kansas, 1995); Altmeyer, *Formative Years*. For state-centered interpretation of the evolution of social reform, see Theda Skocpol, *Protecting Soldiers and Mothers: The Political Origins of Social Policy in the United States* (Cambridge: Belknap Press of Harvard University Press, 1992); Weir, Orloff, and Skocpol, eds., *Politics of Social Policy*.

42. Harry Truman to Congress, Sept. 6, 1945, *Congressional Record* 91 (1945): 8368 (Roosevelt quotation); Truman, "A National Health Program: Message from the President," *Social Security Bulletin* 8 (1945): 7 (quotation), 7–12.

43. Truman, "National Health Program," 9 (quotation), 11 (quotations), 7.

44. Arthur Altmeyer, "How Can We Assure Adequate Health Service for All the People?" *Social Security Bulletin* 8 (1945): 14 (quotation), 12–17; Thomas Parran, "A National Health Program—American Style," Dec. 12, 1945, 3 (quotation), 1 (quotation), Parran Papers, box 47, folder 717; Editorial, "The President's National Health Program and the New Wagner Bill," *JAMA* 129 (1945): 950 (quotation), 950–53

45. U.S. Senate, Committee on Education and Labor, *National Health Program: Hearings . . . on S. 1606*, 79th Cong., 2d sess., 1946 (Washington: GPO, 1946), 47 (Taft quotation), 47–52. In I. S. Falk's recollection, Murray and Taft "quarreled almost to the point where Senator Taft had to be led out by the police." Falk, "Reminiscences," 269 (quotation).

46. Senate, *National Health Program*, 499 (Lowe quotation), 736 (Boas quotation), 443 (Lawless quotation), 136, 438, 442–43, 453, 458, 501–7, 787, 790–94, 2725–33. On the cosmopolitan secularism of American Jewish intellectuals, see David Hollinger, *Science, Jews, and Secular Culture: Studies in Mid-Twentieth-Century American Intellectual History* (Princeton: Princeton University Press, 1996); Lila Corwin Berman, "Measuring Up," Pennsylvania State University Modern History Workshop, Feb. 27, 2004. On the NMA's gravitation into the Wagner-Murray-Dingell camp, see John Givens, "The President's Plan for Medical Care," *JNMA* 38 (1946): 33; H. A. C[allis], "The People's Health," ibid., 33–34; W. Montague Cobb, *Medical Care and the Plight of the Negro* (New York: NAACP, 1947), 31–32.

47. Senate, *National Health Program*, 142 (Mountin quotation), 459 (McMichael quotation), 134–68, 458–59. On exemptions from the insurance provisions of Wagner-Murray-Dingell and the separate health-care arrangements for the "needy," see ibid., 16–19, 29–31, 57, 184–85, 190, 200–202. For the debate pitting the Social Security Board against the PHS and the Children's Bureau, see Commissioner for Social Security and

Surgeon General to [Federal Security] Administrator, Nov. 6, 1946, Cohen Papers, box 27, folder 5.

48. Senate, *National Health Program*, 468 (Green quotation), 2698 (Davis quotation), 58, 108–110, 172, 467–69, 491, 740, 744, 2196.

49. Ibid., 552 (Senserich quotation), 1820 (O'Grady quotation), 551–604, 623–30, 794–816, 929–32, 1667–88, 1770–1845, 2337–60; Poen, *Truman versus Medical Lobby*, 88–92. For further evidence of the equivocal position of McGowan's group, see Administrative Board and Assistant Bishops of the National Catholic Welfare Conference, "Statement on Church and Social Order," Feb. 7, 1940, in *Justice in the Marketplace: Collected Statements of the Vatican and the United States Bishops on Economic Policy, 1891–1984*, ed. David M. Byers (Washington: United States Catholic Conference, 1985), 432–35. In formally reaffirming its commitment to universal access to care in 1944, the AMA made voluntary insurance the primary means to that end. See "Council on Medical Service," *JAMA* 125 (1944): 501; House of Delegates, AMA, "Proceedings of the Chicago Session," ibid., 566–67, 574–76, 651–52. Although she did not apply this line of reasoning directly to the case of health reform, Social Security official Rose McHugh in 1939 offered an explicitly Catholic interpretation of New Deal social policy that embraced John Ryan's position that needs created rights. See Dorothy M. Brown and Elizabeth McKeown, *The Poor Belong to Us: Catholic Charities and American Welfare* (Cambridge: Harvard University Press, 1997), 179. Retired, in declining health, and preoccupied with other social-justice issues, Ryan himself played no significant part in the health-reform drive of the 1940s. He died in 1945, at age seventy-six. See Francis L. Broderick, *Right Reverend New Dealer: John A. Ryan* (New York: Macmillan, 1963), 248–76; John A. Ryan, *Social Doctrine in Action: A Personal History* (New York: Harper and Brothers, 1941), 277–90.

50. Brinkley, *End of Reform*, 10 (quotation), 3–14. For expressions of the needs-centered rationale for reform, see Perrott, "Health Problems of Low Income Families," 488–95; AFL, *Next Steps in Social Insurance* ([Washington]: AFL, 1939); Margaret Klem, "Medical Care Insurance and the Nurse," *American Journal of Nursing* 46 (1946): 387; Senate, *National Health Program*, 501–507. For renditions of the human-capital argument, see Interdepartmental Committee, *National Health Conference*, 11, 14; CIO, *Daily Proceedings of the Fourth Constitutional Convention, 1941* (n.p., n.d.), 111–12; CIO, *For the Nation's Security*, [rev. ed.] (n.p., [1945]), 13; Senate, *National Health Program*, 393–98; Franz Goldmann, "Health Bills Pending in Congress: Part Four," *NEJM* 234 (1946): 749.

51. Senate, *National Health Program*, 527–31, 750, 2023–24, 2690; Nelson Cruikshank, "What Labor Expects from Medicine," *Connecticut State Medical Journal* 10 (1946): 302. On contributory financing, see Mark Leff, "Taxing the 'Forgotten Man': The Politics of Social Security Finance in the New Deal," *JAH* 70 (1983): 359–81.

52. Thomas Parran, "Health Goals," *JNMA* 38 (1946): 214 (quotations); Ernst Boas, "The Need for a National Health Program," ibid. 41 (1949): 170 (quotation), 170–72; "Magna Carta for Health," *Survey*, Oct. 1946, 264. Eight years earlier, Parran detected the beginnings of a "world movement for health." See Parran, "Health of the Nation," 1380 (quotation). On the international human-rights movement, see Paul Lauren, *The Evolution of International Human Rights: Visions Seen* (Philadelphia: University of Pennsylvania Press, 1998); Kenneth Cmiel, "The Recent History of Human Rights," *AHR* 109 (2004): 117–35.

53. Franz Goldmann, *Public Medical Care: Principles and Problems* (New York: Columbia University Press, 1945), v (quotation); Franz Goldmann, "The Right to Medical Care," *Social Service Review* 20 (1946): 28 (quotation), 19.

54. Georges Gurvitch, *The Bill of Social Rights* (New York: International Universities Press, 1946), 85 (quotation), 12–29, 75–76, 90, 94–95. On the health-rights recommendation of the 1944 International Labor Conference, see International Labor Organization, *International Labor Conventions and Recommendations, 1919–1981* (Geneva: International Labor Office, 1982), 567–78; International Labor Conference, *Social Security: Principles, and Problems Arising Out of the War*, 2 pts. (Montreal: International Labor Office, 1944), 1: 57–115, esp. 103–4.

55. Franz Goldmann, "Health Bills Pending in Congress: Part One," *NEJM* 234 (1946): 660 (quotation), 657 (quotation), 657–60; Franz Goldmann, "Health Bills Pending in Congress: Part Two," ibid., 689–90; Rorty, *American Medicine Mobilizes*, 51 (quotation), 228; Henry Sigerist, *Medicine and Human Welfare* (New Haven: Yale University Press, 1941), 101 (quotation), 101–4; Goldmann, *Public Medical Care*, 197; Senate, *National Health Program*, 472–74, 787, 790–94; Alan Derickson, " 'Take Health from the List of Luxuries': Labor and the Right to Health Care, 1915–1949," *Labor History* 41 (2000): 182–84. For the claim that in Jefferson's mind "happiness" required security, see Pauline Maier, *American Scripture: Making the Declaration of Independence* (New York: Vintage Books, 1997), 134. Franz Goldmann was not the only proponent of pure egalitarianism. See United Auto Workers, *Proceedings of the Tenth Convention, 1946* (n.p., n.d.), 33.

56. Conference of Labor Research Group, "Summarized Proceedings," Dec. 10, 1946, 15 (Goodman quotation), United Steelworkers of America Archives, Research Department Records, box 65, folder 7, Historical Collections and Labor Archives, Paterno Library, Pennsylvania State University, University Park; Senate, *National Health Program*, 452 (McMichael quotation), 458; John Kingsbury, *Health in Handcuffs* (New York: Modern Age Books, 1939), 195; CIO, *For the Nation's Security*, 7–8; Ernst Boas, *Why Do We Need National Health Insurance?* (New York: New York Society for Ethical Culture, 1945), 3–4; Parran, "Health Program—American Style," 3–4; CIO, *Final Proceedings of the Eighth Constitutional Convention, 1946* (Washington: n.pub., n.d.), 81.

57. Senate, *To Establish*, 110 (Wagner quoting Greenberg); T. H. Marshall, "Citizenship and Social Class," in Marshall, *Citizenship and Social Class, and Other Essays* (Cambridge: Cambridge University Press, 1950), 1–85. For incisive analyses of Marshall's essay, see Nancy Fraser and Linda Gordon, "Contract versus Charity: Why Is There No Social Citizenship in the United States?" *Socialist Review* 22 (1992): 45–67; Tom Bottomore, "Citizenship and Social Class, Forty Years On, " in *Citizenship and Social Class*, ed. T. H. Marshall and Tom Bottomore (London: Pluto Press, 1992), 55–93; Bryan S. Turner, "Citizenship Studies: A General Theory," *Citizenship Studies* 1 (1997): 5–18; Alice Kessler-Harris, *In Pursuit of Equity: Women, Men, and the Quest for Economic Citizenship in 20th-Century America* (New York: Oxford University Press, 2001), passim, esp. 10–14. On women and the discourses of rights and needs, see Linda Gordon, "Social Insurance and Public Assistance: The Influence of Gender in Welfare Thought in the United States, 1890–1935," *AHR* 97 (1992): 31–33; Lisa Peattie and Martin Rein, *Women's Claims: A Study in Political Economy* (New York: Oxford University Press, 1983), 81–86.

CHAPTER FIVE: Well on the Way

Epigraph: Rita R. Campbell and W. Glenn Campbell, *Voluntary Health Insurance in the United States* (Washington: American Enterprise Association, 1960), 1.

1. Among the most helpful studies of this period are Monte Poen, *Harry S. Truman versus the Medical Lobby: The Genesis of Medicare* (Columbia: University of Missouri Press, 1979); Raymond Munts, *Bargaining for Health: Labor Unions, Health Insurance, and Medical Care* (Madison: University of Wisconsin Press, 1967), 3–79; Paul Starr, *The Social Transformation of American Medicine* (New York: Basic Books, 1982), 280–334; Daniel M. Fox, *Health Policies, Health Politics: The British and American Experience, 1911–1965* (Princeton: Princeton University Press, 1986), 149–68, 188–206; Beth Stevens, "Blurring the Boundaries: How the Federal Government Has Influenced Welfare Benefits in the Private Sector," in *The Politics of Social Policy in the United States*, ed. Margaret Weir, Ann Shola Orloff, and Theda Skocpol (Princeton: Princeton University Press, 1988), 123–48; Beth Stevens, "Labor Unions, Employee Benefits, and the Privatization of the American Welfare State," *Journal of Policy History* 2 (1990): 233–60; Jacob Hacker, *The Divided Welfare State: The Battle over Public and Private Social Benefits in the United States* (Cambridge: Cambridge University Press, 2002), 221–69; Jennifer Klein, *For All These Rights: Business, Labor, and the Shaping of America's Public-Private Welfare State* (Princeton: Princeton University Press, 2003), 162–257; Colin Gordon, *Dead on Arrrival: The Politics of Health Care in Twentieth-Century America* (Princeton: Princeton University Press, 2003), 57–82, 112–16, 219–42.

2. James T. Patterson, *Grand Expectations: The United States, 1945–1974* (New York: Oxford University Press, 1996), vii–viii, 137–41; William Beveridge, *Social Insurance and Allied Services* (New York: Macmillan, 1942); Edwin Witte, "American Post-War Social Security Proposals," *American Economic Review* 33 (1943): 825–38.

3. Alonzo Hamby, *Beyond the New Deal: Harry S. Truman and American Liberalism* (New York: Columbia University Press, 1973), 145 (quotation), 137–45; David McCullough, *Truman* (New York: Simon and Schuster, 1993), 475–506, 523–24. On labor's declining popularity, see George Gallup, *The Gallup Poll: Public Opinion, 1935–1971*, 3 vols. (New York: Random House, 1972), 1: 519, 532, 621; Gilbert Gall, *The Politics of Right to Work: The Labor Federations as Special Interests, 1943–1979* (New York: Greenwood Press, 1988), 27, 33–36.

4. Commissioner for Social Security and Surgeon General to [Federal Security] Administrator, Nov. 6, 1946 (quotation), Wilbur Cohen Papers, box 27, folder 5, Archives Division, Wisconsin Historical Society, Madison; Milton Roemer to George Perrott, Nov. 22, 1946 (quotations), ibid. In California, Governor Earl Warren unsuccessfully promoted inclusive hospital-insurance measures in 1945 and 1946. See Daniel J. Mitchell, "Earl Warren's California Health Insurance Plan: What Might Have Been," *Southern California Quarterly* 85 (2003): 220–22.

5. Michael Davis, "CNH Platform," Dec. 5, 1946, Cohen Papers, box 27, folder 5; I. S. Falk to Harry Rosenfield, Dec. 23, 1946, ibid.; I. S. Falk to Wilbur Cohen, Dec. 5, 1946, RG 47, Records of the Social Security Administration, Division of Research and Statistics, General Correspondence, 1946–50, box 3, folder 32, National Archives, Washington; Falk to C.-E. A. Winslow, Dec. 31, 1946, ibid.; Executive Committee, CNH, "Minutes," Nov. 17, 1946, Michael Davis Papers, box 54, folder: "Executive Committee Minutes—1946," Historical Collections, New York Academy of Medicine Library, New

York; Ernst Boas to Margaret Stein, Nov. 29, 1946, Ernst Boas Papers, series I, box: Co-E, folder: "Committee for the Nation's Health," American Philosophical Society Library, Philadelphia.

6. Wilbur Cohen to John Thurston, May 5, 1947, Cohen Papers, box 27, folder 7; W. L. Mitchell to Watson Miller, May 12, 1947, RG 47, Records of the Social Security Administration, Division of Research and Statistics, General Correspondence, 1946–50, box 2, folder 31.

7. Conference of Labor Research Group, "Summarized Proceedings," Dec. 11, 1946, 25 (quotation), 26 (quotation), and passim, United Steelworkers of America Archives, Research Department Records, box 65, folder 7, Historical Collections and Labor Archives, Paterno Library, Pennsylvania State University, University Park; Arthur Altmeyer, "Social Security and Welfare Funds," in National Industrial Conference Board, *Union Health and Welfare Funds: A Symposium on Evolution and Problems, Operations and Experience* (n.p.: The Board, 1947), 22–25; Hacker, *Divided Welfare State*, 26, 213–14, 220, 232. For evidence that the public basic-private supplemental relationship was accepted (except for health care) across the ideological spectrum, see Chamber of Commerce of the United States, "Policy Declarations of the Chamber of Commerce of the United States on Social Security," *American Economic Security*, Jan.–Feb. 1949, 4, 8, 9; Sanford Jacoby, "Employers and the Welfare State: The Role of Marion B. Folsom," *JAH* 80 (1993): 525–56.

8. Nelson Cruikshank, "Issues in Social Security," *American Federationist*, Feb. 1947, 28 (quotation); CIO, *Proceedings of the Eleventh Constitutional Convention, 1949* (Washington: n.pub., n.d.), 108 (Murray quotation); U.S. Senate, Committee on Labor and Public Welfare, Subcommittee on Health, *National Health Program: Hearings . . . on S. 545 . . . and S. 1320*, 80th Cong., 1st and 2d sess., 1947–48 (Washington: GPO, 1947–48), 48–49, 2798, and passim.

9. Ibid., chart facing 1706 (Shearon quotation), 935–36, 1110–11, 1162, 1206–8, 1218–20, 1338–39, 1693–1921, 1921–2125, 2217–2665; Alan Derickson, "The House of Falk: The Paranoid Style in American Health Politics," *AJPH* 87 (1997): 1836–43; Marjorie Shearon, "ILO Social Security Program Is World-Wide and Covers All Aspects of Our Lives," *American Medicine and the Political Scene*, June 18, 1948, 3; "The Man behind the Wagner Bill," *Medical Economics*, Nov. 1947, 46–51, 127–47; I. S. Falk to Editors, *Medical Economics*, Nov. 14, 1947, I. S. Falk Papers, box 50, folder 359, Manuscripts and Archives, Yale University Library, New Haven; [I. S. Falk], "ILO," July 11, 1947, ibid., box 49, folder 352; I. S. Falk to E. A. Park, Apr. 30, 1948, ibid., box 45, folder 293. For the ILO position, see International Labor Conference, *Social Security: Principles, and Problems Arising Out of the War*, 2 pts. (Montreal: International Labor Office, 1944), 1: 103–4. On Robert Taft's highly partisan tendencies, see James T. Patterson, *Mr. Republican: A Biography of Robert A. Taft* (Boston: Houghton Mifflin, 1972), 324, 335–51, 442–43.

10. Walter B. Martin, "Compulsory Federal Sickness Insurance," *Virginia Medical Monthly* 73 (1946): 308 (quotation), 305–6; W. C. Caudill, "American Medicine Must Remain Free," ibid. 77 (1950): 569 (quotation), 568–70; Julian Rawls, "The Physician's Responsibility to His Community," ibid. 73 (1946): 489–91; Harvey B. Stone, "Politics and Medicine," ibid. 76 (1949): 159–60; Walter B. Martin, "Local Responsibility or Federal Control of Medicine," ibid., 1–2; Donald B. Johnson, comp., *National Party Platforms*, rev. ed., 2 vols. (Urbana: University of Illinois Press, 1978), 1:466–68; U.S. Senate, Committee on Education and Labor, *National Health Program: Hearings . . . on S. 1606*,

79th Cong., 2d sess., 1946 (Washington: GPO, 1946), 784–86; Felix Underwood, "Health and Our Neighbors," *Southern Medical Journal* 37 (1944): 284–86; George Dame, "Local Health Services," ibid. 43 (1950): 10–16. For federal innovations that unsettled powerful agricultural and medical interests, see Michael R. Grey, *New Deal Medicine: The Rural Health Programs of the Farm Security Administration* (Baltimore: Johns Hopkins University Press, 1999). On the discriminatory implementation of New Deal social policy by state and local authorities and, more broadly, the inequalities inscribed in the policy itself, see Robert Lieberman, *Shifting the Color Line: Race and the American Welfare State* (Cambridge: Harvard University Press, 1998); Jill Quadagno, *The Color of Welfare: How Racism Undermined the War on Poverty* (New York: Oxford University Press, 1995), 19–24; Lee Alston and Joseph Ferrie, *Southern Paternalism and the American Welfare State: Economics, Politics, and Institutions in the South, 1865–1965* (Cambridge: Cambridge University Press, 1999), 49–98; Nan Woodruff, *American Congo: The African American Freedom Struggle in the Delta* (Cambridge: Harvard University Press, 2003), 155–227. (Woodruff stresses mounting black resistance to the manipulation of relief and other federal programs by cotton planters in the Mississippi Delta.) On racial disparities in health care throughout the nation at this time, see W. Montague Cobb, *Medical Care and the Plight of the Negro* (New York: NAACP, 1947); W. Montague Cobb, "Medical Care for Minority Groups," *Annals of the American Academy of Political and Social Science* 273 (1951): 169–75; Paul Cornely, "Segregation and Discrimination in Medical Care in the United States," *AJPH* 46 (1956): 1074–81; David McBride, *Integrating the City of Medicine: Blacks in Philadelphia Health Care, 1910–1965* (Philadelphia: Temple University Press, 1989), 85–186; W. Michael Byrd and Linda A. Clayton, *An American Dilemma*, vol. 2: *Race, Medicine, and Health Care in the United States, 1900–2000* (New York: Routledge, 2002), 195–290.

11. Paul Hawley, address, in *John B. Andrews Memorial Symposium on Labor Legislation and Social Security, 1949*, ed. Edwin Witte et al. (n.p., n.d.), 157 (quotation), 158–59 (quotation); Ernest Irons, "Medicine and Economics," *JAMA* 134 (1947): 1021–23; Senate, *National Health Program* (1947–48), 259; Chamber of Commerce of the United States, "Present Policies of the Chamber of Commerce of the United States," *American Economic Security*, Apr.–May 1947, 9; Ronald Numbers, "The Specter of Socialized Medicine: American Physicians and Compulsory Health Insurance," in *Compulsory Health Insurance: The Continuing American Debate*, ed. Ronald Numbers (Westport, Conn.: Greenwood Press, 1982), 9–11; Poen, *Truman versus Medical Lobby*, 102ff; Starr, *Social Transformation*, 280–86.

12. Leslie Perry to Roy Wilkins, May 22, 1947 (quotation), National Association for the Advancement of Colored People Records, pt. II, series A, box 116, folder: "Health Bills, 1947–50," Manuscript Division, Library of Congress, Washington; Oscar Ewing, address, in AFL, *Report of Proceedings of the Sixty-Eighth Convention, 1949* (n.p., n.d.), 411 (quotation), 410–14; Joseph Louchheim to Michael Davis, Sept. 25, 1947 (quotation), Boas Papers, series I, box: Co-E, folder: "Committee for the Nation's Health"; George D. Cannon, "Adequate Medical Care of the Individual and Family," *JNMA* 41 (1949): 18–20.

13. Editorial, "Facing the Facts of Life," *AJPH* 39 (1949): 529 (quotation); United Nations General Assembly, "Universal Declaration of Human Rights," in Amnesty International USA, *The Universal Declaration of Human Rights, 1948–1988: Human Rights, the United Nations, and Amnesty International* (New York: Amnesty International USA Legal Support Network, 1988), 115 (quotation), 111–16; AFL, *Proceedings,*

*1949*, 414; Mary Ann Glendon, *A World Made New: Eleanor Roosevelt and the Universal Declaration of Human Rights* (New York: Random House, 2001), 42–43, 115–17, 156–57, 165, 176; Johannes Morsink, *The Universal Declaration of Human Rights: Origins, Drafting, and Intent* (Philadelphia: University of Pennsylvania Press, 1999), 192–99. For later application of the U.N. declaration, see Cathy Albisa, "Welfare Reform as a Human Rights Issue," *AJPH* 89 (1999): 1476–78; Cheryl Easley et al., "The Challenge and Place of International Human Rights in Public Health," ibid. 91 (2001): 1922–25.

14. Senate, *National Health Program* (1947–48), 2798 (Stephenson quotation); Oscar Ewing, *The Nation's Health: A Report to the President* (Washington: GPO, 1948), xi (quotation), 87 (quotation), 18 (quotation), 1, 3, 8–9, 63, 69, 77, 85–87, 91–102.

15. C.-E. A. Winslow to Isidore [Falk], May 16, 1949 (quotation), C.-E. A. Winslow Papers, box 10, folder 250, Manuscripts and Archives, Yale University Library, New Haven; Barkev Sanders to I. S. Falk, Jan. 26, 1949, RG 47, Records of the Social Security Administration, Division of Research and Statistics, General Correspondence, 1946–50, box 2, folder 28; I. S. Falk to Mr. [George] Perrott, Feb. 7, 1949, ibid.; Federal Security Agency, Health Insurance Committee, "Minutes," Jan. 26, 1949, Harry Becker Papers, box 3, folder: "Activities—1946–50," Division of Rare and Manuscript Collections, Olin Library, Cornell University, Ithaca; C.-E. A. Winslow, "Directed Gradualism in the Field of Medical Care," *AJPH* 40 (1950): 77–78; I. S. Falk, "Draft of a 'Policy' for the Administrator," Jan. 28, 1949, Cohen Papers, box 28, folder 7; I. S. Falk to Arthur Altmeyer, Jan. 31, 1949, ibid.; Legislative Committee, CNH, "Meeting," July 12, 1949, Davis Papers, box 54, folder: "Minutes of Executive Committee Meetings—1949." On the services covered by the administration bill, see U.S. Senate, Committee on Labor and Public Welfare, *National Health Program, 1949: Hearings . . . on S. 1106, S. 1456, S. 1581, and S. 1679*, 81st Cong., 1st sess., 1949 (Washington: GPO, 1949), 60–61.

16. Poen, *Truman versus Medical Lobby*, 142–51; Starr, *Social Transformation*, 282–85; James Burrow, *AMA: Voice of American Medicine* (Baltimore: Johns Hopkins Press, 1963), 361–64; Editorial, "The Drift toward Socialist Democracy," *JAMA* 139 (1949): 156–57; Editorial, "AMA Advertising Program," ibid. 143 (1950): 744; Senate, *National Health Program, 1949*, 221–29, 811–19; Michael Davis, *Medical Care for Tomorrow* (New York: Harper and Brothers, 1955), 287–91; Chamber of Commerce of the United States, *You and Socialized Medicine: The Basic Facts and a Call to Action* (Washington: The Chamber, [1949?]); A. D. Marshall, "Health Progress in the United States," *American Economic Security*, June 1949, 7–10.

17. Franz Goldmann, "Labor's Attitude toward Health Insurance," *Industrial and Labor Relations Review* 2 (1948): 91–92; Sanford Jacoby, *Modern Manors: Welfare Capitalism since the New Deal* (Princeton: Princeton University Press, 1997); Howell Harris, *The Right to Manage: Industrial Relations Policies of American Business in the 1940s* (Madison: University of Wisconsin Press, 1982), 168–75; Elizabeth Fones-Wolf, *Selling Free Enterprise: The Business Assault on Labor and Liberalism, 1945–1960* (Urbana: University of Illinois Press, 1994); Hacker, *Divided Welfare State*. On health programs of welfare capitalists in the late nineteenth and early twentieth centuries, see Stuart Brandes, *American Welfare Capitalism, 1880–1940* (Chicago: University of Chicago Press, 1976), 92–102; Alan Derickson, *Workers' Health, Workers' Democracy: The Western Miners' Struggle, 1891–1925* (Ithaca: Cornell University Press, 1988), 88–89, 104–8, 189–219; U.S. Bureau of Labor Statistics, *Health and Recreation Activities in Industrial Establishments, 1926*, Bulletin 458 (Washington: GPO, 1928).

18. Walter Reuther, "Announcement of UAW-CIO Social Security Program," Nov. 15, 1946, quoted in Frank Dickinson, "The Trend toward Labor Health and Welfare Programs," *JAMA* 133 (1947): 1286 (quotation), 1285–86; Hamby, *Beyond the New Deal*, 137; Helen Baker and Dorothy Dahl, *Group Health Insurance and Sickness Benefits in Collective Bargaining* (Princeton: Industrial Relations Section, Princeton University, 1945); Florence Peterson, Everett Kassalow, and Jean Nelson, "Health-Benefit Programs Established through Collective Bargaining," *Monthly Labor Review* 61 (1945): 191–209; U.S. Bureau of Labor Statistics, *Analysis of Health and Insurance Plans under Collective Bargaining, Late 1955*, Bulletin 1221 (Washington: GPO, 1957), iii; National Industrial Conference Board, *Company Group Insurance Plans* (New York: The Board, 1945), 22; Stevens, "Labor Unions, 233–60; Stevens, "Blurring the Boundaries," 123–48; Hacker, *Divided Welfare State*, 217–19.

19. CIO, *Proceedings, 1949*, 186 (McDonald quotation), 187 (Pollock quotation), 181–88. On the pattern of readjustment into which health bargaining fit, see Nelson Lichtenstein, "Labor in the Truman Era: Origins of the 'Private Welfare State,'" in *The Truman Presidency*, ed. Michael J. Lacey (Cambridge: Cambridge University Press, 1989), 128–55; Nelson Lichtenstein, "From Corporatism to Collective Bargaining: Organized Labor and the Eclipse of Social Democracy in the Postwar Era," in *The Rise and Fall of the New Deal Order, 1930–1980*, ed. Steve Fraser and Gary Gerstle (Princeton: Princeton University Press, 1989), 122–52; David Brody, *Workers in Industrial America: Essays on the Twentieth-Century Struggle* (New York: Oxford University Press, 1993), 157–98.

20. Robert M. MacDonald, *Collective Bargaining in the Automobile Industry: A Study of Wage Structure and Competitive Relations* (New Haven: Yale University Press, 1963), 75 (quotation), 30–31; Alan Derickson, "Health Security for All? Social Unionism and Universal Health Insurance, 1935–1958," *JAH* 80 (1994): 1345–50; Alan Derickson, "Part of the Yellow Dog: U.S. Coal Miners' Opposition to the Company Doctor System, 1936–1946," *International Journal of Health Services* 19 (1989): 709–20; Ivana Krajcinovic, *From Company Doctors to Managed Care: The United Mine Workers' Noble Experiment* (Ithaca: ILR Press of Cornell University Press, 1997), 1–129; Richard Mulcahy, *A Social Contract for the Coal Fields: The Rise and Fall of the United Mine Workers of America Welfare and Retirement Fund* (Knoxville: University of Tennessee Press, 2000), 1–127; Alan Derickson, "The United Steelworkers of America and Health Insurance, 1937–1962," in *American Labor in the Era of World War II*, ed. Sally Miller and Daniel Cornford (Westport, Conn.: Greenwood Press, 1995), 69–85.

21. Derickson, "Health Security," 1350–52; U.S. Senate, Committee on Labor and Public Welfare, Subcommittee on Welfare and Pension Funds, *Welfare and Pension Plans Investigation: Final Report*, 84th Cong., 2d sess., 1956 (Washington: GPO, 1956), 123; Evan Rowe, "Employee-Benefit Plans under Collective Bargaining, Mid-1950," *Monthly Labor Review* 72 (1951): 156–62, esp. 156; "Company Pension and Group-Insurance Plans," ibid. 70 (1950): 298–99; Sumner Slichter, James Healy, and E. Robert Livernash, *The Impact of Collective Bargaining on Management* (Washington: Brookings Institution, 1960), 402–3, 427n10; Joseph Garbarino, *Health Plans and Collective Bargaining* (Berkeley: University of California Press, 1960); Munts, *Bargaining for Health*; Stevens, "Labor Unions," 233–60; Rickey Hendricks, "Liberal Default, Labor Support, and Conservative Neutrality: The Kaiser Permanente Medical Care Program after World War II," *Journal of Policy History* 1 (1989): 156–57, 169–72; National Industrial

Conference Board, *Mutual Benefit Associations* (New York: The Board, 1938), 11–12, 15; Conference Board, *Company Group Insurance Plans*, 3–9, 15–30.

22. National Industrial Conference Board, *Company Group Insurance Plans* [rev. ed.] (New York: The Board, 1951); Jacoby, *Modern Manors*, 45, 219–20; Jacoby, "Employers," 531–37, 545n47, 551–52.

23. Franz Goldmann, *Voluntary Medical Care Insurance in the United States* (New York: Columbia University Press, 1948); Robert Cunningham III and Robert Cunningham Jr., *The Blues: A History of the Blue Cross and Blue Shield System* (DeKalb: Northern Illinois University Press, 1997), 3–117; Rosemary Stevens, *In Sickness and in Wealth: American Hospitals in the Twentieth Century* (New York: Basic Books, 1989), 171–99, 256–83; Odin Anderson, *Blue Cross since 1929: Accountability and the Public Trust* (Cambridge, Mass.: Ballinger Publishing, 1975), 1–83; Editorial, "Experimenting with State Medical Society Plans," *JAMA* 113 (1939): 2421–22; Morton D. Miller, "Voluntary Health Insurance on the National Scene: The Program of the Insurance Companies," *AJPH* 40 (1950): 1125–28; Jennifer Klein, "The Business of Health Security: Employee Health Benefits, Commercial Insurers, and the Reconstruction of Welfare Capitalism, 1945–1960," *International Labor and Working-Class History* 58 (2000): 293–313; Starr, *Social Transformation*, 290–334.

24. U.S. Bureau of the Census, *Historical Statistics of the United States, Colonial Times to 1970*, 2 vols. (Washington: GPO, 1975), 1:55; Fox, *Health Policies, Health Politics*, 149–53, 158–68, 188–206; Herman Somers and Anne Somers, *Doctors, Patients, and Health Insurance: The Organization and Financing of Medical Care* (Washington: Brookings Institution, 1961); Monroe Lerner and Odin Anderson, *Health Progress in the United States, 1900–1960: A Report of Health Information Foundation* (Chicago: University of Chicago Press, 1963); Stephen Strickland, *Politics, Science and Dread Disease: A Short History of United States Medical Research Policy* (Cambridge: Harvard University Press, 1972); Rosemary Stevens, *American Medicine and the Public Interest* (New Haven: Yale University Press, 1971), 293–414; Starr, *Social Transformation*, 335–63; Stanley Reiser, *Medicine and the Reign of Technology* (Cambridge: Cambridge University Press, 1978), 158–73, 219–21; Julie Fairman, "Economically Practical and Critically Necessary? The Development of Intensive Care at Chestnut Hill Hospital," *Bulletin of the History of Medicine* 74 (2000): 80–106; Bert Hansen, "Medical History for the Masses: How American Comic Books Celebrated Heroes of Medicine in the 1940s," ibid. 78 (2004): 148–91.

25. U.S. Senate, Committee on Labor and Public Welfare, *Health Insurance Plans in the United States: Report . . . Pursuant to S. Res. 273 and S. Res. 39*, 82d Cong., 1st sess., 1951, Senate Report 359, 3 pts. (Washington: GPO, 1951), 1: x (quotation), x–xi, 1–3, and passim; Stevens, *In Sickness*, 259; U.S. Public Health Service, *Blue Cross and Medical Service Plans*, by Louis Reed (Washington: GPO, 1947), 12; Hawley, address, in *Andrews Symposium*, 156; Margaret Klem, "Voluntary Health Insurance on the National Scene: The Present Status of Voluntary Health Insurance," *AJPH* 40 (1950): 260–67; Saxon Graham, "Socio-Economic Status, Illness, and the Use of Medical Services," *Milbank Memorial Fund Quarterly* 35 (1957): 58–66; Somers and Somers, *Doctors, Patients*, 167–87.

26. Thomas Parran and Leslie Falk, "Collective Bargaining for Medical Care Benefits: A Recent Development in the USA," *British Journal of Preventive and Social Medicine* 7 (1953): 87, 92; Harry Becker, "The Changing Scene in Health Care Economics," *New York State Journal of Medicine* 59 (1959): 2044; Herbert Northrup, "Union-

Management Welfare and Pension Plans: Their Current Status," in *Employee Welfare and Benefit Programs* (Dubuque, Iowa: William C. Brown, 1950), 6.

27. Deborah A. Stone, "The Struggle for the Soul of Health Insurance," *Journal of Health Policy, Politics and Law* 18 (1993): 301 (quotation), 300–301; John Hayes, "Hospitals and Compulsory Health Insurance," *American Economic Security*, Aug.–Sept. 1946, 24 (quotation), 22 (quotation), 17–24; E. A. Van Steenwyk, "Recent Developments in the Use of Blue Cross and Blue Shield Plans," *AJPH* 41 (1951): 149 (quotation), 147–51; David Rothman, "The Public Presentation of Blue Cross, 1935–1965," *Journal of Health Policy, Politics and Law* 16 (1991): 680–81; George Bugbee, "The New Wagner-Murray-Dingell Bill and S. 191," *Hospitals*, July 1945, 37; Editorial, "Blue Cross Proceeds Alone," ibid., Jan. 1949, 61.

28. Editorial, "Costs of Medical Care Often Burdensome," *Pennsylvania Medical Journal* 49 (1946): 654 (quotations); James McCann, "Medical Society Prepayment Programs: Lessons Learned from Experience in Massachusetts," *JAMA* 126 (1944): 343 (quotation), 341–43; Editorial, "Still the American Way," *NEJM* 240 (1949): 784 (quotations); Leland McKittrick, "Medical Care in Our Free Society," ibid. 236 (1947): 921–27; McKittrick, "Medical Care for the American People: Is Compulsory Health Insurance the Solution?," ibid. 240 (1949): 998–99; Ernest Irons, "Epochs in Medicine: The Improvement of Medical Service to Labor," *JAMA* 127 (1945): 622; Carl Strow and Gerhard Hirschfeld, "Health Insurance," ibid. 128 (1945): 870–78. On the Hill-Aiken and Flanders-Ives proposals, their inability to attain universal protection, and Truman's opposition to them, see Poen, *Truman versus Medical Lobby*, 165–73, 228–29; Senate, *National Health Program, 1949*, 4–9, 86, 284, 970, 974, 981.

29. Earle Muntz, *The National Health Program Scheme: An Analysis of the Wagner-Murray Bill (S. 1606)* (New York: American Enterprise Association, 1946), 31 (quotation), 31–32; A. L. Kirkpatrick, "The Extent of Voluntary Health Insurance," *American Economic Security*, Aug.–Sept. 1948, 26 (quotation); Health Insurance Council, *Accident and Health Coverage in the United States as of December 31, 1952* (Chicago: The Council, 1953), 5 (quotation), 5–12; E. J. Faulkner, "Health Insurance and the American People," *Harper's Magazine*, Apr. 1957, 21 (quotation); Chamber of Commerce of the United States, "Revised Policy Declarations," *American Economic Security*, July–Aug. 1949, 31–32; Northrup, "Union-Management Plans," 6; C. L. Walker, "Shield against Health Hazards," *Nation's Business*, Feb. 1945, 34–40.

30. Harry Becker, "Financing Hospital Care—Prepayment Planning for Tomorrow," Mar. 24, 1953, 6 (quotation), Becker Papers, box 4, folder: "Speeches—1953"; E. Dwight Barnett, "Positive Action to Strengthen Blue Cross," *Hospitals*, Sept. 1954, 79 (quotation), 80–81 (quotation); Commission on Financing of Hospital Care, "Discussion Outline for Workshop Conference," Apr. 15, 1953, Becker Papers, box 5, folder: "Activities—1953"; A. D. Marshall, "Conclusion," in *A Look at Modern Health Insurance*, ed. Chamber of Commerce of the United States (Washington: The Chamber, 1954), 176; Walter Lear, "Medical-Care Insurance for Industrial Workers," *Monthly Labor Review* 73 (1951): 251, 257; Arthur Altmeyer, *The Formative Years of Social Security* (Madison: University of Wisconsin Press, 1966), 237; W. Palmer Dearing, "The Prepayment Challenge," *Public Health Reports* 72 (1957): 110–14; Industrial Relations Department, National Association of Manufacturers, "Health Insurance," Jan. 19, 1955, National Association of Manufacturers Records, series II, box 426, folder 55–247, Manuscripts and Archives Department, Hagley Museum and Library, Greenville,

Del.; J. F. Follmann Jr., "Four Years of Progress in Health Insurance," *AJPH* 47 (1957): 1388–89.

31. Anson Lowitz, "To Ward Off Compulsion—Make It Unnecessary," *Hospitals*, Aug. 1949, 50 (quotation), 49–50; Stevens, *In Sickness*, 140–255; Rothman, "Presentation of Blue Cross," 671–93, esp. 681–84; Chamber of Commerce, "Toward Sound Social Security," 25–26; Cunningham and Cunningham, *The Blues*, 68–70. On labor's changing attitude toward Blue Cross, see Harry Becker, "Reminiscences," interview by Peter Corning, Nov. 21, 1967, transcript, 12–15, Oral History Collection, Oral History Research Office, Butler Library, Columbia University, New York; Harry Becker, "Organized Labor and the Problem of Medical Care," *Annals of the American Academy of Political and Social Science* 273 (1951): 126–29; Derickson, "Steelworkers and Insurance," 76–79; Gerald Markowitz and David Rosner, "Seeking Common Ground: A History of Labor and Blue Cross," *Journal of Health Politics, Policy and Law* 16 (1991): 695–718.

32. Brody, *Workers in Industrial America*, 170 (quotation); Conference Board, *Company Group Insurance Plans* (1945), 21 (quotation), 6; Herbert Northrup, *Boulwarism: The Labor Relations Policies of the General Electric Company, Their Implications for Public Policy and Management Action* (Ann Arbor: Bureau of Industrial Relations, University of Michigan, 1964); Faulkner, "Health Insurance," 21.

33. Dickinson, address, in *Andrews Symposium*, 162 (quotation); Emerson Schmidt, "Our Capacity to Meet Existing Unmet Health Needs," in *Look at Insurance*, ed. Chamber of Commerce, 60 (quotation), 67 (quotation), 60–62, 66–67; R. O. Smith, "The Economics of Medical Care," *Virginia Medical Monthly* 89 (1962): 143–48, esp. 144. On consumerism, see Lizabeth Cohen, *A Consumers' Republic: The Politics of Mass Consumption in Postwar America* (New York: Alfred A. Knopf, 2003); Gary Cross, *An All-Consuming Century: Why Commercialism Won in Modern America* (New York: Columbia University Press, 2000), 82–109. On preliminary cultural change in this direction, see Nancy Tomes, "Merchants of Health: Medicine and Consumer Culture in the United States, 1900–1940," *JAH* 88 (2001): 519–48.

34. Editorial, "Misinterpretation of 'Needs' for Medical Care," *JAMA* 148 (1952): 848 (quotation), 849 (quotation); George W. Cooley, "The Potentialities of Voluntary Health Insurance," ibid. 151 (1953): 1025 (quotation); E. T. Wentworth, "Building America's Health, II," *New York State Journal of Medicine* 53 (1953): 648.

35. U.S. President's Commission on the Health Needs of the Nation, *Building America's Health: A Report to the President*, 5 vols. (Washington: GPO, 1952–53), 1: 3 (quotation), 3–4; Editorial, "The Health Needs of the Nation," *NEJM* 248 (1953): 77 (quotation); Editorial, "Report of the President's Commission on the Health Needs of the Nation," *Journal of the Louisiana State Medical Society* 105 (1953): 35 (quotation); Board of Trustees, AMA, "Statement of the Board of Trustees on Report of the Truman Commission on the Health Needs of the Nation," *JAMA* 151 (1953): 302–3; cf. Editorial, "Health Needs of the Nation," *AJPH* 43 (1953): 335–37.

36. Health Insurance Association of America, *Source Book of Health Insurance Data—1991* (Washington: The Association, 1991), 62; Munts, *Bargaining for Health*, 87, 93–100; President's Commission, *Building America's Health;* Commission on Financing of Hospital Care, *Financing Hospital Care in the United States*, 3 vols. (New York: Blakiston, 1955); Rosemary Stevens, *American Medicine and the Public Interest* (New Haven: Yale University Press, 1971), 418; cf. Starr, "Transformation in Defeat: The Changing

Objectives of National Health Insurance, 1915–1980," *AJPH* 72 (1982): 84–86. Another indication that the "haves" had discrete concerns from the "have-nots" was the appearance of the term "under-insurance." See Klem, "Voluntary Health Insurance," 263.

37. Harry Becker, "The Changing Scene in Health Care Economics," *New York State Journal of Medicine* 59 (1959): 2047 (quotation), 2044–49.

38. Senate, *National Health Program* (1947–48), 1292 (quotation); Nelson Cruikshank, "Issues in Social Security," *American Federationist*, Feb. 1947, 28 (quotation); Goldmann, "Labor's Attitude," 91 (quotation), 90–98; Cruikshank, remarks, *Andrews Symposium*, 144; Rosenthal, "Welfare Plans," 86–87; "Collective Bargaining and Industrial Relations," *Monthly Labor Review* 68 (1949): 146; Wilbur Cohen to Katherine Ellickson, Jan. 6, 1949, Cohen Papers, box 28, folder 7; Becker, "Labor and Medical Care," 129–30.

39. President's Commission, *Building America's Health*, 4: 116 (quotation), 116–20, 1: 47 (quotation), 47–49; Commission on Financing of Hospital Care, *Financing Hospital Care in the United States: Recommendations of the Commission on Financing of Hospital Care* (n.p., 1954), 54 (Ruttenberg quotation), vi–vii, 53–56; Jane Brickman, " 'Medical McCarthyism': The Physicians Forum and the Cold War," *Journal of the History of Medicine and Allied Sciences* 49 (1994): 380–418; Elizabeth Fee, "The Pleasures and Perils of Prophetic Advocacy: Socialized Medicine and the Politics of American Medical Reform," in *Making Medical History: The Life and Times of Henry E. Sigerist*, ed. Elizabeth Fee and Theodore M. Brown (Baltimore: Johns Hopkins University Press, 1997), 216–17; Derickson, "Health Security for All," 1354–56; Derickson, "Steelworkers and Insurance," 73–80; Leonard Woodcock, "Where Are We Going in Public Health?" *AJPH* 46 (1956): 281–82.

40. Wilbur Cohen, "Extent of Medical Care Coverage," in National Conference on Labor Health Services, *Papers and Proceedings* (Washington: American Labor Health Association, 1958), 28 (quotation), 29 (quotation), 28–34; Davis, *Medical Care for Tomorrow*, 267 (quotations), 238–47; United Auto Workers, *Proceedings, Nineteenth Constitutional Convention, 1964* (n.p., n.d.), 119; I. S. Falk, "A Formulation of Labor's Views," in Industrial Relations Research Association, *Proceedings of the Twelfth Annual Meeting, 1959* (Madison, Wis.: The Association, 1960), 56–69, esp. 60–61; Franz Goldmann, "Voluntary Medical Insurance: Achievements and Shortcomings," *JNMA* 46 (1954): 224; CNH, *Health Needs and What to Do about Them* (Washington: The Committee, 1953), 1, 9; Louis Reed, "Group Payment since the Committee on the Costs of Medical Care," *AJPH* 48 (1958): 992–93.

41. Lee F. Block, "Annual Administrative Reviews: Prepayment," *Hospitals*, Apr. 16, 1961, 150; Anne Somers, "Some Basic Determinants of Medical Care and Health Policy: An Overview of Trends and Issues," *Milbank Memorial Fund Quarterly* 46 (1968): 25–26. On the rare explicit commitment of one major investigatory group to "identify non-covered groups and evaluate possibilities and techniques for accomplishing their coverage," see Commission on Financing of Hospital Care, "Proposed Studies and Reports," Nov. 26, 1952, Becker Papers, box 5, folder: "Activities—1952."

42. Senate, *Health Insurance Plans*, 1: vii–ix, 7–9, 13. Neither the Clark study nor subsequent analyses reported any sizable difference in insurance status by gender. A 1957 study by the Health Insurance Association of America found that 69 percent of men, 67 percent of women, and 66 percent of children had voluntary health insurance. See J. F. Follmann Jr. , *Medical Care and Health Insurance: A Study in Social Progress* (Homewood, Ill.: Richard D. Irwin, 1963), 204. For evidence that female employees

received less generous health benefits than their male counterparts, see Alice Kessler-Harris, *In Pursuit of Equity: Women, Men, and the Quest for Economic Citizenship in 20th-Century America* (New York: Oxford University Press, 2001), 246–47.

43. Follmann, "Four Years of Progress," 1387 (quotation), 1384–89; Senate, *Health Insurance Plans*, 1: 9, 2: 6; New York Department of Labor, *Health Benefit Coverage of the Labor Force in New York State, December 1958* (New York: The Department, 1960), 1, 18–19, 42; Health Information Foundation, "Voluntary Health Insurance for the Individual Subscriber—Its Problems, Progress and Promise," *Progress in Health Services*, Mar. 1953, 1–3; Odin Anderson and Jacob Feldman, *Family Medical Costs and Voluntary Health Insurance: A Nationwide Survey* (New York: McGraw-Hill, 1956), 16–17; Goldmann, "Voluntary Medical Care Insurance," 227; J. Henry Smith, "Group Health Insurance," in Chamber of Commerce, *Modern Health Insurance*, 103; Health Insurance Institute, *A Profile of the Health Insurance Public: A National Study of the Pattern of Health Insurance Coverage, Public Attitudes and Knowledge* (New York: The Institute, 1959), 12; Solomon Levine, Odin Anderson, and Gerald Gordon, *Non-Group Enrollment for Health Insurance: A Study of Administrative Approaches of Blue Cross Plans* (Cambridge: Harvard University Press, 1957). On the extremely low levels of private insurance in rural areas prior to postwar expansion, see Michael R. Grey, *New Deal Medicine: The Rural Health Programs of the Farm Security Administration* (Baltimore: Johns Hopkins University Press, 1999), 148–50.

44. Health Information Foundation, "Insurance for the Individual," 1–3; Follmann, *Medical Care and Health Insurance*, 185–202.

45. Senate, *Health Insurance Plans*, 1: 89; U.S. Bureau of the Census, *Historical Statistics of the United States, Colonial Times to 1970*, 2 pts. (Washington: GPO, 1975), 1: 126–27; John Steinle and Associates, "Health Insurance Coverage of the Unemployed in New York State," Sept. 1958, Becker Papers, box 61, folder: "Unemployed Health Insurance Coverage Survey"; Commission on Financing of Hospital Care, *Recommendations*, 31; Follmann, *Medical Care and Health Insurance*, 208–14; Barnett, "Positive Action," 81.

46. Dorothy McCamman and Agnes Brewster, "Voluntary Health Insurance Coverage of Aged Beneficiaries of Old-Age and Survivors Insurance," *Social Security Bulletin* 17 (1954): 3 (quotation), 3–11; Follmann, *Medical Care and Health Insurance*, 150–66, 170–71; Goldmann, "Voluntary Medical Care Insurance," 227.

47. Louis Bauer, "The President's Page: A Monthly Message," *JAMA* 150 (1952): 1675 (quotation); Health Insurance Association of America, "A Statement of Policy," May 3, 1959, 2 (quotation), 2–3, National Association of Manufacturers Records, series II, box 575, folder 59–3758; Smith, "Group Health Insurance," 103; Harry Becker, "Blue Cross and the Community," Dec. 6, 1957, 6–7, Becker Papers, box 136; Faulkner, "Health Insurance," 24; Follmann, *Medical Care and Health Insurance*, 151, 166–84; Campbell and Campbell, *Voluntary Health Insurance*, 26, 32, 40–43; Munts, *Bargaining for Health*, 90–91; Dorothy Greene and Harry Davis, "Changes in Selected Health and Insurance Plans, 1954 to 1958," *Monthly Labor Review* 81 (1958): 1246–48; Walter Polner, "New Experiments to Provide Voluntary Health Insurance," *JAMA* 168 (1958): 194–96.

48. Senate, *Health Insurance Plans*, 1: 9 (quotation); Steinle and Associates, "Coverage of Unemployed," 9; Somers, "Some Basic Determinants," 25; Byrd and Clayton, *American Dilemma*, 2: 210–14; Commission on Financing of Hospital Care, *Recommendations*, 54, 56; Health Information Foundation, "The People without Health Insurance," *Progress in Health Services*, Oct. 1961, 2–6.

49. Follmann, *Medical Care and Health Insurance*, 72–75, 81–88, 217–18; Faulkner, "Health Insurance," 24; Commission on Financing of Hospital Care, *Financing Hospital Care in the United States*, vol. 3: *Financing Hospital Care for Nonwage and Low-Income Groups*, ed. Harry Becker (New York: Blakiston, 1955); 52–60; Robert Stevens and Rosemary Stevens, *Welfare Medicine in America: A Case Study of Medicaid* (New York: Free Press, 1974), 21–41; Harry F. Dowling, *City Hospitals: The Undercare of the Underprivileged* (Cambridge: Harvard University Press, 1982), 173–89; Sandra Opdycke, *No One Was Turned Away: The Role of Public Hospitals in New York City since 1900* (New York: Oxford University Press, 1999), 99–129; Sidney Fine, "The Kerr-Mills Act: Medical Care for the Indigent in Michigan, 1960–1965," *Journal of the History of Medicine and Allied Sciences* 53 (1998): 285–316.

50. U.S. President's Commission on the Health Needs of the Nation, *Public Hearing*, 8 vols. (Washington: Ward and Paul, 1952), 1: 6672, 8: 50; President's Commission, *Building America's Health*, 1: 44; Anderson and Feldman, *Family Medical Costs*, 14–15; Health Information Foundation, "People without Insurance," 1–6; Health Insurance Institute, *Profile*, 12; Campbell and Campbell, *Voluntary Health Insurance*, 12; Follmann, *Medical Care and Health Insurance*, 218–20; Gordon, *Dead on Arrival*, 78.

51. Editorial, "The Health Needs of the Nation," *NEJM* 248 (1953): 77 (quotation), 77–78; President's Commission, *Building America's Health*, 1: 44–45; Commission on Financing of Hospital Care, *Financing Hospital Care*, 3: passim, esp. ix, xiv–xv, 44–52; U.S. Senate and U.S. House of Representatives, Joint Committee on the Economic Report, *A Program for the Low-Income Population at Substandard Levels of Living: A Report of the Joint Committee on the Economic Report to the Congress of the United States*, 84th Cong., 2d sess., 1956, Senate Report 1311 (Washington: GPO, 1956), 6; Health Information Foundation, "People without Insurance," 3–6; Follmann, *Medical Care and Health Insurance*, 215, 221–25; George Bugbee, "Insuring the Uninsured," *Progress in Health Services*, Oct. 1961, 6.

52. President's Commission, *Public Hearing*, 1: 6832–33 (Block quotation), 6838 (Block quotation), 6831–40; Michael Harrington, *The Other America: Poverty in the United States* (New York: Macmillan, 1962), 169 (quotation), 2, 4, 6, 9, 11, 15, 115–19, 121–38; Bureau of the Census, *Historical Statistics*, 1: 82; Editorial, "The Denver Meeting," *JAMA* 150 (1952): 1672; C. Rufus Rorem, "The Case of Mr. X," *Hospitals*, May 1953, 78–80; Commission on the Financing of Hospital Care, *Financing Hospital Care*, 3: xv; Stevens, *In Sickness*, 269–70; Starr, *Social Transformation*, 350.

53. Walter Kolodrubetz, "Two Decades of Employee-Benefit Plans: A Review," *Social Security Bulletin* 35 (1972): 17; Klein, "Business of Health Security," 293–99; Jacoby, *Modern Manors*, 4, 39–40, 46, 50–53; Fones-Wolf, *Selling Free Enterprise*, 67–107.

54. Martha Eliot, "Next Steps," in National Conference, *Papers and Proceedings*, 179 (quotation), 177–89; Alan Draper, *A Rope of Sand: The AFL-CIO Committee on Political Education, 1955–1967* (New York: Praeger Publishers, 1989), 56, 141; Derickson, "Health Security," 1356; Lichtenstein, "From Corporatism," 144–45.

CHAPTER SIX: As Much a Birthright as Education

Epigraphs: Richard Nixon, *Health: A Message from the President of the United States Relative to Building a National Health Strategy*, 92d Cong., 1st sess., 1971, House Document 92–49 (Washington: GPO, 1971), 2; George Pickett (president, APHA), "The Basics of Health Policy: Rights and Privileges," *AJPH* 68 (1978): 236.

1. Richard Titmuss, *Social Policy: An Introduction*, ed. Brian Abel-Smith and Kay Titmuss (New York: Pantheon Books, 1975), 30 (quotation) and passim. Among those who have built on this concept is Gosta Esping-Andersen, *The Three Worlds of Welfare Capitalism* (Princeton: Princeton University Press, 1990).

2. Theodore Marmor, *The Politics of Medicare*, 2d ed. (New York: Aldine de Gruyter, 2000), 1–92; Theodore Marmor, "The Right to Health Care: Reflections on Its History and Politics," in *Rights to Health Care*, ed. Thomas Bole III and William Bondeson (Dordrecht, Neth.: Kluwer Academic Publishers, 1991), 23–49; Richard O. Harris, *A Sacred Trust* (New York: New American Library, 1966); Nelson Polsby, *Political Innovation in America: The Politics of Policy Initiation* (New Haven: Yale University Press, 1984), 112–28; Martha Derthick, *Policymaking for Social Security* (Washington: Brookings Institution, 1979), 316–38.

3. Robert Stevens and Rosemary Stevens, *Welfare Medicine in America: A Case Study of Medicaid* (New York: Free Press, 1974) 61 (quotation) and passim, esp. 51–81; James T. Patterson, *America's Struggle against Poverty in the Twentieth Century* (Cambridge: Harvard University Press, 2000), 164–65; Jane Orient, "The Arizona Health Care Cost Containment System: A Prepayment Model for a National Health Service?" *Western Journal of Medicine* 145 (1986): 114; Health Insurance Association of America, *Source Book of Health Insurance Data, 1991* (Washington: The Association, 1991), 42–43.

4. Edward Annis, "Government Health Care: First the Aged, Then Everyone," *Current History* 45 (1963): 104, 106, 109, 119; Robert M. Ball, "What Medicare's Architects Had in Mind," *Health Affairs* 14: 4 (1995): 62–64; Stevens and Stevens, *Welfare Medicine*, 52–53; Lawrence R. Jacobs, *The Health of Nations: Public Opinion and the Making of American and British Health Policy* (Ithaca: Cornell University Press, 1993), 137–64, 190–236, esp. 160–61.

5. Lyndon Johnson, "Remarks in San Antonio at the Signing of the Medicare Extension Bill," Apr. 8, 1966, in Johnson, *Public Papers of the Presidents of the United States: Containing the Public Messages, Speeches, and Statements of the President, 1966*, 2 vols. (Washington: GPO, 1967), 1: 408 (quotation), 409 (quotation); Jaap Kooijman, . . . *And the Pursuit of National Health: The Incremental Strategy toward National Health Insurance in the United States of America* (Amsterdam: Rodopi, 1999), 205–6.

6. Eveline M. Burns, "Policy Decisions Facing the United States in Financing and Organizing Health Care," *Public Health Reports* 81 (1966): 680 (quotation), 679 (quotation), 675–83. While still preoccupied with making appeals on behalf of children and their mothers, some maternalists had long ago moved beyond a particularist perspective. For the universalizing influence of Katharine Lenroot and Martha Eliot of the Children's Bureau, see U.S. Committee on Economic Security, *Social Security in America: The Factual Background of the Social Security Act as Summarized from Staff Reports to the Committee on Economic Security*, Social Security Board Publication 20 (Washington: GPO, 1937), 227–98, esp. 229–31, 259–60; Kriste Lindemeyer, *"A Right to Childhood": The U.S. Children's Bureau and Child Welfare, 1912–46* (Urbana: University of Illinois Press, 1997), 179–202.

7. Lyndon B. Johnson, "The State of the Union—Address by the President of the United States," *Congressional Record* 114 (1968): 142 (quotation); U.S. Senate, Commit-

tee on Government Operations, Subcommittee on Executive Reorganization, *Health Care in America: Hearings*, 90th Cong., 2d sess., 1968 (Washington: GPO, 1969), 490 (Cohen quotation), 494 (Cohen quotation), 489–94; Eveline Burns, "Health Services for All: Is Health Insurance the Answer?" *AJPH* 59: suppl. (1969): 13 (quotation), 17; Wilbur Cohen, "Health Care for the Nation's Children," *Bulletin of Pediatric Practice* 1 (1967): 3–4, 8; Wilbur Cohen, "Next Steps for Children," *Child Welfare* 47 (1968): 442. On Cohen's agile incrementalism, see Edward Berkowitz, *Mr. Social Security: The Life of Wilbur J. Cohen* (Lawrence: University Press of Kansas, 1995), 138–284, esp. 265, 270; Theodore R. Marmor and Philip Fellman, "Entrepreneurship in Public Management: Wilbur Cohen and Robert Ball," in *Leadership and Innovation: A Biographical Perspective on Entrepreneurs in Government*, ed. Jameson Doig and Erwin Hargrove (Baltimore: Johns Hopkins University Press, 1987), 246–81. On the incrementalist tradition, see Kooijman, *Pursuit of National Health*.

8. *NYT*, Aug. 15, 1968, 30 (quotations), 1; Philip R. Lee, "HCFA [U.S. Health Care Financing Administration] Oral History Interview," by Edward Berkowitz, Nov. 27, 1995, Washington Social Security Administration History Archives, online at http://www.ssa.gov/history/LEE.html, accessed Apr. 23, 2003; Donald B. Johnson, comp., *National Party Platforms*, rev. ed., 2 vols. (Urbana: University of Illinois Press, 1978), 2: 737.

9. U.S. Department of Health, Education, and Welfare, *Health, Education, and Welfare: Accomplishments, 1963–1968, Problems and Challenges, and a Look to the Future: A Report to President Lyndon B. Johnson*, by Wilbur Cohen (Washington: The Department, 1968), 64, 99, 115; Eveline Burns, "Discussion," *AJPH* 59 (1969): 619–23; "President Johnson Proposes Increased Medical Spending," *JAMA* 203 (1968): 53–54; Lester Breslow, "Some Essentials in a National Health Program for Child Health," *Pediatrics* 44 (1969): 327–32; [CNHI], "Ten Reasons Why 'Kidicare' Won't Work," [1969?], CNHI Collection, box 46, folder 6, Archives of Labor and Urban Affairs, Reuther Library, Wayne State University, Detroit; Edward M. Kennedy to Max Fine, Sept. 25, 1973, Isidore S. Falk Papers, box 144, folder 2097, Manuscripts and Archives, Yale University Library, New Haven; *NYT*, Jan. 15, 1977, 21; Arthur Coleman, "The 'Kiddy Care' Program," *JNMA* 69 (1977): 93; Wilbur Cohen, "The Father of Medicare Looks at National Health Insurance," *Medical Economics*, Sept. 5, 1977, 226.

10. Editorial, "Forward Step in Health," *NYT*, May 1, 1966, sec. 4, 10 (quotation); Editorial, "Hospitals: Light of Reason," ibid., Apr. 12, 1965, 34; Editorial, "Patchwork Health Plans," ibid., Feb. 25, 1966, 26; Editorial, "Program for Health," ibid., Mar. 2, 1966, 40; United States, *United States Statutes at Large*, 89th Cong., 2d sess., 1966, vol. 80, pt. 1 (Washington: GPO, 1967), 1180; Joshua B. Freeman, *Working-Class New York: Life and Labor since World War II* (New York: New Press, 2000), 139; *Philadelphia Inquirer*, Jan. 23, 1967, 5.

11. I. S. Falk, "Medicare: Where Do We Go from Here?" *Modern Hospital*, June 1966, 99 (quotation), 98–99; *NYT*, Jan. 5, 1967, 26; Anne R. Somers, "Some Basic Determinants of Medical Care and Health Policy: An Overview of Trends and Issues," *Milbank Memorial Fund Quarterly* 46 (1968): 26; I. S. Falk, "Beyond Medicare," *AJPH* 59 (1969): 608 (quotation), 608–19. Just the prospect of Medicare stirred one agitator for social justice to reopen the question of universal health security. See Michael Harrington, *The Other America: Poverty in the United States* (New York: Macmillan, 1962), 169.

12. James T. Patterson, *Grand Expectations: The United States, 1945–1974* (New York: Oxford University Press, 1996), 443 (quotation), 442–662, esp. 525, 562–91; David

Chalmers, *And the Crooked Places Made Straight: The Struggle for Social Change in the 1960s* (Baltimore: Johns Hopkins University Press, 1991); Maurice Isserman and Michael Kazin, *America Divided: The Civil War of the 1960s* (New York: Oxford University Press, 2000); Hugh Davis Graham, "Legacies of the 1960s: The American 'Rights Revolution' in an Era of Divided Governance," *Journal of Policy History* 10 (1998): 267–88; Michael B. Katz, *The Undeserving Poor: From the War on Poverty to the War on Welfare* (New York:: Pantheon Books, 1989), 106–12, 114; Felecia Kornbluh, "To Fulfill Their 'Rightly Needs': Consumerism and the National Welfare Rights Movement," *Radical History Review* 69 (1997): 76–113.

13. A. Philip Randolph Institute, *A "Freedom Budget" for All Americans: Budgeting Our Resources, 1966–1975, to Achieve "Freedom from Want"* (New York: The Institute, 1966), 3 (quotation), 58 (quotation), 19 (quotation), 1–3, 12, 15; Paula Pfeffer, *A. Philip Randolph, Pioneer of the Civil Rights Movement* (Baton Rouge: Louisiana State University Press, 1996), 281–83, 286–91; Daniel S. Levine, *Bayard Rustin and the Civil Rights Movement* (New Brunswick: Rutgers University Press, 2000), 187–93; Jervis Anderson, *Bayard Rustin: Troubles I've Seen* (New York: HarperCollins, 1997), 286–90. For the thinking behind the Freedom Budget, see Bayard Rustin, "From Protest to Politics: The Future of the Civil Rights Movement," *Commentary*, Feb. 1965, 25–31.

14. Martha Eliot, "Next Steps," in National Conference on Labor Health Services, *Papers and Proceedings* (Washington: American Labor Health Association, 1958), 180; Walter Reuther, "The Health Care Crisis: Where Do We Go from Here?" *AJPH* 59 (1969): 14 (quotations), 12–15. On Reuther's social unionism and its complications, see Nelson Lichtenstein, *Walter Reuther: The Most Dangerous Man in Detroit* (Urbana: University of Illinois Press, 1997); Nelson Lichtenstein, "From Corporatism to Collective Bargaining: Organized Labor and the Eclipse of Social Democracy in the Postwar Era," in *The Rise and Fall of the New Deal Order, 1930–1980* (Princeton: Princeton University Press, 1989), 122–52; Victor Reuther, *The Brothers Reuther and the Story of the UAW: A Memoir* (Boston: Houghton Mifflin, 1979), passim, esp. 356–57. For Reuther's effort to increase the AFL-CIO's involvement in universalistic reform in the wake of the passage of Medicare, see AFL-CIO, *Proceedings of the Sixth Constitutional Convention, 1965*, 2 vols. (Washington: AFL-CIO, n.d.), 1: 512–14.

15. Reuther, "Health Care Crisis," 16 (quotation), 15 (quotation), 15–20; Editorial, "The Health Crisis—What to Do?" *AJPH* 59 (1969): 1–3; David C. Jacobs, "The United Auto Workers and the Campaign for National Health Insurance: A Case Study of Labor in Politics" (Ph.D. diss., Cornell University, 1983); David C. Jacobs, "The UAW and the Committee for National Health Insurance: The Contours of Social Unionism," in *Advances in Industrial and Labor Relations*, ed. David Lewin, David Lipsky, and Donna Sockell (Greenwich, Conn.: JAI Press, 1987), 119–40. The UAW had sown the seeds of the CNHI much earlier. See Melvin Glasser to I. S. Falk, Nov. 25, 1963, Falk Papers, box 26, folder 547; I. S. Falk to Melvin Glasser, Jan. 7, 1964, ibid., folder 548; United Auto Workers, *Proceedings, Nineteenth Constitutional Convention, 1964* (n.p., n.d.), 119–20; I. S. Falk, "Proposals for National Health Insurance in the USA: Origins and Evolution, and Some Perceptions for the Future," *Milbank Memorial Fund Quarterly* 55 (1977): 173–74.

16. Burns, "Policy Decisions," 683 (quotation), 679; Reuther, "Health Care Crisis," 20 (CNHI quotation); Falk, "Beyond Medicare," 611 (quotation), 608–19. For a reminder that Johnson's devotion to equal opportunity stopped short of the pursuit of equal social conditions, see Patterson, *Grand Expectations*, 590–92; Gareth Davies,

*From Opportunity to Entitlement: The Transformation and Decline of Great Society Liberalism* (Lawrence: University Press of Kansas, 1996), 32–34, 40–41, 155, 161.

17. Peter Rogatz, "Basic Wrongs and Basic Rights in Health Care," *Hospitals*, Nov. 1, 1966, 118 (quotation), 43–45; Wilbur Cohen, "Challenge and Opportunity: Meeting the Health Needs of the Nation," *Public Health Reports* 82 (1967): 574 (quotation), 565–67; David Rothman, *Beginnings Count: The Technological Imperative in American Health Care* (New York: Oxford University Press, 1997), 67–86; Wilbur Cohen, "Health Care for All Americans," Aug. 19, 1967, 1–6, 29–30, Wilbur Cohen Papers, box 259, folder 7, Archives Division, Wisconsin Historical Society; *NYT*, May 9, 1967, 31. For two veteran reformers uncomfortable with rights assertions, see I. S. Falk, "Medical Care and Social Policy," *AJPH* 54 (1964): 522–28; Michael M. Davis, "Reminiscences," interview by Peter Corning, Feb. 18, 1966, transcript, 41, Oral History Collection, Oral History Research Office, Butler Library, Columbia University, New York. During the Medicare debate, HEW secretary Anthony Celebrezze denied that the elderly had any right to health care beyond that established by their own financial contributions. See U.S. House of Representatives, Committee on Ways and Means, *Medical Care for the Aged: Hearings . . . on H.R. 3920*, 88th Cong., 1st and 2d sess., 1963–64 (Washington: GPO, 1964), 31–33, 158–59.

18. U.S. Senate, Committee on Government Operations, Subcommittee on Executive Reorganization, *Health Care in America: Hearings*, 90th Cong., 2d sess., 1968 (Washington: GPO, 1969), 1 (Ribicoff quotation), 408 (Rockefeller quotations), 20, 40–42, 119, 413, 415, 430; *NYT*, May 17, 1968, 23 (McCarthy quotation), Apr. 25, 1968, 26, July 31, 1968, 23, Oct. 16, 1968, 18; Abraham Ribicoff and Paul Danaceau, *The American Medical Machine* (New York: Saturday Review Press, 1972), 10, 139, 142–43, 147–48.

19. Harry Becker, "The Future of Blue Cross: Or What?" May 1, 1967, 4 (quotation), 9, Falk Papers, box 3, folder 50; Benjamin I. Page and Robert Y. Shapiro, *The Rational Public: Fifty Years of Trends in Americans' Policy Preferences* (Chicago: University of Chicago Press, 1992), 129.

20. AMA, *Proceedings of the House of Delegates, 118th Annual Convention, 1969* (Chicago: AMA, 1969), 296 (quotations), 361–62; Wiley Armstrong, "The Health Crisis in America and the National Medical Association," *JNMA* 63 (1971): 469 (quotation); *NYT*, Jan. 27, 1970, 33; Melvin Glasser, "Meeting with American Medical Association Representatives," Jan. 8, 1970, CNHI Collection, box 16, folder 1.

21. Senate, *Health Care in America*, 444–45 (Smith quotations); Governing Council, APHA, "A Medical Care Program for the Nation," *AJPH* 60 (1970): 189 (quotation), 189–90; *NYT*, Nov. 24, 1970, 28 (American Hospital Association committee quotation), July 19, 1969, 7, May 11, 1971, 28, May 28, 1971, 37; L. F. Detwiller, "The Right to Health," *Hospitals*, Feb. 16, 1971, 64; Frank Furstenberg, "National Health Care Is a Citizen's Right," *Baltimore Sun*, July 19, 1970, K2; Interreligious Task Force on Health Care, *The Need for a New Health Care Policy in the United States* (Washington: Board of Church and Society, 1972).

22. Health Insurance Association of America, *Program for Healthcare in the 1970s* (n.p: The Association, 1970), 21 (quotation), 1, and passim; *NYT*, Oct. 14, 1971, 23 (Annis quotations); Nixon, *Health: A Message;* Robert Sade, "Medical Care as a Right: A Refutation," *NEJM* 285 (1971): 1288–92.

23. Russell Roth, "Second Lecture," in John R. Price, Frank Furstenberg, and Russell Roth, *National Health Insurance* (Washington: American Enterprise Institute for

Public Policy Research, 1972), 23 (quotation); *NYT*, July 18, 1969, 38 (CNHI quotation); William Curran, "The Right to Health in National and International Law," *NEJM* 284 (1971): 1258–59; Paul Starr, *The Social Transformation of American Medicine* (New York: Basic Books, 1982), 388–89.

24. Health Insurance Association of America, *Program for 1970s*, 4 (quotation); Herman Somers and Anne Somers, "Major Issues in National Health Insurance," *Milbank Memorial Fund Quarterly* 50 (1972): 177, 181; Bert Seidman to John M. Martin Jr., Feb. 6, 1970, AFL, CIO, and AFL-CIO Department of Legislation Records, box 25, folder 23, George Meany Memorial Archives, Silver Spring, Md.; *Congressional Record* 116 (1970): 30142; *NYT*, Aug. 9, 1971, 20, Jan. 1, 1972, 30.

25. J. Martin Stone, "National Compulsory Health Insurance: Time for a Positive Program," *Hospitals*, May 1, 1969, 58 (quotation), 58–62; *NYT*, Sept. 9, 1969, 21; Gerald Dorman, "President's Report to the House of Delegates," *JAMA* 213 (1970): 269.

26. Walter Reuther, "America's Challenge: A National System to Organize and Finance Personal Health Services to Meet the Nation's Health Needs," Oct. 14, 1969, repr. in *Congressional Record* 115 (1969): 31329 (quotation), 31329–30; Sylvester Berki, "National Health Insurance: An Idea Whose Time Has Come?" *Annals of the American Academy of Political and Social Science* 399 (1972): 128: "'Medical care is a right' is the cliché of the year. Judging by the disparity between stated objectives and observed actions, it is hypocrisy as well."

27. *Congressional Record* 116 (1970): 30142 (Kennedy quotation), 30142–66, 115 (1969): 31330–32; CNHI, "Specifications for National Health Insurance," [Oct. 1969?], CNHI Collection, box 17, folder 4; [CNHI], "Position Paper on Universal Coverage," [1969?], ibid., box 29, folder 29; Edward M. Kennedy, *In Critical Condition: The Crisis in America's Health Care* (New York: Simon and Schuster, 1972), 241–54; Adam Clymer, *Edward M. Kennedy: A Biography* (New York: William Morrow, 1999), 159–60.

28. Berki, "National Health Insurance," 129; Somers and Somers, "Major Issues," 188–98; Conference on National Health Insurance, *National Health Insurance: Proceedings of the Conference on National Health Insurance, 1970*, ed. Robert Eilers and Sue Moyerman (Homewood, Ill.: Richard D. Irwin, 1971), 287–336; *NYT*, Oct. 3, 1969, 4, Nov. 4, 1969, 12; Sharon Bills, "National Health Insurance: The Battle Takes Shape," *Hospitals*, Apr. 16, 1971, 126–29.

29. George Meany to Raymond Corbett, Mar. 4, 1970, AFL-CIO Legislation Records, box 25, folder 23; Bert Seidman and Dick Shoemaker to Andy Biemiller et al., July 13, 1973, ibid., folder 34; Melvin Glasser, "Meeting with American Medical Association Representatives," Jan. 8, 1970, CNHI Collection, box 16, folder 1; Emerson Walden, "NMA Comments on National Health Insurance Plans," *JNMA* 63 (1971): 503–6; *NYT*, Nov. 10, 1969, 27; Rashi Fein, "National Health Insurance," *AJPH* 61 (1971): 1072–74; Bruce C. Stuart, "National Health Insurance and the Poor," ibid. 62 (1972): 1258.

30. Somers and Somers, "Major Issues," 181 (quotation), 186–89.

31. Intellectual egalitarianism may have reflected, in part, an awareness of an underlying strain of societal egalitarianism regarding health protection. A 1972 survey found that a solid majority of Americans favored equal benefits for all participants in national health insurance. See Stephen Strickland, *U.S. Health Care: What's Right and What's Wrong* (New York: Universe Books, 1972), 71–72.

32. George Silver, "Insurance Is Not Enough," *Nation*, June 8, 1970, 682 (quotation; italics in original), 680–83. For other analyses that presumed that universal-insurance

legislation would not automatically make care accessible to all Americans, see Charles E. Lewis, Rashi Fein, and David Mechanic, *A Right to Health: The Problem of Access to Primary Medical Care* (New York: John Wiley and Sons, 1976); Somers and Somers, "Major Issues," 208–10.

33. George Silver, "Is National Health Insurance the Question?" *AJPH* 60 (1970): 1889 (quotation; italics in original), 1890 (quotation), 1887–90 (and repr. in *Church and Society*, Mar.–Apr. 1971, 11–14); George Silver, "Fair Shares: The U.S.A. Is Ready for a National Health Service," *Pharos* 36 (1973): 95–100; George Silver to Wilbur Cohen, Oct. 1, 1973, Cohen Papers, box 234, folder 3. For Silver's inspiration, see Eveline Burns, "Health Services for All: Is Health Insurance the Answer?" *AJPH* 69: suppl. (1969): 9–18. Even while advocating a national health service, Silver offered qualified support for Edward Kennedy's version of national insurance. See George Silver, "National Health Insurance, National Health Policy, and the National Health," *American Journal of Nursing* 71 (1971): 1730–34.

34. Alice Sardell, *The U.S. Experiment in Social Medicine: The Community Health Center Program, 1965–1986* (Pittsburgh: University of Pittsburgh Press, 1988), 50ff; Karen Davis and Cathy Schoen, *Health and the War on Poverty: A Ten-Year Appraisal* (Washington: Brookings Institution, 1978), 161–202; Lisle Carter Jr., "Health and the War on Poverty," *JNMA* 58 (1966): 176–77; Seymour Bellin and H. Jack Geiger, "Actual Public Acceptance of the Neighborhood Health Center by the Urban Poor," *JAMA* 214 (1970): 2147–53; Roger A. Reynolds, "Improving Access to Health Care among the Poor—The Neighborhood Health Center Experience," *Milbank Memorial Fund Quarterly* 54 (1976): 47–82; Patricia Bauman, "The Formulation and Evolution of the Health Maintenance Organization Policy, 1970–1973," *Social Science and Medicine* 10 (1976): 129–42; Starr, *Social Transformation*, 395–97, 400–401. For an avowedly universalistic proposal to expand community health facilities presented on the eve of the passage of the Economic Opportunity Act, see APHA, "The Organization of Medical Care and the Health of the Nation," *AJPH* 54 (1964): 147–52. For other efforts to empower the poor, see Frances Fox Piven and Richard Cloward, *Poor People's Movements: Why They Succeed, How They Fail* (New York: Vintage Books, 1979), 264–361; Martha F. Davis, *Brutal Need: Lawyers and the Welfare Rights Movement, 1960–1973* (New Haven: Yale University Press, 1993), 30–33.

35. Sardell, *Experiment in Social Medicine*, 3–4 (quotation); Medical Committee for Human Rights, *Preliminary Position Paper on National Health Care* (Chicago: The Committee, 1971), 1 (quotation), 1–4; Thomas Bodenheimer, "The Hoax of National Health Insurance," *AJPH* 62 (1972): 1324 (quotation), 1324–27; Charles Willie, "Comprehensive Community Health Centers," ibid. 61 (1971): 1931–32; Herbert Abrams, "Neighborhood Health Centers," ibid., 2236–39; Lily Hoffman, *The Politics of Knowledge: Activist Movements in Medicine and Planning* (Albany: State University of New York Press, 1989), 70–79. For an offshoot of MCHR with a similar brand of New Left activism, see Naomi Rogers, " 'Caution: The AMA May Be Dangerous to Your Health': The Student Health Organization (SHO) and American Medicine, 1965–1970," *Radical History Review* 80 (2001): 5–34.

36. Ronald Dellums and H. Lee Halterman, *Lying Down with the Lions: A Public Life from the Streets of Oakland to the Halls of Power* (Boston: Beacon Press, 2000), 70 (quotation), 68–70; Milton Roemer and S. J. Axelrod, "A National Health Service and Social Security," *AJPH* 67 (1977): 465 (quotation), 462–65; Governing Council, APHA,

"Establishment of a National Health Service," ibid., 86–87; Milton Terris et al., "The Case for a National Health Service," ibid., 1183–85.

37. Leon Kass, "Regarding the End of Medicine and the Pursuit of Health," *Public Interest* 40 (1975): 39 (quotation), 35–39; Daniel Callahan, "Health and Society: Some Ethical Imperatives," in *Doing Better and Feeling Worse: Health in the United States*, ed. John H. Knowles (New York: W. W. Norton, 1977), 30 (quotation), 30–33; Robert Veatch, "What Is a 'Just' Health Care Delivery?" in *Ethics and Health Policy*, ed. Veatch and Roy Branson (Cambridge, Mass.: Ballinger Publishing, 1976), 133 (quotation), 127–42; Johnson, *National Party Platforms*, 2: 795. On the rise of the academic specialty of bioethics, see Albert Jonsen, *The Birth of Bioethics* (New York: Oxford University Press, 1998). For assertions of a right to health itself, see CNHI, "Ten Reasons for National Health Insurance," [1975?], 1, CNHI Collection, box 52, folder 16; Arthur Coleman, "United States Health Care in Transition," *JNMA* 69 (1977): 725. The source of Veatch's interpretation was John Rawls, *A Theory of Justice* (Cambridge: Harvard University Press, 1971).

38. William Blackstone, "On Health Care as a Legal Right: An Exploration of Legal and Moral Grounds," *Georgia Law Review* 10 (1976): 410 (quotation), 409 (quotation), 391–418; Callahan, "Health and Society," 28 (quotations), 30–33; Louis F. Buckley, "Catholic Social Thought Concerning the Right to Health and to Health Care," *Linacre Quarterly* 37 (1970): 74 (quotation), 72–84; Pope John XXIII, "Peace on Earth: Encyclical Letter," in *Social Justice: The Catholic Position*, ed. Vincent Mainelli (Washington: Consortium Press, 1975), sec. 276; Robert Veatch, "Just Social Institutions and the Right to Health Care," *Journal of Medicine and Philosophy* 4 (1979): 172–73; Gene Outka, "Social Justice and Equal Access to Health Care," in *Ethics and Health Policy*, 79–98, esp. 82–83, 89–91. For ethicists' attempts to use moral obligation, not right, as the basis for guaranteeing health care to a limited extent, see Tom Beauchamp and Ruth Faden, "The Right to Health and the Right to Health Care," *Journal of Medicine and Philosophy* 4 (1979): 118–31, esp. 128; James Childress, "A Right to Health Care," ibid., 132–47, esp. 143, 145.

39. Veatch, " 'Just' Health Care Delivery," 141–52; Blackstone, "Care as Legal Right," 416; Kass, "End of Medicine," 41–43; Outka, "Social Justice," 93–94. For religious support for national health insurance, see Editorial, "National Health Insurance: Proposals and Prospects," *Christian Century*, May 8, 1974, 494–95; House, *National Health Insurance*, 3080–85, 3223–27, 3263–67, 3370–3404.

40. Health Insurance Association of America, *Source Book of Health Insurance Data, 1991* (Washington: The Association, 1991), 62–63; U.S. Department of Health, Education, and Welfare, *A Report to the President on Medical Care Prices* (Washington: GPO, 1967); Robert Eilers, "National Health Insurance: What Kind and How Much," *NEJM* 284 (1971): 881–86; Paul Starr, "Transformation in Defeat: The Changing Objectives of National Health Insurance, 1915–1980," *AJPH* 72 (1982): 84–86; Charlie Schultze and Jim McIntyre to the President, May 31, 1978, Records of the Domestic Policy Staff, Stuart Eizenstat's Subject File, 1976–81, box 241, folder: "National Health Insurance, May 1978," Jimmy Carter Library, Atlanta; James McIntyre and Charlie Schultze to the President, [June 1978?], ibid., box 242, folder: "National Health Insurance, June 1978"; Economic Policy Group, "EPG Issue Paper: Welfare Reform and National Health Plan," Nov. 27, 1978, RG 220, Records of Temporary Committees, Commissions, and Boards, Council of Economic Advisors Files, box 110, folder: "Economic Policy Group

Meeting, Nov. 28, 1978," Jimmy Carter Library, Atlanta. For the ways that the uncontrolled costs of Medicare and Medicaid helped to subvert demands for universal insurance, see Rick Mayes, *Universal Coverage: The Elusive Quest for National Health Insurance* (Lanham, Md.: Lexington Books, 2001), 81–137. On the Carter economic advisors' preoccupation with inflation, see W. Carl Biven, *Jimmy Carter's Economy: Policy in an Age of Limits* (Chapel Hill: University of North Carolina Press, 2002).

41. *NYT*, Mar. 30, 1973, 78 (Johnson quotation), Jan. 7, 1972, 12, May 30, 1972, 36; House, *National Health Insurance*, 3393 (McDaniel quotation), 3393–94; Starr, *Social Transformation*, 396, 405.

42. Expenditure Process Subcommittee, Government Operations/Expenditures Committee, National Association of Manufacturers, "Health Care and Delivery: Report and Position Paper," Sept. 19, 1970, National Association of Manufacturers Records, series II, box 800, folder 70–1095, Manuscripts and Archives Department, Hagley Museum and Library, Greenville, Del.; Nixon, *Health: A Message*, 3; *NYT*, Feb. 11, 1972, 1, 12, Apr. 30, 1973, 13; Martin Feldstein, "A New Approach to National Health Insurance," *Public Interest* 23 (1971): 93–105; Alain Enthoven to Joseph Califano, Sept. 22, 1977, Records of the Domestic Policy Staff, Stuart Eizenstat's Subject File, 1976–81, box 240, folder: "National Health Insurance"; Alain Enthoven, "Consumer-Choice Health Plan," *NEJM* 298 (1978): 650–58, 709–20; Alain Enthoven, *Health Plan: The Only Practical Solution to the Soaring Cost of Medical Care* (Reading, Mass.: Addison-Wesley, 1980).

43. Aaron Wildavsky, "Doing Better and Feeling Worse: The Political Pathology of Health Policy," in *Doing Better*, ed. Knowles, 105 (quotation), 106 (quotation), 105–23; Jim McIntyre to the President, Apr. 5 1978 (quotation), Records of the Office of the Staff Secretary, Handwriting File, box 79, folder: "Apr. 6, 1978 (1)"; Califano, *Governing America*, 110 (Champion quotation), 110–11; James T. McIntyre and Charlie Schultze to the President, [June 1978?], Records of the Domestic Policy Staff, Stuart Eizenstat's Subject File, 1976–81, box 242, folder: "National Health Insurance, June 1978"; Ivan Illich, *Medical Nemesis: The Expropriation of Health* (New York: Pantheon Books, 1976); Robert Morison, "Rights and Responsibilities: Redressing the Uneasy Balance," *Hastings Center Report*, Apr. 1974, 1–4; Kass, "End of Medicine," 39; Starr, *Social Transformation*, 410. For a more measured skepticism, see Paula Diehr et al., "Increased Access to Medical Care: The Impact on Health," *Medical Care* 17 (1979): 989–99. For an interpretation that acknowledged the importance of lifestyle, environment, and other nonmedical factors but regarded health care as a significant factor in health status, see Melvin Glasser, "Health as a Right—The Human and Political Dimensions," in National Conference on Social Welfare, *The Social Welfare Forum, 1975: Official Proceedings, 102d Annual Forum* (New York: Columbia University Press, 1976), 3–17.

44. Peter Bourne to Stu Eizenstat, Feb. 4, 1978, Office of the Chief of Staff Files, Deputy Chief of Staff Subject File, box 116, folder: "National Health Insurance, Apr. 16, 1976–Apr. 17, 1978," Jimmy Carter Library, Atlanta; Joe Onek et al. to Stu Eizenstat and Landon Butler, Mar. 13, 1978, ibid.; Lane Kirkland, "The Uniquely American Solution," *American Federationist*, Sept. 1976, 18–19; Starr, *Social Transformation*, 379–419; Jacobs, "Auto Workers and National Health Insurance"; Mayes, *Universal Coverage*, 88–100; Colin Gordon, *Dead on Arrival: The Politics of Health Care in Twentieth-Century America* (Princeton: Princeton University Press, 2003), 243–50. For an account that criticizes labor for excessive flexibility on the question of mandated private benefits in the 1970s and beyond, see Marie Gottschalk, *The Shadow Welfare State: Labor, Business, and the*

*Politics of Health Care in the United States* (Ithaca: ILR Press of Cornell University Press, 2000), 65–85.

45. Joint Technical Drafting Committee, AFL-CIO and CNHI, minutes, Nov. 7, 1970, 3 (quotation), CNHI Collection, box 20, folder 6; Starr, *Social Transformation*, 405 (quotation), 404–5; Executive Committee, CNHI, and Executive Board, Health Security Action Council, "Joint Meeting," Jan. 4, 1974, CNHI Collection, box 20, folder 23; Executive Committee, CNHI, and Executive Board, Health Security Action Council, "Joint Meeting," Apr. 15, 1974, ibid., folder 2; U.S. House of Representatives, Committee on Ways and Means, *National Health Insurance: Hearings . . . on the Subject of National Health Insurance*, 93d Cong., 2d sess., 1974 (Washington: GPO, 1974), 1155–56, 1170; [Health Security Action Council], "National Health Security Action Council," list of 68 participating organizations, June 1974, AFL-CIO Legislation Records, box 25, folder 38; Alfred Lewis to Andrew Biemiller, July 23, 1974, ibid.; Edward Kennedy to Max Fine, Sept. 25, 1973, Isidore S. Falk Papers, box 144, folder 2097; Edward Kennedy to Richard Lowyer, Apr. 1, 1974, ibid.; *NYT*, Apr. 3, 1974, 1, 18, Aug. 23, 1974, 28, Sept. 19, 1974, 42; Hazel Erskine, "The Polls: Health Insurance," *Public Opinion Quarterly* 39 (1975): 143. On Mills, see Julian Zelizer, *Taxing America: Wilbur D. Mills, Congress, and the State, 1945–1975* (Cambridge: Cambridge University Press, 1998).

46. Theodore Marmor, "A National Health Insurance Proposal," *NYT*, Jan. 15, 1977, 21 (quotation); Lisbeth Bamberger Schorr, "Memorandum," Mar. 17, 1978, Records of the Office of Peter Bourne, White House Office Subject File, 1977–78, box 41, folder: "National Health Insurance, Oct. 28, 1977–July 7, 1978," Jimmy Carter Library, Atlanta; Arthur Coleman, "The 'Kiddy Care' Program," *JNMA* 69 (1977): 93; Wilbur Cohen, "The Father of Medicare Looks at National Health Insurance," *Medical Economics*, Sept. 5, 1977, 226; Wilbur Cohen to Stuart Eizenstat, Dec. 21, 1978, Records of the Domestic Policy Staff, Stuart Eizenstat's Subject File, 1976–81, box 241, folder: "National Health Insurance"; Arthur Altmeyer to Ig [Falk], Dec. 24, 1970, CNHI Collection, box 5, folder 1; Dick Shoemaker to Bert Seidman, Nov. 21, 1974, AFL-CIO Legislation Records, box 25, folder 39; Subcommittee of [CNHI] Technical Committee, "Meeting," Nov. 22, 1974, ibid.; Bert Seidman, interview by author, Oct. 26, 1990, audio tape in author's possession.

47. Falk, "Beyond Medicare," 609 (quotation), 611–12; I. S. Falk to Joseph Duffy, Oct. 20, 1976 (quotation), Falk Papers, box 144, folder 2088; CNHI, "Statement," July 28, 1978, 2 (quotation), 1–2, CNHI Collection, box 50, folder 16; CNHI, "Report, First Meeting," Feb. 13, 1969, 1–2, ibid., box 17, folder 3; Reuther, "Health Care Crisis," 20; I. S. Falk, "Report from the Technical Committee," Aug. 2, 1974, AFL-CIO Legislation Records, box 25, folder 38; Falk, "Proposals for National Health Insurance," 177; Edward Kennedy, "Statement on National Health Insurance," July 28, 1978, Records of the Domestic Policy Staff, Stuart Eizenstat's Subject File, 1976–81, box 242, folder: "National Health Insurance, July 1978"; Douglas Fraser, news release, July 28, 1978, CNHI Collection, box 50, folder 16; *NYT*, July 29, 1978, 20.

48. Peter Bourne to Hamilton Jordan and Landon Butler, Apr. 17, 1978 (quotation), Chief of Staff Files, Deputy Chief Subject File, box 116, folder: "National Health Insurance, Apr. 16, 1976–Apr. 17, 1978"; Joseph Califano Jr., "Remarks," May 8, 1978, 1 (quotation) and passim, esp. 12, Speechwriters Files, Subject File, box 10, folder: "Health, Jan. 16–Aug. 29, 1978," Jimmy Carter Library, Atlanta; Peter Bourne to Landon Butler, Mar. 16, 1978, Chief of Staff Files, Deputy Chief Subject File, box 116, folder: "National

Health Insurance, Apr. 16, 1976–Apr. 17, 1978"; Jimmy Carter, "Address by Jimmy Carter on National Health Policy before the Student National Medical Association," Apr. 16, 1976, Records of Peter Bourne, White House Office Subject File, 1977–78, box 41, folder: "National Health Insurance, Apr. 16, 1976–Nov. 9, 1977"; Jimmy Carter, "Department of Health, Education, and Welfare: Remarks and a Question-and-Answer Session with Department Employees," Feb. 16, 1977, 159, 162, in Jimmy Carter, *Public Papers of the Presidents of the United States: Jimmy Carter, 1977*, 2 vols. (Washington: GPO, 1977), 1: 887–95; Jimmy Carter, "United Auto Workers: Remarks at the Union's Convention in Los Angeles," May 17, 1977, ibid., 887–95; Jimmy Carter, "Presidential Directive/DPS-3 to the Secretary of Health, Education and Welfare," July 29, 1978, Records of the Domestic Policy Staff, Stuart Eizenstat's Subject File, 1976–81, box 242, folder: "National Health Insurance, July 1978"; Joseph Califano Jr., "Statement," July 29, 1978, CNHI Collection, box 50, folder 16; Stuart Eizenstat, "Remarks," July 29, 1978, ibid.; *NYT*, Apr. 17, 1976, 1, 6, July 29, 1978, 20; Joseph Califano Jr., *Governing America: An Insider's Report from the White House and the Cabinet* (New York: Simon and Schuster, 1981), 88–135, esp. 92, 107–19; Clymer, *Kennedy*, 246, 253–56, 269–70; Martin Halpern, "Jimmy Carter and the UAW: Failure of an Alliance," *Presidential Studies Quarterly* 26 (1996): 755–77, esp. 757, 764–66. The Carter administration's refusal to make rights claims did not reflect the viewpoint of Secretary Califano and Peter Bourne, who urged the president to present universal access to basic care as a fundamental right. See Joe Califano to the President, June 14, 1978, Tab A, 1, Records of the Domestic Policy Staff, Stuart Eizenstat's Subject File, 1976–81, box 242, folder: "National Health Insurance, June 1978"; Peter Bourne to Hamilton Jordan and Landon Butler, Apr. 17, 1978, Chief of Staff Files, Deputy Chief Subject File, box 116, folder: "National Health Insurance, Apr. 16, 1976–Apr. 17, 1978." For the development of human-rights policy and practice, see Joshua Muravchik, *The Uncertain Crusade: Jimmy Carter and the Dilemma of Human Rights Policy* (Lanham, Md.: Hamilton Press, 1986); Jimmy Carter, "Universal Declaration of Human Rights: Remarks at a White House Meeting Commemorating the Thirtieth Anniversary of the Declaration's Signing," Dec. 6, 1978, in Jimmy Carter, *Public Papers of the Presidents of the United States: Jimmy Carter, 1978*, 2 vols. (Washington: GPO, 1979), 2: 2161–65, esp. 2164; Kenneth Cmiel, "The Emergence of Human Rights Politics in the United States," *JAH* 86 (1999): 1231–50.

49. Joseph Boyle Jr., "The Concept of Health and the Right to Health Care," *Social Thought* 3 (1977): 14 (quotation), 5–17; Gerald Rosenthal and Daniel Fox, "A Right to What? Toward Adequate Minimum Standards for Personal Health Services," *Milbank Memorial Fund Quarterly* 56 (1978): 2 (quotations, italics in original), 1–6; Amy Gutmann, "For and against Equal Access to Health Care," ibid. 59 (1981): 559 (quotation), 556–57; Brian Abel-Smith, "Minimum Adequate Levels of Personal Health Care: History and Justification," ibid. 56 (1978): 7–21; Callahan, "Health and Society," 31–33; Eli Ginzberg, *The Limits of Health Reform: The Search for Realism* (New York: Basic Books, 1977), 113–28, 212–13; Victor Fuchs, *Who Shall Live? Health, Economics, and Social Choice* (New York: Basic Books, 1975), 149–50. For a prescient voice of moderation in this regard, see David Mechanic, "Trends in the Delivery of Health Services: Some Issues and Problems," *Inquiry* 8 (1971): 7. On growing antipathy to entitlements, see Davies, *From Opportunity to Entitlement*, 145–243.

50. White House Press Office, Office of Media Liaison, "National Health Plan: Background Report," June 15, 1979, 2 (quotation) and passim; Chief of Staff Files,

Deputy Chief Subject File, box 116, folder: "National Health Insurance, Apr. 16, 1976–Apr. 17, 1978"; Califano, *Governing America*, 135 (quotation), 133–35; Nelson Cruikshank, "Address," June 28, 1979, 7 (quotation), passim, CNHI Collection, box 2, folder 33; Tim Foley to Nelson Cruikshank, July 18, 1979, ibid.; Senate, *Health Care in America*, 27; Sharon Bills, "National Health Insurance: The Battle Takes Shape," *Hospitals*, Apr. 16, 1971, 127; Jimmy Carter to Congress of the United States, June 12, 1979, Records of the Domestic Policy Staff, Stuart Eizenstat's Subject File, 1976–81, box 241, folder: "National Health Insurance"; Office of the White House Press Secretary, "Press Briefing by Joseph A. Califano and Stuart E. Eizenstat," June 12, 1979, Speechwriters Files, Subject File, box 10, folder: "Health Issues, Jan. 1, 1979–Aug. 31, 1980"; I. S. Falk, "Some Lessons from the Fifty Years since the CCMC Final Report, 1932," *Journal of Public Health Policy* 4 (1983): 150–51; Starr, *Social Transformation*, 413–14.

51. Leda Judd, "National Health Insurance—What Is It," Aug. 1, 1975, CNHI Collection, box 24, folder 52; Karen Davis, *National Health Insurance: Benefits, Costs, and Consequences* (Washington: Brookings Institution, 1975), 34–36; Karen Davis, Marsha Gold, and Diane Makuc, "Access to Health Care for the Poor: Does the Gap Remain?" *Annual Review of Public Health* 2 (1981): 159–82; Pennsylvania Insurance Commissioner's Advisory Task Force on Women's Insurance Problems, *Final Report and Recommendations* (Harrisburg: Pennsylvania Insurance Department, 1974), 9–17; Deborah A. Lewis, "Women and National Health Insurance: Issues and Solutions," *Medical Care* 14 (1976): 549–58; U.S National Center for Health Services Research, *Who Are the Uninsured?* Data Preview 1 (Hyattsville, Md.: The Center, 1980); Julian Roebuck and Robert Quan, "Health-Care Practices in the American Deep South," in *Marginal Medicine*, ed. Roy Wallis and Peter Morley (New York: Free Press, 1974), 141–61. For studies that emphasize the improvements in access following from the implementation of Medicare and Medicaid, see Lu Ann Aday, "The Impact of Health Policy on Access to Medical Care," *Milbank Memorial Fund Quarterly* 54 (1976): 215–33; Robert Wood Johnson Foundation, *A New Survey on Access to Medical Care* (Princeton: The Foundation, 1978). Karen Davis recognized that universal health insurance would not automatically bring universal access, especially for members of racial minorities. See Karen Davis, "Improving the Performance of the U.S. Health Care System," Sept. 1976, Records of the 1976 Campaign to Elect Jimmy Carter, Sam Bleicher's Issues Office Subject Files, 1976, box 35, folder: "Health (4)"; Davis, *National Health Insurance*, 154–59. On the preoccupation of feminist activists in the 1960s and 1970s with community self-help projects as opposed to national policy on access to basic health care, see Sandra Morgen, *Into Our Own Hands: The Women's Health Movement in the United States, 1969–1990* (New Brunswick: Rutgers University Press, 2002), 3–180.

52. For the mixture of particularism and universalism within the National Welfare Rights Organization, the leading voice of Medicaid beneficiaries, see House, *National Health Insurance*, 3099–3110; Joseph D'Oronzio, "A Human Right to Healthcare Access: Returning to the Origins of the Patients' Rights Movement," *Cambridge Quarterly of Healthcare Ethics* 10 (2001): 285–98. On defensive particularism in groups representing Medicare beneficiaries, see Henry J. Pratt, *The Gray Lobby* (Chicago: University of Chicago Press, 1976); W. Andrew Achenbaum, "The History of Federal Policies toward the Aged," in *Federal Social Policy: The Historical Dimension*, ed. Donald Critchlow and Ellis Hawley (University Park: Pennsylvania State University Press, 1988), 43.

EPILOGUE: Alone among the Developed Nations

Epigraph: John Iglehart, "The American Health Care System," *NEJM* 326 (1992): 962; Nicole Lurie, Steven Miles, and David Haugen, "Now Is the Time: Physician Involvement in Health Care Reform," *Annals of Internal Medicine* 118 (1993): 226.

1. On the lure of Canadian and other foreign models, see Robert Dickman et al., "An End to Patchwork Reform of Health Care," *NEJM* 317 (1987): 1087–88; Robert Blendon et al., "Satisfaction with Health Systems in Ten Nations," *Health Affairs* 9: 2 (1990): 185–92; Theodore Marmor and Jerry Mashaw, "Canada's Health Insurance and Ours: The Real Lessons, the Big Choices," *American Prospect*, Fall 1990, 18–29; Pat Armstrong and Hugh Armstrong, *Universal Health Care: What the United States Can Learn from the Canadian Experience* (New York: New Press, 1999); William Glaser, "Universal Health Insurance That Really Works: Foreign Lessons for the United States," *Journal of Health Politics, Policy and Law* 18 (1993): 695–722; Victor Rodwin, "The Health Care System under French National Health Insurance: Lessons for Health Reform in the United States," *AJPH* 93 (2003): 31–37; Christa Altenstetter, "Insights from Health Care in Germany," ibid., 38–44; Paulo Elias and Amelia Cohn, "Health Reform in Brazil: Lessons to Consider," ibid., 44–48; Lawrence D. Brown, "Comparing Health Systems in Four Countries: Lessons for the United States," ibid., 52–56. On comparative health status and health-care performance, see Organization for Economic Cooperation and Development, *Health at a Glance: OECD Indicators, 2003* (Paris: The Organization, 2003).

2. Craig Renner and Vicente Navarro, "Why Is Our Population of Uninsured and Underinsured Persons Growing? The Consequences of 'Deindustrialization' of America," *Annual Review of Public Health* 10 (1989): 85–94; Deborah Chollet, "Employer-Based Health Insurance in a Changing Work Force," *Health Affairs* 13: 1 (1994): 315–26; Richard Kronick and Todd Gilmer, "Explaining the Decline in Health Insurance Coverage, 1979–1995," ibid. 18: 2 (1999): 30–47; Jon Gabel, "Job-Based Health Insurance, 1977–1998: The Accidental Health System under Scrutiny," ibid. 18: 6 (1999): 62–74; Jon Gabel et al., "Job-Based Health Benefits in 2002: Some Important Trends," ibid. 21: 5 (2002), 143–51; James Maxwell, Peter Temin, and Saminaz Zaman, "The Benefits Divide: Health Care Purchasing in Retail versus Other Sectors," ibid., 224–33; Gerard Anderson et al., "It's the Prices, Stupid: Why the United States Is So Different from Other Countries," ibid. 22: 3 (2003): 89–105; Allyson G. Hall, Karen Collins, and Sherry Glied, *Employer-Sponsored Health Insurance: Implications for Minority Workers* (New York: Commonwealth Fund, 1999); U.S. Bureau of Labor Statistics, "Employee Benefits in Private Industry, 2003," Sept. 17, 2003, 1, 3, online at http://www.bls.gov/news. release/pdf/ebs2.pdf, accessed June 5, 2004; *NYT*, Nov. 25, 2002, A1, A17, Dec. 7, 2002, B1, B3, Sept. 10, 2003, A1, C2, Oct. 19, 2003, sec. 4, 3, Oct. 22, 2003, C1, C2. For some of the underlying forces at work, see William Greider, *One World, Ready or Not: The Manic Logic of Global Capitalism* (New York: Simon and Schuster, 1997); Barry Bluestone and Bennett Harrison, *The Deindustrialization of America: Plant Closings, Community Abandonment, and the Dismantling of Basic Industry* (New York: Basic Books, 1982); David Gordon, *Fat and Mean: The Corporate Squeeze of Working Americans and the Myth of Managerial "Downsizing"* (New York: Free Press, 1996); Arne Kallenberg, Barbara Reskin, and Ken Hudson, "Bad Jobs in America: Standard and Nonstandard Employment Relations and Job Quality in the United States," *American Sociological*

*Review* 65 (2000): 256–78, esp. 264. On faltering unionism, see Nelson Lichtenstein, *State of the Union: A Century of American Labor* (Princeton: Princeton University Press, 2002), 212–45; Kim Moody, *An Injury to All: The Decline of American Unionism* (New York: Routledge, 1997); Thomas Geoghegan, *Which Side Are You On? Trying to Be for Labor When It's Flat on Its Back* (New York: Farrar, Straus and Giroux, 1991).

3. U.S. House of Representatives, Select Committee on Aging, *The Catastrophe of Uninsured and Underinsured Americans: In Search of a U.S. Health Plan*, 99th Cong., 2d sess., 1986 (Washington: GPO, 1986), 73 (Reinhardt quotation), 31–33, 52, 72–116, 119; M. Eugene Moyer, "A Revised Look at the Number of Uninsured Americans," *Health Affairs* 8: 2 (1989): 102–10; U.S. Senate, Committee on Governmental Affairs, Subcommittee on Intergovernmental Relations, *Access to Health Insurance and Health Care: Hearings*, 99th Cong., 2d sess., 1986 (Washington: GPO, 1986), passim, esp. 1; Katherine Swartz, *The Medically Uninsured: Special Focus on Workers* (Washington: Urban Institute Press, 1989); Kaiser Commission on Medicaid and the Uninsured, *Uninsured in America: A Chart Book* (Washington: The Commission, 1998), passim, esp. 4; David Takeuchi, Rita Chung, and Haikang Shen, "Health Insurance Coverage among Chinese Americans in Los Angeles County," *AJPH* 88 (1998): 451–53; Olveen Carrasquillo et al., "Going Bare: Trends in Health Insurance Coverage, 1989 through 1996," ibid. 89 (1999): 36–42; U.S. Congressional Budget Office, *How Many People Lack Health Insurance and for How Long?* (Washington: CBO, 2003); *NYT*, Feb. 26, 1999, A1, A14, Sept. 30, 2003, A1, A19.

4. Karen Davis and Diane Rowland, "Uninsured and Underserved: Inequities in Health Care in the United States," *Milbank Memorial Fund Quarterly* 61 (1983): 149 (quotation), 149–76; Robert Wood Johnson Foundation, *Updated Report on Access to Health Care for the American People* (Princeton: The Foundation, 1983), 4, 6, 8–9; Donald Nutter, "Access to Care and the Evolution of Corporate, For-Profit Medicine," *NEJM* 311 (1984): 917–19; Keith Wrenn, "No Insurance, No Admission," ibid. 312 (1985): 373–74; William Curran, "Economic and Legal Considerations in Emergency Care," ibid., 374–75; Bradford Gray and Walter McNerney, "For-Profit Enterprise in Health Care: The Institute of Medicine Study," ibid. 314 (1986): 1525–28; Howard Freeman et al., "Americans Report on Their Access to Health Care," *Health Affairs* 6: 1 (1987): 6–18, esp. 14–15; American College of Physicians, "Position Paper: Access to Health," *Annals of Internal Medicine* 112 (1990): 645; Judith Feder, Jack Hadley, and Ross Mullner, "Falling through the Cracks: Poverty, Insurance Coverage, and Hospital Care for the Poor, 1980 and 1982," *Milbank Memorial Fund Quarterly* 62 (1984): 544–66; Chris Hafner-Eaton, "Physician Utilization Disparities between the Uninsured and Insured," *JAMA* 269 (1993): 787–92; Patricia A. Butler, *Too Poor to Be Sick: Access to Medical Care for the Uninsured* (Washington: APHA, 1988); U.S. Congress, Office of Technology Assessment and Congressional Research Service, *Universal Health Insurance and Uninsured People: Effects on Use and Costs* (Washington: The Office, 1994), 4–9; Lisa Duchon et al., *Listening to Workers: Findings from the Commonwealth Fund 1999 National Survey of Workers' Health Insurance* (New York: Commonwealth Fund, 2000), 21; John Ayanian et al., "Unmet Health Needs of Uninsured Adults in the United States," *JAMA* 284 (2000): 2061–69; Joseph Sudano Jr. and David W. Baker, "Intermittent Lack of Health Insurance Coverage and Use of Preventive Services," *AJPH* 93 (2003): 130–37; Gay Becker and Edwina Newsom, "Socioeconomic Status and Dissatisfaction with Health Care among Chronically Ill African Americans," ibid., 742–48; John Ayanian

et al., "Undiagnosed Hypertension and Hypercholesterolemia among Uninsured and Insured Adults in the Third National Health and Nutrition Examination Survey," ibid., 2051–54. On the emergence and ambitions of health services research, see Eli Ginzberg, ed., *Health Services Research: Key to Health Policy* (Cambridge: Harvard University Press, 1991).

5. Institute of Medicine, *Access to Health Care in America*, ed. Michael Millman (Washington: National Academy Press, 1993), 3 (quotation), 5–8; Paula Braveman et al., "Adverse Outcomes and Lack of Health Insurance among Newborns in an Eight-County Area of California, 1982–1986," *NEJM* 321 (1989): 508–13; Steven Shea, "Predisposing Factors for Severe, Uncontrolled Hypertension in an Inner-City Minority Population," ibid. 327 (1992): 776–81; Jack Hadley et al., "Comparison of Uninsured and Privately Insured Hospital Patients: Condition on Admission, Resource Use and Outcome," *JAMA* 265 (1991): 374–79; Peter Franks, Carolyn Clancy, and Marthe Gold, "Health Insurance and Mortality: Evidence from a National Cohort," ibid. 270 (1993): 737–41; Joel Weissman et al., "Delayed Access to Health Care: Risk Factors, Reasons, and Consequences," *Annals of Internal Medicine* 114 (1991): 325–31; U.S. Congress, Office of Technology Assessment, *Does Health Insurance Make a Difference? Background Paper* (Washington: GPO, 1992), 20–28; Joel Weissman and Arnold Epstein, *Falling through the Safety Net: Insurance Status and Access to Health Care* (Baltimore: Johns Hopkins University Press, 1994), 99–112; Richard Roetzheim et al., "Effects of Health Insurance and Race on Colorectal Cancer Treatments and Outcomes," *AJPH* 90 (2000): 1746–54; Jack Hadley, "Sicker and Poorer—The Consequences of Being Uninsured: A Review of the Research on the Relationship between Health Insurance, Medical Care Use, Health, Work, and Income," *Medical Care Research and Review* 60: suppl. (2003): 3S–75S, esp. 62S (aggregate mortality estimate); Institute of Medicine, *Care without Coverage: Too Little, Too Late* (Washington: National Academies Press, 2002), passim, esp. 161–65 (aggregate mortality estimate).

6. Linda Bergthold, "The Fat Kid on the Seesaw: American Business and Health Care Cost Containment, 1970–1990," *Annual Review of Public Health* 12 (1991): 157–75; Linda Bergthold, *Purchasing Power in Health: Business, the State, and Health Care Politics* (New Brunswick: Rutgers University Press, 1990); Cardinal John O'Connor, "1985 Labor Day Statement: The Right to Health Care," Sept. 2, 1985, Committee for National Health Insurance Collection, box 57, folder 15, Archives of Labor and Urban Affairs, Reuther Library, Wayne State University, Detroit; Alain Enthoven, "The Competition Strategy: Status and Prospects," *NEJM* 304 (1981): 109–12. On the economic changes convulsing the health-care industries, see Paul Starr, *The Social Transformation of American Medicine* (New York: Basic Books, 1982), 420–49; Robert Kuttner, *Everything for Sale: The Virtues and Limits of Markets* (Chicago: University of Chicago Press, 1999), 110–58; James C. Robinson, *The Corporate Practice of Medicine: Competition and Innovation in Health Care* (Berkeley: University of California Press, 1999). For a facetious interpretation of conservative social policy, see "Republicans Back Universal Lawn-Care Bill," *Onion*, June 22, 2000, 1, 6. On labor's waning political influence, see Thomas Edsall, "The Changing Shape of Power: A Realignment in Public Policy," in *The Rise and Fall of the New Deal Order, 1930–1980*, ed. Steve Fraser and Gary Gerstle (Princeton: Princeton University Press, 1989), 269–93, esp. 276–78, 288–89; Lichtenstein, *State of the Union*, 234–38, 250–55; David Brody, *Workers in Industrial America: Essays on the Twentieth Century Struggle* (New York: Oxford University Press, 1993), 222–39; Gary M.

Fink, "Labor Law Revision and the End of the Postwar Labor Accord," in *Organized Labor and American Politics, 1894–1994: The Labor-Liberal Alliance*, ed. Kevin Boyle (Albany: SUNY Press, 1998), 239–57. On the general political shift, see David Vogel, *Fluctuating Fortunes: The Political Power of Business in America* (New York: Basic Books, 1989), 148–289; Kim McQuaid, *Uneasy Partners: Big Business in American Politics, 1945–1990* (Baltimore: Johns Hopkins University Press, 1994), 151–95; Frances Fox Piven and Richard Cloward, *The Breaking of the American Social Compact* (New York: New Press, 1997); William Berman and Stanley Kutler, *America's Right Turn: From Nixon to Clinton*, 2d ed. (Baltimore: Johns Hopkins University Press, 1998).

7. Nancy Fraser and Linda Gordon, "Contract versus Charity: Why Is There No Social Citizenship in the United States?" *Socialist Review* 22 (1992): 45 (quotation), 45–67; Lawrence Mead, *Beyond Entitlement: The Social Obligations of Citizenship* (New York: Free Press, 1986); U.S. President's Commission for the Study of Ethical Problems in Medicine and Biomedical and Behavioral Research, *Securing Access to Health Care: A Report on the Ethical Implications of Differences in the Availability of Health Services*, 3 vols. (Washington: GPO, 1983), 1: 4–6, 32–35; Albert Jonsen, *The Birth of Bioethics* (New York: Oxford University Press, 1998), 113–15; David Rothman, "Is There a Right to Health Care?" *Constitution* 5 (1993): 30–37; Thomas Bole III and William Bondeson, eds., *Rights to Health Care* (Dordrecht, Netherlands: Kluwer Academic Publishers, 1991); Norman Daniels, *Just Health Care* (Cambridge: Cambridge University Press, 1985); Ruth Roemer, "The Right to Health Care—Gains and Gaps," *AJPH* 78 (1988): 241–47; David Kinzer, "Universal Entitlement to Health Care: Can We Get There from Here?" *NEJM* 322 (1990): 467–70. On health care as an international human right, see World Health Organization, *Health for All in the Twenty-First Century* (Geneva: WHO, 1998), 20; Margaret Whitehead, "Diffusion of Ideas on Social Inequalities in Health: A European Perspective," *Milbank Quarterly* 76 (1998): 469–92, esp. 480, 484; Jonathan M. Mann et al., eds., *Health and Human Rights: A Reader* (New York: Routledge, 1999); Audrey R. Chapman, ed., *Health Care Reform: A Human Rights Approach* (Washington: Georgetown University Press, 1994); Paul Farmer and Nicole Gastineau, "Rethinking Health and Human Rights: Time for a Paradigm Shift," *Journal of Law, Medicine and Ethics* 30 (2002): 655–66; Peter Jacobson and Soheil Soliman, "Co-opting the Health and Human Rights Movement," ibid., 705–15. For a critique of the presidential ethics commission's aversion to rights, see Dan W. Brock, "The President's Commission on the Right to Health Care," in ibid., 65–83. On the culturally limited value of American rights rhetoric, see Kimberle Crenshaw, "Were the Critics Right about Rights? Reassessing the American Debate about Rights in the Post-Reform Era," in *Beyond Rights Talk and Culture Talk: Comparative Essays on the Politics of Rights and Culture*, ed. Mahmood Mamdani (New York: St. Martin's Press, 2000), 61–74. On the limits of human-rights discourse, see Kenneth Cmiel, "The Emergence of Human Rights Politics in the United States," *JAH* 86 (1999): 1231–50, esp. 1250.

8. *Congressional Record* 137 (1991): S14708 (Wofford quotation), S14856–58; Haynes Johnson and David Broder, *The System: The American Way of Politics at the Breaking Point* (Boston: Little, Brown, 1997), 93 (Rockefeller quotation), 92–93; *Philadelphia Inquirer*, Sept. 14, 1991, 2-B, Sept. 27, 1991, 6-B, Oct. 18, 1991, 1-B, 2-B, Nov. 3, 1991, 1-A, 12-A, Nov. 6, 1991, 1-A, 8-A; Robert Blendon et al., "The 1991 Pennsylvania Senate Race and National Health Insurance," *Journal of American Health Policy* 2 (1992): 21–23; John Iglehart, "The American Health Care System," *NEJM* 326 (1992): 964; Robert Blendon

et al., "The Beliefs and Values Shaping Today's Health Reform Debate," *Health Affairs* 13: 1 (1994): 274–84. On the paucity of social rights in the U.S., see, among many others, Herbert Gans, *The War against the Poor: The Underclass and Antipoverty Policy* (New York: Basic Books, 1995); Sonya Michel, *Children's Interests/Mothers' Rights: The Shaping of America's Child Care Policy* (New Haven: Yale University Press, 1999); Philip Harvey, *Securing the Right to Employment: Social Welfare Policy and the Unemployed in the United States* (Princeton: Princeton University Press, 1989); Gwendolyn Mink, *Welfare's End* (Ithaca: Cornell University Press, 1998); Alice Kessler-Harris, *In Pursuit of Equity: Women, Men, and the Quest for Economic Citizenship in 20th-Century America* (New York: Oxford University Press, 2000). By the 1990s, opponents of a right to health care were adopting an offensive stance. See David Kelley, "Is There a Right to Health Care?" Nov. 1993, online at http://suif.stanford.edu/~rfrench/political/health-right1.txt, accessed June 5, 2003; Richard A. Epstein, *Mortal Peril: Our Inalienable Right to Health Care?* (Reading, Mass.: Addison-Wesley, 1997).

9. Emily Friedman, "The Uninsured: From Dilemma to Crisis," *JAMA* 265 (1991): 2495 (quotation), 2491–95; Senate, *Access*, 50; Edward Kennedy, "Ensuring Access to Essential Health Care," *Hospitals*, Jan. 20, 1987, 120; "Universal Coverage: The Elusive Goal," ibid., Aug. 5, 1990, 42; "Emergency Action Needed on Gaping Health Coverage," *AFL-CIO News*, Feb. 28, 1987, 1, 2; James Todd, "It Is Time for Universal Access, Not Universal Insurance," *NEJM* 321 (1989): 46–47; David Himmelstein, Steffie Woolhandler, and Writing Committee [of Physicians for a National Health Program], "A National Health Program for the United States," ibid. 320 (1989): 102–7; Arnold Relman, "American Medicine at the Crossroads: Signs from Canada," ibid., 590–91; Alain Enthoven and Richard Kronick, "A Consumer-Choice Health Plan for the 1990s: Universal Health Insurance in a System Designed to Promote Quality and Economy," ibid., 29–37, 94–101; Alan Monheit and Pamela Farley Short, "Mandating Health Coverage for Working Americans," *Health Affairs* 8: 4 (1989): 22–38; David Jacobs, "Labor and the Strategy of Mandated Health Benefits," *Labor Studies Journal* 14 (1989): 23–33; Kenneth Frisof, "The Case for Universal Health Insurance," *Journal of Family Practice* 30 (1990): 465–67; U.S. Bipartisan Commission on Comprehensive Health Care, *A Call for Action: Final Report* (Washington: GPO, 1990), 53–86; Gordon T. Moore, "Let's Provide Primary Care to All Uninsured Americans—Now!" *JAMA* 265 (1991): 2108–9; Karen Davis, "Expanding Medicare and Employer Plans to Achieve Universal Health Insurance," ibid., 2525–28; John Holahan et al., "An American Approach to Health System Reform," ibid., 2537–40; Robert Blendon and Jennifer Edwards, "Caring for the Uninsured: Choices for Reform," ibid., 2563–65; Paul Starr, *The Logic of Health Care Reform: Transforming American Medicine for the Better* (Knoxville, Tenn.: Whittle Books, 1992); Paul Starr, "Healthy Compromise: Universal Coverage and Managed Competition under a Cap," *American Prospect*, Winter 1993, 44–52. Eagerness to dismiss the experience of other countries seldom led to serious consideration of Hawaiian experience with a virtually universal system that centered on requiring employers to insure their workers. On this neglected precedent, see Emily Friedman, "Mandatory Insurance: A Cure for Indigence," *Hospitals*, June 5, 1986, 46–48; John Lewin and Peter Sybinsky, "Hawaii's Employer Mandate and Its Contribution to Universal Access," *JAMA* 269 (1993): 2538–43. On similar legislation enacted (but never fully implemented) in Massachusetts, see Susan Goldberger, "The Politics of Universal Access: The Massachusetts Health Security Act of 1988," *Journal of Health Politics, Policy and Law* 15 (1990): 857–85;

Robert Blendon et al., "The Uninsured and the Debate over the Repeal of the Massachusetts Universal Health Care Law," *JAMA* 267 (1992): 1113–17.

10. On the Clinton initiative, see Johnson and Broder, *System*; Theda Skocpol, *Boomerang: Clinton's Health Security Effort and the Turn against Government in U.S. Politics* (New York: W. W. Norton, 1996); Nicholas Laham, *A Lost Cause: Bill Clinton's Campaign for National Health Insurance* (Westport, Conn.: Praeger, 1996); Jacob Hacker, *The Road to Nowhere: The Genesis of President Clinton's Plan for Health Security* (Princeton: Princeton University Press, 1997); Dan Beauchamp, *Health Care Reform and the Battle for the Body Politic* (Philadelphia: Temple University Press, 1996), 75–111; "Roundtable on the Defeat of Reform," *Journal of Health Politics, Policy and Law* 20 (1995): 391–494. For the Clintons' rejection of Canadian-style reform, see Tom Hamburger and Ted Marmor, "Dead on Arrival: Why Washington's Power Elites Won't Consider Single Payer Health Reform," *Washington Monthly*, Sept. 1993, 27–28; Hillary Rodham Clinton, *Living History* (New York: Simon and Schuster, 2003), 150.

11. Working Group 17, "Preamble: A New Health Care System," Apr. 1, 1993, 3 (quotation), 1–7, U.S. White House Health Care Interdepartmental Working Group Records, box 306, Archives I, National Archives and Records Administration, Washington; Working Group 17, "Ethical Foundations Briefing Book," [May 1993?], ibid., box 2274; [Working Group on Low-Income Coverage], "Protecting Low-Income Populations," [Apr. 1993?], ibid., box 1105; Coalition for National Health Reform and Access to Care for the Underserved to Ira Magaziner, May 5, 1993, ibid., box 2272; Working Group on Low-Income Coverage, "Briefing Book on Low Income Coverage," [June 1993?], ibid., box 2276. On the creation and operation of the much-ridiculed task force and its army of expert advisors, see Johnson and Broder, *System*, 96–146; Hacker, *Road to Nowhere*, 122–29.

12. William Clinton, "Address to a Joint Session of Congress on Health Care Reform," Sept. 22, 1993, in *Public Papers of the Presidents of the United States: William J. Clinton, 1993*, 2 vols. (Washington: GPO, 1994), 2: 1557 (quotation), 1556–65; U.S. President, White House Domestic Policy Council, *Health Security: The President's Report to the American People* (Washington: The Council, 1993), 17 (Koop quotation), iii–iv, 1–5, 33–46, 85–87; Johnson and Broder, *System*, 170. On promoting universalism to those already insured, see Skocpol, *Boomerang*, 117–19; Johnson and Broder, *System*, 153–54, 506; Hacker, *Road to Nowhere*, 140; *NYT*, Apr. 7, 1993, A1, A21, July 16, 1994, 9; Lawrence R. Jacobs, "Health Reform Impasse: The Politics of American Ambivalence toward Government," *Journal of Health Politics, Policy and Law* 18 (1993): 633. On the religious roots of Koop's universalism, see "The Ethics of Health Care: An Interview with C. Everett Koop," *Christian Century*, Jan. 26, 1994, 79.

13. *NYT*, Jan. 22, 1994, 9 (quotation), Jan. 4, 1994, A1, A12, May 26, 1994, D21, June 22, 1994, A1, A18, June 30, 1994, A1, B10, July 16, 1994, 9, July 20, 1994, A1, A12, July 21, 1994, A22, B9, July 31, 1994, 1, 24, Oct. 3, 1994, A12; William F. May, "The Ethical Foundations of Health Care Reform," *Christian Century*, June 1–8, 1994, 576; Johnson and Broder, *System*, 200–202, 369, 375–93, 402, 438–40, 456; Clinton, *Living History*, 219, 230–31.

14. *NYT*, Nov. 11, 1996, A1, A12, Feb. 7, 1997, A25, May 26, 1997, A8, Sept. 21, 1997, sec. 1, 1, 32; U.S General Accounting Office, *Health Insurance for Children: Private Insurance Coverage Continues to Decline* (Washington: GAO, 1996); Marian Wright Edelman to Editors and Editorial Writers, Jan. 10, 1997, online at http://www.childrensdefense.org/insurememo.html, accessed May 5, 1997; Families USA, *One out of Three: Kids without Health Insurance, 1995–1996* (Washington: Families USA, 1997); Paul Newacheck, Dana

Hughes, and Jeffrey Stoddard, "Children's Access to Primary Care: Differences by Race, Income, and Insurance Status," *Pediatrics* 97 (1996): 26–32; Paul Newacheck et al., "Adolescent Health Insurance Coverage: Recent Changes and Access to Care," ibid. 104 (1999): 195–202; Peter Cunningham, "SCHIP Making Progress: Increased Take-Up Contributes to Coverage Gains," *Health Affairs* 22: 4 (2003): 163–72; John Holahan, Lisa Dubay, and Genevieve Kenney, "Which Children Are Uninsured and Why," *Future of Children* 13 (2003): 55; "Millions of Children Still Lack Health Coverage," *Nation's Health*, Oct. 2003, 7. On incremental reforms to aid adults, see Karen Davis, "Uninsured in an Era of Managed Care," *Health Services Research* 31 (1997): 641–49; Jacob Hacker and Theda Skocpol, "The New Politics of U.S. Health Policy," *Journal of Health Politics, Policy and Law* 22 (1997): 315–38; John McDonough, Christie Hager, and Brian Rosman, "Health Reform Stages a Comeback in Massachusetts," *NEJM* 336 (1997): 148–51; Robert Kuttner, "The Kassebaum-Kennedy Bill: The Limits of Incrementalism," *NEJM* 337 (1997): 64–67; Peter Budetti, "Health Insurance for Children: A Model for Incremental Health Reform?" ibid. 338 (1998): 541–42; *NYT*, July 2, 1995, sec. 1, 1, 20, Nov. 24, 1997, A1, A18, Aug. 9, 1998, sec. 1, 1, 22, Jan. 3, 1999, 1, 18, June 14, 2003, A10, Jan. 20, 2004, C1, C8; Deborah Chollet and Lori Achman, *Approaching Universal Coverage: Minnesota's Health Insurance Programs* (New York: Commonwealth Fund, 2003); Andrew Bindman and David Haggstrom, "Small Steps or a Giant Leap for the Uninsured?" *JAMA* 290 (2003): 816–18.

15. Vicente Navarro, "Policy without Politics: The Limits of Social Engineering," *AJPH* 93 (2003): 64–67; Beatrix Hoffman, "Health Care Reform and Social Movements in the United States," ibid., 75–85; Alan Derickson, "The House of Falk: The Paranoid Style in American Health Politics," ibid. 87 (1997): 1836–43. For signs of recent activism, see Jobs with Justice, "March 2004 Update," online at http://www.jwj.org/updates/2004/03–04.htm, accessed Apr. 8, 2004; "Unions, Health Care Reform Advocates Stage Nationwide Day of Action Events," *Labor Relations Week*, Mar. 11, 2004, 357; Universal Health Care Action Network, "National Campaigns for Universal Health Care," online at http://www.uhcan.org, accessed Apr. 8, 2004; Pennsylvanians United for Single-Payer Healthcare, *The Health Care Crisis: People's Lives and Health Are at Risk* (n.p.: Pennsylvanians United, [2004]); *Philadelphia Inquirer*, Feb. 9, 2000, A1, A12; "Impassioned Call for a Single-Payer National Health System Rings Out from Chicago," *Nation's Health*, Sept. 1998, 1, 10; *Labor Unity*, July–Aug. 1991, 12, May–June 1993, 16; Health Access Foundation, *Health Access Pursues Universal Access for '92* (San Francisco: The Foundation, 1991); *USA Today*, June 3, 1991, 1B, 2B; Camille Colatosi, "Health Care Activists Target Insurance Industry," *Labor Notes*, July 1991, 3, 15. On movements and their moving ideas, Peter Coclanis and Stuart Bruchey, eds., *Ideas, Ideologies, and Social Movements: The United States Experience since 1800* (Columbia: University of South Carolina Press, 1999); Sidney Tarrow, *Power in Movement: Social Movements and Contentious Politics* (Cambridge: Cambridge University Press, 1998), 106–22; David A. Snow and Robert Benford, "Master Frames and Cycles of Protest," in *Frontiers in Social Movement Theory*, ed. Aldon Morris and Carol McClurg Mueller (New Haven: Yale University Press, 1992), 133–55; E. P. Thompson, "The Moral Economy of the English Crowd in the Eighteenth Century," *Past and Present* 50 (1971): 76–136. For examples of improbable social movements, see Jacqueline Vaughn Switzer, *Disabled Rights: American Disability Policy and the Fight for Equality* (Washington: Georgetown University Press, 2003), passim, esp. 68–89; Renee Anspach, "From Stigma to Identity Politics:

Political Activism among the Physically Disabled and Former Mental Patients," *Social Science and Medicine* 13A (1979): 765–73; Steven Epstein, *Impure Science: AIDS, Activism, and the Politics of Knowledge* (Berkeley: University of California Press, 1996); Alan Derickson, *Black Lung: Anatomy of a Public Health Disaster* (Ithaca: Cornell University Press, 1998), passim, esp. 143–82; Steven Hahn, *A Nation under Our Feet: Black Political Struggles in the Rural South from Slavery to the Great Migration* (Cambridge: Belknap Press of Harvard University Press, 2003); John Dittmer, *Local People: The Struggle for Civil Rights in Mississippi* (Urbana: University of Illinois Press, 1994); J. Craig Jenkins and Charles Perrow, "Insurgency of the Powerless: Farm Worker Movements (1946–1972)," *American Sociological Review* 42 (1977): 249–68; Frances Fox Piven and Richard Cloward, *Poor People's Movements: Why They Succeed, How They Fail* (New York: Vintage Books, 1979); Abraham Hoffman, *The Townsend Movement: A Political Analysis* (New York: Octagon Books, 1975); Edwin Amenta, Bruce Carruthers, and Yvonne Zylan, "A Hero for the Aged? The Townsend Movement, the Political Mediation Model, and U.S. Old-Age Policy, 1934–1950," *American Journal of Sociology* 98 (1992): 308–39; Paul Longmore and David Goldberger, "The League of the Physically Handicapped and the Great Depression," *JAH* 87 (2000): 888–921.

16. Rosemary Stevens, "Public Roles for the Medical Profession in the United States: Beyond Theories of Decline and Fall," *Milbank Quarterly* 79 (2001): 346 (quotation), 327–53; Norton Greenberger et al., "Universal Access to Health Care in America: A Moral and Medical Imperative," *Annals of Internal Medicine* 112 (1990): 637–39; American College of Physicians, "Universal Insurance for American Health Care: A Proposal of the American College of Physicians," ibid. 117 (1992): 511–19; American College of Physicians, *Universal Coverage: Renewing the Call to Action* (Philadelphia: The College, 1996); American College of Physicians–American Society of Internal Medicine, "Providing Access to Care for All Americans: A Statement of Core Policy Principles," Oct. 29, 2000, American College of Physicians–American Society of Internal Medicine Records, Position Paper Series, ACP-ASIM Archives, Philadelphia; American College of Physician–American Society of Internal Medicine, "Achieving Affordable Health Insurance Coverage for All within Seven Years: A Proposal from America's Internists," Apr. 9, 2002, ibid.; Physicians' Working Group for Single-Payer National Health Insurance, "Proposal of the Physicians' Working Group for Single-Payer National Health Insurance," *JAMA* 290 (2003): 798–805; Deborah A. Stone, "AIDS and the Moral Economy of Insurance," *American Prospect*, Spring 1990, 62–73; *NYT*, Nov. 17, 2003, A15; Marian Wright Edelman, "Keynote Address [at the Fourth Annual Margaret E. Mahoney Symposium]," *Journal of Urban Health* 75 (1998): 623–33; Young-Hee Yoon et al., *Women's Access to Health Insurance* (Washington: Institute for Women's Policy Research, 1994). On reform coalitions that bridged class divisions, see Kathryn Kish Sklar, *Florence Kelley and the Nation's Work: The Rise of Women's Political Culture, 1830–1900* (New Haven: Yale University Press, 1995); Walter Trattner, *Crusade for the Children: A History of the National Child Labor Committee and Child Labor Reform in America* (Chicago: Quadrangle Books, 1970); Elizabeth Payne, *Reform, Labor, and Feminism: Margaret Dreier Robins and the Women's Trade Union League* (Urbana: University of Illinois Press, 1988); Theda Skocpol, *The Missing Middle: Working Families and the Future of American Social Policy* (New York: W. W. Norton, 2000), passim, esp. 30–32. For recent advocacy of universal care as a matter of fairness to racial and ethnic minorities, see Marsha Lillie-Blanton and Ana Alfaro-Correa, *In the Nation's Interest:*

*Equity in Access to Health* (Washington: Joint Center for Political and Economic Studies, 1995), passim, esp. v; Carrasquillo et al., "Going Bare," 36–42; William Julius Wilson, *When Work Disappears: The World of the New Urban Poor* (New York: Vintage Books, 1997), 207–38, esp. 234–38. On the consequences of the widespread lack of insurance in the minority population, see Robin Weinick, Samuel Zuvekas, and Joel Cohen, "Racial and Ethnic Differences in Access to and Use of Health Care Services, 1977 to 1996," *Medical Care Research and Review* 57: suppl. 1 (2000): 36–54; E. Richard Brown et al., *Racial and Ethnic Disparities in Access to Health Insurance and Health Care* (Los Angeles: UCLA Center for Health Policy Research and Henry J. Kaiser Family Foundation, 2000); Morehouse Medical Treatment Effectiveness Center, *Racial and Ethnic Differences in Access to Medical Care: A Synthesis of the Literature* (Menlo Park, Calif.: Henry J. Kaiser Family Foundation, 1999); American College of Physicians–American Society of Internal Medicine, *No Health Insurance? It's Enough to Make You Sick: Latino Community at Great Risk* (Philadelphia: American College of Physicians–American Society of Internal Medicine, 2000); Natalie Freeman, Dona Schneider, and Patricia McGarvey, "The Relationship of Health Insurance to the Diagnosis and Management of Asthma and Respiratory Problems in Children in a Predominantly Hispanic Urban Community," *AJPH* 93 (2003): 1316–20.

17. Larry Churchill, *Self-Interest and Universal Health Care: Why Well-Insured Americans Should Support Coverage for Everyone* (Cambridge: Harvard University Press, 1994), 51 (quotation), and passim; David Rothman, "A Century of Failure: Health Care Reform in America," *Journal of Health Politics, Policy and Law* 18 (1993): 273 (quotation), 273–74; Institute of Medicine, *A Shared Destiny: Community Effects of Uninsurance* (Washington: National Academies Press, 2003); Inder Verma, "SARS: Fear of a Global Pandemic," *Molecular Therapy* 7 (2003): 711; U.S. Centers for Disease Control and Prevention, "Updated Interim Surveillance Case Definition for Severe Acute Respiratory Syndrome (SARS)—United States, Apr. 29, 2003," *JAMA* 289 (2003): 2637–39; *NYT*, Mar. 2, 2004, D1, D6; Laurie Garrett, *The Coming Plague: Newly Emerging Diseases in a World Out of Balance* (New York: Penguin Books, 1995); Judith Walzer Leavitt, *Typhoid Mary: Captive to the Public's Health* (Boston: Beacon Press, 1996); Alan Kraut, *Silent Travelers: Germs, Genes, and the "Immigrant Menace"* (New York: Basic Books, 1994); Amy Fairchild, *Science at the Borders: Immigrant Medical Inspection and the Shaping of the Modern Industrial Labor Force, 1891 to 1930* (Baltimore: Johns Hopkins University Press, 2003); Tera Hunter, *To 'Joy My Freedom: Southern Black Women's Lives and Labors after the Civil War* (Cambridge: Harvard University Press, 1997), 186–218. On the disproportionate share of recent immigrants without insurance, see Olveen Carrasquillo, Angeles Carrasquillo, and Steven Shea, "Health Insurance Coverage of Immigrants Living in the United States: Differences by Citizenship Status and Country of Origin," *AJPH* 90 (2000): 917–23; E. Richard Brown et al., *Undocumented Immigrants: Changes in Health Insurance Coverage with Legalized Immigration Status* (Los Angeles: UCLA Center for Health Policy Research, 1999). On the societal costs associated with the uninsured, see Institute of Medicine, *Hidden Cost, Value Lost: Uninsurance in America* (Washington: National Academies Press, 2003).

18. For signs of discouragement, see Uwe Reinhardt, "Is There Hope for the Uninsured? *Health Affairs Web Exclusives* W3 (2003): 376–90; Colin Gordon, *Dead on Arrival: The Politics of Health Care in Twentieth-Century America* (Princeton: Princeton University Press, 2003), passim, esp. 297–301.

# Index

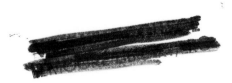